Hand Hygiene

Hospital Medicine: Current Concepts

Scott A. Flanders and Sanjay Saint, Series Editors

Hand Hygiene
A Handbook for Medical Professionals

Edited by

Didier Pittet
Infection Control Program and WHO Collaborating Centre on Patient Safety,
University of Geneva Hospitals and Faculty of Medicine,
Geneva, Switzerland

John M. Boyce
Hospital Epidemiology and Infection Control, Yale-New Haven Hospital,
and Yale University School of Medicine,
New Haven, CT, USA

Benedetta Allegranzi
Infection Prevention and Control Global Unit,
Department of Service Delivery and Safety,
World Health Organization, and Faculty of Medicine, University of Geneva,
Geneva, Switzerland

Series Editors

Scott A. Flanders, MD, MHM
Sanjay Saint, MD, MPH, FRCP

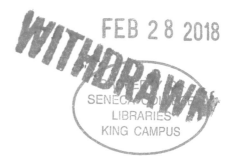
WILEY Blackwell

This edition first published 2017 ©2017 by John Wiley & Sons, Inc

Registered office: John Wiley & Sons, Ltd, The Atrium, Southern Gate, Chichester, West Sussex, PO19 8SQ, UK

Editorial offices: 9600 Garsington Road, Oxford, OX4 2DQ, UK
        The Atrium, Southern Gate, Chichester, West Sussex, PO19 8SQ, UK
        111 River Street, Hoboken, NJ 07030-5774, USA

For details of our global editorial offices, for customer services and for information about how to apply for permission to reuse the copyright material in this book please see our website at www.wiley.com/wiley-blackwell

Library of Congress Cataloging-in-Publication Data

Names: Pittet, Didier, 1957- editor. | Boyce, John M., editor. | Allegranzi, Benedetta, editor.
Title: Hand hygiene : a handbook for medical professionals / edited by Didier Pittet, John M. Boyce, Benedetta Allegranzi.
Other titles: Hand hygiene (Pittet) | Hospital medicine, current concepts.
Description: Chichester, West Sussex, UK ; Hoboken, NJ : John Wiley & Sons, Ltd., 2016.
| Series: Hospital medicine : current concepts | Includes bibliographical references and index.
Identifiers: LCCN 2016016293 (print) | LCCN 2016017182 (ebook) | ISBN 9781118846865 (pbk.) | ISBN 9781118846803 (pdf) | ISBN 9781118846858 (epub)
Subjects: | MESH: Hand Hygiene
Classification: LCC RA776.95 (print) | LCC RA776.95 (ebook) | NLM WA 110 | DDC 613–dc23
LC record available at https://lccn.loc.gov/2016016293

A catalogue record for this book is available from the British Library.

Wiley also publishes its books in a variety of electronic formats. Some content that appears in print may not be available in electronic books.

Cover design: Wiley
Cover images: (Top) © monkeybusinessimages/Gettyimages; (Middle) © CNRI/Science Photo Library/Corbis; (Bottom) © Antagain/Gettyimages

Typeset in 9/12pt MeridienLTStd by SPi Global, Chennai, India

Printed in the United States of America.

10 9 8 7 6 5 4 3 2 1

Contents

Contributors

Benedetta Allegranzi, Infection Prevention and Control Global Unit, Department of Service Delivery and Safety, World Health Organization, and Faculty of Medicine, University of Geneva, Geneva, Switzerland

Jaffar A. Al-Tawfiq, Saudi Aramco Medical Services Organization, Dhahran, Saudi Arabia

Hanan H. Balkhy, Infection Prevention and Control Department, King Saud bin Abdulaziz University for Health Sciences, Riyadh, Saudi Arabia

Fernando Bellissimo-Rodrigues, Infection Control Program and WHO Collaborating Centre on Patient Safety, University of Geneva Hospitals and Faculty of Medicine, Geneva, Switzerland

Anne Marie Benedicto, The Joint Commission, Oakbrook Terrace, USA

Pascal Bonnabry, University of Geneva Hospitals and Faculty of Medicine, and Univeristy of Lausanne, Geneva and Lausanne, Switzerland

John M. Boyce, Hospital Epidemiology and Infection Control, Yale-New Haven Hospital, and Yale University School of Medicine, New Haven, USA

Barbara I. Braun, The Joint Commission, Oakbrook Terrace, USA

Enrique Castro-Sánchez, National Institute for Health Research, Health Protection Research Unit in Healthcare Associated Infection and Antimicrobial Resistance, Imperial College London, London, UK

Mark R. Chassin, The Joint Commission, Oakbrook Terrace, USA

Marie-Noëlle Chraïti, Infection Control Program and WHO Collaborating Centre on Patient Safety, University of Geneva Hospitals, Geneva, Switzerland

Lauren Clack, Division of Infectious Diseases and Infection Control, University Hospitals of Zurich, Zürich, Switzerland

Ben S. Cooper, Mahidol-Oxford Tropical Medicine Research Unit, Faculty of Tropical Medicine, Mahidol University, Bangkok, Thailand and Centre for Tropical Medicine and Global Health, Nuffield Department of Clinical Medicine, University of Oxford, Oxford, UK

Benjamin J. Cowling, Department of Pathology, Hong Kong Baptist Hospital, Kowloon Tong, Hong Kong SAR, China

Nizam Damani, Infection Prevention and Control, Southern Health and Social Care Trust, Portadown, and Queen's University, Belfast, UK

Katherine Ellingson, Oregon Health Authority, Public Health Division, Healthcare-Associated Infections Program, Portland, USA

Angèle Gayet-Ageron, Infection Control Program and WHO Collaborating Centre on Patient Safety, University of Geneva Hospitals and Faculty of Medicine, Geneva, Switzerland

Nicholas Graves, School of Public Health and Institute of Health and Biomedical Innovation, Queensland University of Technology, Brisbane, Australia

M. Lindsay Grayson, Infectious Diseases Department, Austin Hospital and University of Melbourne, Melbourne, Australia

Stephan Harbarth, Infection Control Program and WHO Collaborating Centre on Patient Safety, University of Geneva Hospitals and Faculty of Medicine, Geneva, Switzerland

Alison Holmes, National Institute for Health Research, Health Protection Research Unit in Healthcare Associated Infection and Antimicrobial Resistance, Imperial College London, London, UK

Gürkan Kaya, Dermatology and Venereology Service, University of Geneva Hospitals and Faculty of Medicine, Geneva, Switzerland

Claire Kilpatrick, Infection Prevention and Control Global Unit, Department of Service Delivery and Safety, World Health Organization, Geneva, Switzerland

Caroline Landelle, Infection Control Unit, Centre Hospitalier Universitaire Grenoble Alpes, and University Grenoble Alpes/CNRS, THEMAS TIM-C UMR 5525, Grenoble, France

Elaine Larson, Columbia University School of Nursing, New York, USA

Yves Longtin, Infection Control and Prevention Unit, Jewish General Hospital, and McGill University, Montreal, Canada

Nantasit Luangasanatip, Mahidol-Oxford Tropical Medicine Research Unit, Faculty of Tropical Medicine, Mahidol University, Bangkok, and School of Public Health, Queensland University of Technology, Brisbane, Australia

Jean-Christophe Lucet, Infection Control Unit, Bichat-Claude Bernard Hospital, Paris, France

Maryanne McGuckin, Patient-Centered Outcomes Research Institute, Washington, USA

Mary-Louise McLaws, Healthcare Infection and Infectious Diseases Control, University of New South Wales, Sydney, Australia

Shaheen Mehtar, Unit for Infection Prevention and Control, Division of Community Health, Stellenbosch University, Cape Town, South Africa

Ziad A. Memish, Former Deputy Health Minister, College of Medicine, Alfaisal University, Riyadh, Kingdom of Saudi Arabia

Maria Luisa Moro, Health and Social Agency Emilia-Romagna Region, Bologna, Italy

Eleanor Murray, Saïd Business School, University of Oxford, Oxford, UK

Sepideh Bagheri Nejad, Department of Service Delivery and Safety, World Health Organization, Geneva, Switzerland

Eli Perencevich, Department of Internal Medicine, University of Iowa, Carver College of Medicine, Iowa City, USA

Daniela Pires, Infection Control Programme and WHO Collaborating Centre on Patient Safety, University of Geneva Hospitals and Faculty of Medicine, Geneva, Switzerland

Didier Pittet, Infection Control Program and WHO Collaborating Centre on Patient Safety, University of Geneva Hospitals and Faculty of Medicine, Geneva, Switzerland

Peter Pronovost, Armstrong Institute for Patient Safety and Quality, Johns Hopkins, and Patient Safety and Quality, The Johns Hopkins University School of Medicine, Baltimore, USA

Manfred L. Rotter, Institute of Hygiene and Applied Immunology, Medical University of Vienna, Vienna, Austria

Philip L. Russo, Hand Hygiene Australia, Melbourne, Australia

Matthew Samore, Department of Epidemiology, University of Utah School of Medicine, Salt Lake City, USA

Syed A. Sattar, Department of Biochemistry, Microbiology and Immunology, Faculty of Medicine, University of Ottawa, Ottawa, Canada

Hugo Sax, Division of Infectious Diseases and Infection Control, University Hospital of Zurich, Zürich, Switzerland

Wing-Hong Seto, World Health Organization Collaborating Centre for Infectious Disease, Epidemiology and Control, School of Public Health, The University of Hong Kong, Hong Kong SAR, China

Susan E. Sheridan, World Alliance for Patient Safety, World Health Organization, Geneva, Switzerland

Joseph Solomkin, University of Cincinnati College of Medicine, Cincinnati, USA

François Stéphan, Réanimation Adulte, Centre Chirurgical Marie Lannelongue, Le Plessis Robinson, France

Andrew J. Stewardson, Infectious Diseases Department, Austin Health and Hand Hygiene Australia, Melbourne, Australia and Infection Control Program and WHO Collaborating Centre on Patient Safety, University of Geneva Hospitals and Faculty of Medicine, Geneva, Switzerland

Julie Storr, Infection Prevention and Control Global Unit, Department of Service Delivery and Safety, World Health Organization, Geneva, Switzerland

Miranda Suchomel, Institute of Hygiene and Applied Immunology, Medical University of Vienna, Vienna, Austria

Andreas Voss, Radboud University Medical Centre and Canisius-Wilhelmina Hospital, Nijmegen, The Netherlands

Robert M. Wachter, Department of Medicine, University of California, and University of California San Francisco Medical Center, San Francisco, USA

Andreas F. Widmer, Division of Infectious Diseases and Hospital Epidemiology, University Hospital of Basel, Basel, Switzerland

Walter Zingg, Infection Control Program and WHO Collaborating Centre on Patient Safety, University of Geneva Hospitals and Faculty of Medicine, Geneva, Switzerland

Preface

Do we need another medical textbook?

Does a textbook of hand hygiene exist?

Does hand hygiene deserve a textbook?

These are some of the questions I asked myself when I was invited to consider such a project. I write "project," when, in fact, I mean "journey." Editing *Hand Hygiene* was a journey; in the same way, hand hygiene promotion is a journey. But what a fantastic journey it is!

Together with my dear friends and colleagues John M. Boyce and Benedetta Allegranzi, we have had the unique privilege to ask the world's pre-eminent scholars and clinicians on hand hygiene, infection control, and patient safety to contribute to the first comprehensive, single-source overview of best practices in hand hygiene. *Hand Hygiene* fully integrates the World Health Organization (WHO) guidelines and policies, and offers a global perspective in tackling challenges in both developed and developing countries. A total of fifty-five chapters includes coverage of basic and highly complex clinical applications of hand hygiene practices, and considers novel and unusual issues in hand hygiene, such as religious and cultural aspects, social marketing, campaigning, and patient participation. It also provides guidance on the best approaches to achieve behavioral change in healthcare workers that can also be applied in fields other than hand hygiene.

We asked authors to be concise, to review the evidence as well as what is unknown, and to highlight unique research perspectives in their own field. Each chapter reads easily and contains major issues summarized as bullet points, key figures, and tables. These are also available for download by accessing the e-version of *Hand Hygiene*, together with all of the instruments referenced in the book. My co-editors and I are extremely pleased by the work and commitment of the authors in this team effort, and take this opportunity to warmly thank them all.

Excellence is an attitude and excellence in hand hygiene, a journey.

May *Hand Hygiene* drive excellence in hand hygiene practices, research, and attitudes for many years to come, and contribute to save many more millions of lives every year worldwide.

Professor Didier Pittet, MD, MS, CBE
Infection Control Programme and World Health Organization
Collaborating Centre on Patient Safety,
The University of Geneva Hospitals and Faculty of Medicine,
Geneva, Switzerland

Foreword

Hand hygiene in healthcare settings seems like a pretty simple act. One places an antiseptic agent on the hands, rubs the hands together to reduce the transient microorganisms, dries the hands or lets them dry, and thereby reduces the risk of transmission of pathogens to patients and to the healthcare worker. In *Hand Hygiene*, Drs Pittet, Boyce, and Allegranzi, and their esteemed colleagues, show us how complicated – yet essential – hand hygiene really is.

The book encompasses all the important aspects of hand hygiene. Each chapter has a simple-to-read format: key messages; what we know – the scientific evidence; what we don't know; and the research that needs to be done to fill these gaps. The authors begin by providing a summary of the current status of data on healthcare-associated infections (HAIs) in both developed and resource-limited countries. These data show the enormous impact that HAIs have throughout the world, including morbidity, mortality, and cost. This chapter also illustrates how even now – over thirty-five years since the Centers for Disease Control and Prevention's (CDC) Study of the Efficacy of Nosocomial Infection Control (SENIC) programs documented the preventive impact of HAI surveillance and prevention intervention programs – many countries still do not have adequate surveillance systems in place to even answer what their HAI rates are, much less evaluate the impact of prevention interventions.

Next, the authors describe the history of hand hygiene from the time of Semmelweis, discuss the flora and physiology of skin, describe the dynamics of pathogen transmission from the skin, and culminate in three chapters on mathematical models of hand-borne pathogen transmission, methodological issues in hand hygiene science, and statistical issues in hand hygiene research. These last three chapters highlight the many gaps in our knowledge about hand hygiene, illustrate the weaknesses in many if not most of our current studies, and point out that conducting the studies that are necessary may be more difficult than Semmelweis's challenge of convincing clinicians that hand hygiene should be done at all. Essential issues include antiseptic agent volume, method of application, duration of application, agent formulation, and when these are all optimized, and what percentage of HAIs are prevented by best practices. These methodological chapters are particularly important, as they illustrate that if our Guidelines are supposed to depend solely upon well-designed randomized controlled trials (RCTs) of hand hygiene – rather than on the entire body of epidemiologic data – such RCTs do not and probably never will exist, and hand hygiene will be relegated to an unresolved issue. These methodological issues also should be kept in mind as one reads the rest of this book (or other published literature) in which many studies are referenced that suffer from these methodological design flaws.

The next three chapters discuss the various available hand hygiene agents, the methods for evaluating their efficacy and the hand hygiene technique. These chapters are incredibly important and discuss issues often not known or understood in the infection control/patient safety community. Data show that formulation of alcohol-based hand hygiene agents matters. The chapter on evaluating efficacy illustrates the differences between North American and European standards – that is American Society for Testing Methods (ASTM) vs. Comité Européen de Normalisation (CEN or EN) standard methods. Everyone in infection control should understand the different methods used, what these tests do and do not tell us about efficacy, how in vivo testing does or does not relate to clinical practice, and the importance of demanding that all manufacturers provide such data to us when we are comparing products. Formulation matters, and such testing can document this.

This leads to several chapters on compliance with hand hygiene best practices, barriers to compliance, and a discussion of physicians and the almost universal finding that they are the worst compliers with hand hygiene recommendations of all healthcare workers. We must ask ourselves exactly what compliance with hand hygiene best practices is. Is it as mentioned at the beginning of this foreward simply applying some agent (formulation and amount irrelevant) and rubbing our hands together (duration and method irrelevant)? Or does compliance with hand hygiene *best practices* mean using a *formulation* documented to be effective, using the correct *volume* of that specific product documented in the ASTM or EN standard testing (realizing that volume will differ by product and for gels, foams vs. rubs), applying the product in a specific *manner* (such as recommended by the World Health Organization [WHO]), for the correct *duration*, at each of the WHO *five moments*? With current visual observation of hand hygiene "compliance," how many healthcare workers pay any attention to the volume of agent used, the method of application, the duration of application, and so on. All of these are critical elements in hand hygiene best practices, yet they are often ignored. We need more precise definitions of what hand hygiene best practices are and when they should be done and measured. From the patient's perspective, moments 1 and 2 are most important. From the healthcare worker's perspective, moments 3, 4, and 5 are most important. These chapters also raise questions about who should monitor hand hygiene compliance (self-reporting appears to generally be inaccurate), when and how.

The next general area includes a discussion of behavior and hand hygiene, hand hygiene promotion strategies, the WHO five moments for hand hygiene, system change, and education of healthcare professionals. These chapters illustrate the continual struggle that those of us in infection control/quality improvement have trying to educate our healthcare workers about the importance of hand hygiene and methods to improve behavior, reduce barriers to compliance, and try to change our systems. Do we continue to invest enormous resources (time, personnel, and funding) to these activities to try to get our healthcare "professionals" to comply with hand hygiene best practices, or do we follow the dictates of the chapter on "Personal Accountability for Hand Hygiene"? As we have learned in the United States, if we do not regulate ourselves (e.g., through mandatory reporting of HAI rates, reduced funding for preventable HAIs), outside regulatory agencies will (i.e., the government). We all agree that proper performance of hand hygiene will reduce HAIs and improve patient safety. Then why do we accept noncompliance?

The chapter on monitoring hand hygiene compliance is critical. What should the gold standard be for measuring hand hygiene compliance? The majority of those measuring hand hygiene compliance (and/or publishing such studies) use "trained observer" visual observation. This chapter describes some flaws in such an approach: it is prone to bias, overestimates true performance, often captures <1% of hand hygiene opportunities at the time in the institution (yet is generalized to the entire facility), has large inter-rater variation, etc. As these authors state, "Today, a unique reliable and robust method to measure hand hygiene performance does not exist." We know that indirect and less costly (time, personnel, etc.) methods for estimating hand hygiene compliance, such as measuring the amount of agent used, are not accurate. We know that merely measuring hand hygiene compliance on patient room entry or exit does not predict in-room practices (which are most important for the prevention of pathogen transmission to the patient). We know that self-reporting is grossly inaccurate. However, at least in developing countries, emerging technologies may be the answer for the future. The question becomes what we want the system to measure. Currently, electronic systems can measure whether hand hygiene is performed. Such systems generally do not assess the volume of the specific product, the method and duration of application, or specific compliance with each of the five moments or with specific invasive procedures. Video systems are just emerging and have the capacity not only to measure all these elements, but also to be a record to play back for healthcare workers who deny their noncompliance. In the future, where our systems truly demand individual accountability, such video/electronic systems may become essential. It does appear that at least in the developing world – as personnel clinician accountability is enforced and systems insist that hand hygiene best practices be a patient safety issue and thus must be complied with, for cost and personnel reasons – electronic or video systems for hand hygiene measure will become integral components of our measuring systems.

The book ends with chapters on national and international campaigns and regulatory/accrediting body approaches. Undoubtedly, such campaigns – whether local, system-wide, state or nationwide or worldwide – have improved hand hygiene awareness, importance, and compliance. Given the large number of elements we have learned in this book are required for true "hand hygiene best practices compliance" – that is, the best agent, the correct volume, application in compliance with the five moments, application in the correct fashion and for the correct duration – it is hard to believe local or national hand hygiene compliance rates of 85%–95% or that such levels – even if they can be achieved – can be sustained.

This book provides the most contemporary comprehensive summary of what we do and do not know about hand hygiene. It is essential reading for all those who are involved in infection control, patient safety, and quality improvement, or who practice clinical medicine. We must realize that until we have a reliable and robust method to measure hand hygiene performance, we really do not know what our hand hygiene compliance rates really are, nor can we calculate what percentage of HAIs actually can be prevented with high hand hygiene compliance rates. It is my hope that through reading this book and understanding the challenges ahead, video or electronic systems for measuring true hand hygiene compliance with best practices will be developed, and that we will require clinician accountability with hand hygiene recommendations. Then, we will be able to calculate what percentage of HAIs are prevented with different levels of hand hygiene compliance (or with higher or lower compliance with different moments of the WHO five moments) and through achievement of high sustainable hand hygiene compliance rates, we will be leaders in a worldwide campaign to improve patient safety and prevent HAIs through this simple intervention – hand hygiene!

William R. Jarvis, MD
Jason and Jarvis Associates, LLC
Hilton Head Island, South Carolina, USA

Chapter 1

The Burden of Healthcare-Associated Infection

Benedetta Allegranzi,[1] Sepideh Bagheri Nejad,[2] and Didier Pittet[3]

[1] *Infection Prevention and Control Global Unit, Department of Service Delivery and Safety, World Health Organization, and Faculty of Medicine, University of Geneva, Geneva, Switzerland*
[2] *Department of Service Delivery and Safety, World Health Organization, Geneva, Switzerland*
[3] *Infection Control Program and WHO Collaborating Centre on Patient Safety, University of Geneva Hospitals and Faculty of Medicine, Geneva, Switzerland*

KEY MESSAGES

- The World Health Organization (WHO) estimates that hundreds of millions of patients are affected by healthcare-associated infection (HAI) worldwide each year, leading to significant mortality and financial losses for health systems, but precise data of the global burden are not available.

- Of every 100 hospitalized patients at any given time, 6 to 7 will acquire at least one HAI in developed countries and 10 in developing countries.

- In low- and middle-income countries, HAI frequency, especially in high-risk patients, is at least two to three times higher than in high-income countries, and device-associated infection densities in intensive care units are up to 13 times higher.

Healthcare-associated infections (HAIs) affect patients in hospitals and other healthcare settings. These infections are not present or incubating at time of admission, but include infections appearing after discharge, and occupational infections among staff. HAIs are one of the most frequent adverse events during healthcare delivery. No institution or country can claim to have solved this problem, despite many efforts. Healthcare workers' (HCWs') hands are the most

Hand Hygiene: A Handbook for Medical Professionals, First Edition.
Edited by Didier Pittet, John M. Boyce and Benedetta Allegranzi.
© 2017 John Wiley & Sons, Inc. Published 2017 by John Wiley & Sons, Inc.

common vehicle of microorganisms causing HAI. The transmission of these pathogens to the patient, the HCW, and the environment can be prevented through hand hygiene best practices.

WHAT WE KNOW – THE EVIDENCE

Although a national HAI surveillance system is in place in most high-income countries, only 23 developing countries (23/147 [15.6%]) reported a functioning system when assessed in 2010.[1] In 2010, all 27 European Union (EU) Member States and Norway contributed to at least one of the four components of the Healthcare-Associated Infections Surveillance Network (HAI-Net), coordinated by the European Centre for Disease Prevention and Control (ECDC). Among these, 25 and 23 countries participated in the point prevalence surveys of HAI and antimicrobial use in long-term care facilities (LTCF) and acute care hospitals, respectively; 13 countries participated in the surveillance of surgical site infections (SSI); 14 in surveillance of HAI in intensive care units (ICUs); and 7 countries contributed to all surveillance components.[2]

Based on a 1995–2010 systematic review and meta-analysis of national and multicenter studies from high-income countries conducted by the WHO, the prevalence of hospitalized patients who acquired at least one HAI ranged from 3.5% to 12%. Pooled HAI prevalence was 7.6 episodes per 100 patients (95% confidence interval [CI], 6.9–8.5) and 7.1 infected patients per 100 patients admitted (95% CI, 6.5–7.8).[1] Very similar data were issued in 2008 by the ECDC based on a review of studies carried out between 1996 and 2007 in 19 countries.[3] Mean HAI prevalence was 7.1%; the annual number of infected patients was estimated at 4,131,000 and the annual number of HAI at 4,544,100.[3] In 2011–2012, a point prevalence study coordinated by ECDC in 29 countries indicated that, on average, 6% (range, 2.3%–10.8%) of admitted patients acquired at least one HAI in acute care hospitals.[4] Based on these data, ECDC estimated that approximately 80,000 patients in Europe on any given day develop at least one HAI for a total annual number of 3.2 million patients (95% CI 1.9–5.2) with a HAI.[4]

The estimated HAI incidence in the United States was 4.5% in 2002, corresponding to 9.3 infections per 1000 patient-days and 1.7 million affected patients.[5] In the United States and Europe, urinary tract infection (UTI) used to be considered the most frequent type of infection hospital-wide (36% and 27%, respectively).[3,5] In the recent European point prevalence study, lower respiratory tract infection (23.4%) was the most frequent HAI, followed by SSI (19.6%) and UTI (19%).[4] According to several studies, the frequency of SSI varies between 1.2% and 5.2% in high-income countries.[1] In European countries, SSI rates varied according to the type of operation; the highest were in colon surgery (9.9%) and the lowest in knee prosthesis (0.7%).[4]

HAI incidence is much higher in severely ill patients. In high-income countries, approximately 30% of ICU patients are affected by at least one episode of

HAI with substantial associated morbidity and mortality.[6] Pooled HAI cumulative incidence density in adult high-risk patients was 17 episodes per 1000 patient-days (range 13.0–20.3) in a meta-analysis performed by WHO.[1] Incidence densities of device-associated infections in ICUs from different studies including WHO reviews are reported in Table 1.1. In a large-scale study conducted in some middle-income countries in Latin America, HAIs were the most common type of incidents occurring in hospitalized patients; the most frequent were pneumonia and SSI.[7]

According to a systematic review, WHO reported that HAIs are at least two to three times more frequent in resource-limited settings than in high-income countries.[1,8] In low- and middle-income countries, HAI prevalence varied between 5.7% and 19.1% with a pooled prevalence of 10.1 per 100 patients (95% CI, 8.4–12.2); the reported prevalence was significantly higher in high- than in low-quality studies (15.5% vs. 8.5%, respectively).[8] In contrast to Europe and the United States, SSI was the leading infection hospital-wide in settings with limited resources, affecting up to one-third of patients exposed to surgery; SSI was the most frequently surveyed HAI in low- and middle-income countries.[1,8] The reported SSI incidence ranged from 0.4 to 30.9 per 100 patients undergoing surgical procedures and from 1.2 to 23.6 per 100 surgical procedures, with pooled rates of 11.8 per 100 patients exposed to surgery (95% CI, 8.6–16.0) and 5.6 per 100 surgical procedures (95% CI, 2.9–10.5).[8] This is up to nine times higher than in high-income countries.

In low- and middle-income countries, the proportion of patients with ICU-HAI ranged from 4.4% to 88.9% with an infection incidence as high as 42.7 episodes per 1000 patient-days (Table 1.1).[1] This is almost three times higher than in high-income countries. The cumulative incidence of specific device-associated HAI in low- and middle-income countries was estimated by WHO and is regularly reported by the International Nosocomial Infection Control Consortium (INICC), a surveillance network comprising ICUs from 36 low- and middle-income countries. Again, the incidence was found to be at least two to three times higher than in high-income countries and even up to 13 times higher in some countries (Table 1.1). Newborns are also at higher risk in low- and middle-income countries with infection rates 3 to 20 times higher than in high-income countries. Among hospital-born babies in developing countries, HAIs are responsible for 4% to 56% of all causes of death in the neonatal period, and as much as 75% in Southeast Asia and Sub-Saharan Africa.[1] HAIs are not limited to the hospital setting. They are a major problem in LTCF and nursing homes with high levels of antimicrobial resistance and can also result from any type of outpatient care (see Chapters 42C and 42D).

According to available data, the burden of endemic HAI is very significant in terms of excess costs, prolonged hospital stay, attributable mortality, and additional complications and related morbidities. European estimates indicate that HAIs cause 16 million extra days of hospital stay and 37,000 attributable deaths annually, but they also contribute to an additional 110,000 deaths; the annual economic impact in Europe is as high as £7 billion.[3] In the United States, around

Table 1.1 Cumulative Incidence Density of HAI and Device-Associated Infections in Adult ICU Patients in High-, and Low/Middle-Income Countries

Surveillance Networks/ Reviews, Study Period, Country	HAI/1000 Patient-Days (95% CI)	Patient-Days	CR-BSI/1000 Central Line-Days (95% CI)	Catheter-Days	CR-UTI/1000 Urinary Catheter-Days (95% CI)	Urinary Catheter-Days	VAP/1000 Ventilator-Days (95% CI)	Ventilator-Days
WHO meta-analysis, high-income countries, 1995–2010	17.0 (14.2–19.8)	32,537,324	3.5 (2.8–4.1)	5,339,322	4.1 (3.7–4.6)	13,614,567	7.9 (5.7–10.1)	5,339,322
NHSN, 2006–2008, USA#	/	/	2.1	699,300	3.4	546,824	2.9	383,068
WHO meta-analysis, low- and middle-income countries, 1995–2010	42.7 (34.8–50.5)	193,139	12.2 (10.5–13.9)	891,220	8.8 (7.4–10.3)	970,710	23.9 (20.7–27.1)	679,950
INICC, 2004–2009, 36 developing countries#†	/	/	6.8 (6.6–7.0)	506,934	7.1 (6.9–7.3)	535,414	18.4 (17.9–18.8)	357,214

Source: Adapted with permission from reference 1.

HAI, healthcare-associated infection; CR-BSI, central-venous catheter-related bloodstream infection; CR-UTI, catheter-related urinary tract infection; VAP, ventilator-associated pneumonia; NHSN, National Healthcare Safety Network; INICC, International Nosocomial Infection Control Consortium.
#Medical/surgical ICUs in major teaching hospitals.
† Argentina, Brazil, Bulgaria, China, Colombia, Costa Rica, Cuba, Dominican Republic, Ecuador, Egypt, Greece, India, Jordan, Kosovo, Lebanon, Lithuania, Macedonia, Malaysia, Mexico, Morocco, Pakistan, Panama, Peru, Philippines, Puerto Rico, El Salvador, Saudi Arabia, Singapore, Sri Lanka, Sudan, Thailand, Tunisia, Turkey, Venezuela, Vietnam, Uruguay. In: Rosenthal VD et al., *Am J Infect Control* 2012;**40**:396–407.

99,000 deaths were attributed to HAI in 2002.[5] According to the Centers for Disease Control and Prevention (CDC), the overall annual direct medical costs of HAI to US hospitals ranges from US$36 to US$45 billion; of these, from US$25 to US$32 billion would be avoidable when considering that up to 70% of HAIs are preventable.[9]

Very limited data are available at the national level to assess the impact of HAI in low- and middle-income countries. According to a WHO review, increased length of stay associated with HAI in low- and middle-income countries varied between 5 and 29.5 days.[1] Crude excess mortality rates of 18.5%, 23.6%, and 29.3% for catheter-related UTI, central venous catheter-related bloodstream infection, and ventilator-associated pneumonia, respectively, were reported by INICC in adult patients in 173 ICUs in Latin America, Asia, Africa, and Europe.[1] Wide variations in cost estimates associated with HAI were observed between countries. Methods used to estimate excess costs associated with HAIs also varied substantially among studies published in different countries. For instance, in Mexican ICUs, the overall average cost of a HAI episode was US$12,155; in Argentina, overall extra-costs for catheter-related bloodstream infection and healthcare-associated pneumonia were US$4,888 and US$2,255 per case, respectively.[1] In a recent case-control study from Brazil, overall costs of hospitalization for methicillin-resistant *Staphylococcus aureus* bacteremia reached US$123,065 for cases *versus* US$40,247 for controls.[10]

WHAT WE DO NOT KNOW – THE UNCERTAIN

Despite dramatic data related to specific countries or regions, HAI is not included in the list of diseases for which the global burden is regularly estimated by WHO or the Institute for Health Metrics and Evaluation. Precise estimates of the number of patients affected by HAI and the number of episodes occurring worldwide every year, or at a certain moment in time, are not available. Similarly, estimating the number of deaths attributable to HAI is extremely difficult because co-morbidities are usually present, and HAIs are seldom reported as the primary cause of death. Disability-adjusted life years estimates attributable to HAI are not available. Indeed, for instance, it is complex to calculate years of life lost due to a HAI in a cancer patient dying of HAI. In addition, little is known about the occurrence of HAI complications and associated temporary or permanent disabilities. Finally, the available information regarding indirect attributable costs associated with HAI is limited, in particular regarding the extent of economic losses potentially avoidable through better infection control.

Although the number of publications on HAI surveillance in settings with limited resources has increased over the last few years, the picture of the endemic burden of HAI and antimicrobial resistance patterns in low- and middle-income countries remains very scattered. Data from these countries are hampered in all the aforementioned areas, and HAI surveillance is not a priority in most countries. There is a need to identify simplified, but reliable protocols and definitions for HAI surveillance in settings with limited resources. In addition, standardized approaches are very much required to facilitate the best use of data to inform policy makers, raise awareness among frontline staff, and identify priority measures.

RESEARCH AGENDA

Further research is needed to:

- Identify reliable and standardized epidemiological models to estimate the global burden of HAI in terms of proportion of affected patients and number of HAI episodes, attributable mortality, length of stay, disability-adjusted life years, and costs per year saved.
- Develop and validate approaches to estimate the HAI incidence and disease burden using International Classification of Diseases codes and additional information available from computerized patient records.
- Develop and validate protocols and definitions suitable for HAI surveillance in settings with limited resources.
- Identify risk factors for HAI, in particular potential differences between high-income and low- and middle-income countries.

REFERENCES

1. Report on the burden of endemic health care-associated infection worldwide. Geneva: WHO, 2011.
2. ECDC, Annual epidemiological report 2012. Reporting on 2010 surveillance data and 2011 epidemic intelligence data. Stockholm: European Centre for Disease Prevention and Control, 2013.
3. ECDC, Annual epidemiological report on communicable diseases in Europe 2008. Report on the state of communicable diseases in the EU and EEA/EFTA countries. Stockholm: European Centre for Disease Prevention and Control, 2008.
4. ECDC, Point prevalence survey of healthcare-associated infections and antimicrobial use in European acute care hospitals. Stockholm: European Centre for Disease Prevention and Control, 2013.
5. Klevens RM, Edwards JR, Richards CL, Jr., et al., Estimating health care-associated infections and deaths in U.S. hospitals, 2002. *Public Health Rep* 2007;**122**:160–166.
6. Vincent JL, Nosocomial infections in adult intensive-care units. *Lancet* 2003;**361**: 2068–2077.
7. IBEAS, A pioneer study on patient safety in Latin America. World Health Organization, Geneva, 2011. Available at www.who.int/patientsafety/research/country_studies/en/index.html. Accessed March 7, 2017.

8. Allegranzi B, Bagheri Nejad S, Christophe Combescure, et al., Burden of endemic health care-associated infection in developing countries: systematic review and meta-analysis. *Lancet* 2011;**377**:228–241.

9. Scott II RD, The direct medical costs of healthcare-associated infections in U.S. hospitals and the benefits of prevention. Centers for Disease Control and Prevention, 2009.

10. Primo MG, Guilarde AO, Martelli CM, et al., Healthcare-associated Staphylococcus aureus bloodstream infection: length of stay, attributable mortality, and additional direct costs. *Braz J Infect Dis* 2012;**16**:503–509.

Chapter 2

Historical Perspectives

Andrew J. Stewardson[1, 2] and Didier Pittet[2]

[1] Infectious Diseases Department, Austin Health and Hand Hygiene Australia, Melbourne, Australia

[2] Infection Control Program and WHO Collaborating Centre on Patient Safety, University of Geneva Hospitals and Faculty of Medicine, Geneva, Switzerland

One could reasonably consider that the modern era of hand hygiene in healthcare started in the mid-nineteenth century with the work of Ignaz Semmelweis (1818–1865).[1,2] Semmelweis was employed as assistant in obstetrics at the Vienna General Hospital in 1846, and he quickly became concerned about the high maternal mortality rate due to puerperal fever. At the time, women were admitted to one of two obstetric wards on the basis of alternating days: one ward staffed by doctors and medical students, and the other by midwives. In what was a landmark achievement in hospital epidemiology, this setting combined with Semmelweis's careful surveillance of maternal mortality enabled him to dismiss contemporary hypotheses regarding the cause of the disease, such as miasma or patient-level factors. He concluded that the cause was a factor unique to the ward staffed by doctors and medical students, which had a mortality rate more than double of that staffed by midwives. The clue was provided by the death of his colleague, Jakob Kolletschka, with an illness resembling childbed fever following a scalpel laceration while supervising an autopsy. This led Semmelweis to hypothesize that the elevated mortality rate in the medical ward was due to contamination of medical student hands with "cadaverous particles" during autopsies, a newly popular teaching tool. As a result, Semmelweis instituted a new regimen of hand scrubbing with chlorinated lime. Initially required on entry to the obstetric ward, hand scrubbing was soon extended to between contact with each patient. While this intervention was effective in producing a sustained reduction in maternal mortality, it proved unpopular with students and colleagues, and his contract was not renewed. This failure was likely the result of a combination of the hand irritation caused by chlorinated lime, the absence of a biologic explanatory model, and

Hand Hygiene: A Handbook for Medical Professionals, First Edition.
Edited by Didier Pittet, John M. Boyce and Benedetta Allegranzi.
© 2017 John Wiley & Sons, Inc. Published 2017 by John Wiley & Sons, Inc.

what is commonly described as Semmelweis's abrasive temperament and lack of diplomacy.

Unfortunately, in his day, Semmelweis's work did not lead to widespread changes in practice or appreciation of the significance of hand hygiene (perhaps the notable exception being within the field of surgery, where attention to aseptic technique became established sooner). It wasn't until the mid-twentieth century that rapid progress was made. In the wake of hospital-based clusters of staphylococcal infections in the 1950s in the United States, the 1960s and 1970s were a period of rapid development in the field of infection prevention and control. Several studies in the 1960s confirmed the importance of healthcare workers hands in transmission of *Staphylococcus aureus*. For example, Mortimer et al. found that handwashing after caring for an "index case" neonate colonized by *S. aureus* reduced the risk of colonization of other neonates in the same nursery from 92% to 53%.[3] In 1975, a year after launching the landmark *Study on the Efficacy of Infection Control* (SENIC), the CDC published a review on handwashing in healthcare that began with the statement that "handwashing is generally considered the most important procedure in preventing nosocomial infections." When reported a decade later, the SENIC results established the importance of active infection control interventions beyond passive surveillance.[4] Thus the stage was set for a new phase in hand hygiene promotion. Progress since then can be tracked by the shifts seen in hand hygiene guidelines over the last 30 years as well as the increasing number of publications in the medical literature (see Chapter 45).

By the mid-1980s, handwashing was a central focus of formal CDC guidelines on prevention of healthcare-associated infections.[5] Handwashing with water and soap was the recommended method, with healthcare workers instructed to undertake "vigorous rubbing together of all surfaces of lathered hands for at least 10 seconds, followed by thorough rinsing under a stream of water." These detailed guidelines outlined a stratified approach based on real-time risk assessment by healthcare workers. Plain soap was the preferred product except when caring for newborns, immunocompromised patients, and other high-risk patients, when antimicrobial-containing products were recommended. Healthcare workers were not obliged to perform hand hygiene for "routine, brief patient-care activities involving direct patient contact" unless they fulfilled one of a series of criteria, such as before an invasive procedure, before caring for "particularly susceptible patients," or after activities during which "microbial contamination of hands is likely to occur." These guidelines mentioned waterless foams and rinses, but limited their use to circumstances where handwashing facilities were not available.

The 1990s saw a shift towards wider use of alcohol-based handrubs (ABHRs). Previously, ABHRs were well established in some European countries, particularly Germany. In the mid-1990s, both the Association for Professionals in Infection Control (APIC) and the CDC Healthcare Infection Control Practices Advisory Committee (HICPAC) published hand hygiene guidelines that supported the more widespread use of ABHRs in clinical settings. Their more widespread incorporation into routine care gained momentum following a report from the University of Geneva Hospitals, Switzerland, where implementation of a multimodal strategy for hand hygiene promotion resulted in improved healthcare worker hand hygiene compliance with a simultaneous reduction in the prevalence of healthcare-associated infection and the incidence of methicillin-resistant *Staphylococcus aureus* (MRSA) colonization events.[6] This strategy was repeated elsewhere, and catalyzed a paradigm shift in the approach to hand hygiene.

In 2002, joint guidelines from the Healthcare Infection Control Practices Advisory Committee (HICPAC), the Society for Healthcare Epidemiology of America (SHEA), Association for Professionals in Infection Control (APIC), and the Infectious Diseases Society of America (IDSA) recommended use of ABHRs as the preferred method for hand hygiene, unless hands were visibly soiled.[7] Handwashing with soap and water remained an acceptable alternative. A broader approach was taken to indications for hand hygiene, with healthcare workers now advised to perform hand hygiene before all patient contacts and after contact with objects in the immediate vicinity of patients, in addition to "high risk" procedures. Implementation became a focus, and a multidisciplinary approach to hand hygiene promotion employing aspects of behavior change theory was proposed. This included education, performance feedback and support of institutional leadership.[7,8]

These new directions were further developed in the World Health Organization Guidelines for Hand Hygiene in Healthcare published in 2006 (draft form) and 2009.[9] Access to ABHRs at the point of care was of central importance within a well-defined multimodal strategy for hand hygiene promotion. This strategy included five components: system change, education and training, performance feedback, reminders in the workplace, and safety climate. A new method for conceptualizing indications for hand hygiene was introduced. This method, My Five Moments for Hand Hygiene, completed the transition from the complex list of indications requiring healthcare worker risk assessment seen in earlier guidelines to a condensed group of five "moments" (see also Chapter 20). These guidelines also sought to broaden the scope of hand hygiene promotion by describing a strategy that could be implemented globally, in low-, middle-, and high-income settings.[10] An accompanying suite of tools (available in several languages) was produced to facilitate hand hygiene promotion (see also Chapter 33).

At the current time, hand hygiene has become increasingly embedded within healthcare on clinical, administrative, and political levels. Since 2005, the ministers of health in more than 150 countries have signed the WHO-facilitated pledge to reduce healthcare-associated infections by means including hand hygiene promotion. In many countries, hand hygiene campaigns are coordinated nationally or regionally. Hand hygiene compliance and its surrogate measures, such as ABHR consumption, are widely used as quality indicators, and some countries have set specific targets, implemented public reporting of institutional results, or linked funding with hand hygiene performance. Simultaneously, the last decade has witnessed an explosion in the medical literature related to hand hygiene, including important input from the disciplines of quality improvement and patient safety, behavioral sciences, health economics, human factors design and implementation science, and engineering. Although of clear value in the prevention of healthcare infections and reduced transmission of antimicrobial resistance, these advances have brought with them many new challenges, and the field continues to evolve rapidly.

REFERENCES

1. Nuland SB, *The doctor's plague: germs, childbed fever, and the strange story of Ignác Semmelweis.* New York: WW Norton & Company, 2003.
2. Stewardson A, Pittet D, Ignac Semmelweis—celebrating a flawed pioneer of patient safety. *Lancet* 2011;**378**:22–23.
3. Mortimer EA, Jr., Lipsitz PJ, Wolinsky E, et al., Transmission of staphylococci between newborns. *Am J Dis Child* 1962;**104**:289–295.
4. Haley RW, Culver DH, White JW, et al., The efficacy of infection surveillance and control programs in preventing nosocomial infections in US hospitals. *Am J Epidemiol* 1985;**121**:182–205.
5. Garner JS, Favero MS, Guideline for handwashing and hospital environmental control. Program Center for Infectious Diseases, Centers for Disease Control and Prevention; 1985.
6. Pittet D, Hugonnet S, Harbarth S, et al., Effectiveness of a hospital-wide programme to improve compliance with hand hygiene. *Lancet* 2000;**356**:1307–1312.
7. Boyce JM, Pittet D, Guideline for hand hygiene in health-care settings: recommendations of the Healthcare Infection Control Practices Advisory Committee and the HICPAC/SHEA/APIC/IDSA hand hygiene Task force. *Infect Control Hosp Epidemiol* 2002;**23**(Suppl. 12):S3–S40.
8. Larson EL, Early E, Cloonan P, et al., An organizational climate intervention associated with increased handwashing and decreased nosocomial infections. *Behav Med* 2000;**26**:14–22.
9. World Health Organization, *WHO Guidelines on Hand Hygiene in Health Care.* Geneva: WHO, 2009.
10. Allegranzi B, Gayet-Ageron A, Damani N, et al., Global implementation of WHO's multimodal strategy for improvement of hand hygiene: a quasi-experimental study. *Lancet Infect Dis* 2013;**13**:843–851.

Chapter 3

Flora and Physiology of Normal Skin

Gürkan Kaya[1] and Didier Pittet[2]

[1] *Dermatology and Venereology Service, University of Geneva Hospitals and Faculty of Medicine, Geneva, Switzerland*

[2] *Infection Control Program and WHO Collaborating Centre on Patient Safety, University of Geneva Hospitals and Faculty of Medicine, Geneva, Switzerland*

KEY MESSAGES

- The skin is composed of three layers: the epidermis, dermis, and subcutaneous tissue (hypodermis). The barrier to percutaneous absorption is the *stratum corneum*, the most superficial layer of the epidermis. The function of the *stratum corneum* is to reduce water loss, provide protection against abrasive action, and prevent penetration of infectious agents and chemicals.

- Bacteria recovered from the hands could be divided into two categories, namely resident or transient. Although the count of transient and resident flora varies considerably among individuals, it is often relatively constant for any given individual. Resident flora has two main protective functions: microbial antagonism and competition for nutrients in the ecosystem. Transient flora, which colonizes the superficial layers of the skin, is more amenable to removal by hand hygiene.

- Recent metagenomic studies have shown that the skin contains complex and diverse microbial ecosystems, called the skin microbiome. Interactions between the skin microbiome and hand hygiene agents and their combination deserve further studies.

The skin is the largest organ of the human body and has a surface area between 1.5 and 2 square meters. It accounts for 16% of total body weight. Considered one of the most important organs of the body, the skin functions as a protective

Hand Hygiene: A Handbook for Medical Professionals, First Edition.
Edited by Didier Pittet, John M. Boyce and Benedetta Allegranzi.

barrier against external organisms, maintains temperature control, senses our surroundings, eliminates wastes, and synthesizes vitamin D.

Recent metagenomic studies have shown that the skin contains complex and diverse microbial ecosystems, called the skin microbiome.[1] Metagenomics refers to the amplification of the small subunit prokaryotic ribosomal RNA (16S rRNA) gene by polymerase chain reaction (PCR) from skin samples.[2] In 2007, the National Institutes of Health launched the Human Microbiome Project to develop a reference catalog of microbial genome sequences found in different body areas including the skin.[3] Metagenomic studies using 16S rRNA sequencing revealed that the vast majority of skin bacteria belong to Actinobacteria, Firmicutes, Bacteroidetes, and Proteobacteria phyla.[4] However, thousands of distinct species have been identified within these phyla. The analysis of the palm microbiome revealed 4742 distinct species in 51 healthy subjects.[5]

In 1938 already, Price established that bacteria recovered from the hands could be divided into two categories, namely resident or transient.[6] The resident flora (resident microbiota) consists of microorganisms residing under the superficial cells of the *stratum corneum* and can also be found on the surface of the skin.[7,8] *Staphylococcus epidermidis* is the dominant species,[9] with extraordinarily high oxacillin resistance, particularly among healthcare workers (HCWs).[10] Other resident bacteria include *S. hominis* and other coagulase-negative staphylococci, followed by Actinobacteria (propionibacteria, corynebacteria, and other dermobacteria).[11] Among fungi, the most common genus of the resident skin flora, when present, is *Pityrosporum* (*Malassezia*) spp.[12] Resident flora has two main protective functions: microbial antagonism and the competition for nutrients in the ecosystem.[13] In general, resident flora is less likely to be associated with infections, but may cause infections in sterile body cavities, the eyes, or on non-intact skin.[14]

Transient flora (transient microbiota), which colonizes the superficial layers of the skin, is more amenable to removal by routine hand hygiene. Transient microorganisms do not usually multiply on the skin, but they survive and sporadically multiply on skin surface.[13] They are often acquired by HCWs when in contact with patients or contaminated surfaces adjacent to the patient and are frequently associated with healthcare-associated infections (HAIs). Some types of contact during routine neonatal care are more frequently associated with higher levels of bacterial contamination of HCWs' hands: respiratory secretions, nappy/diaper change, and direct skin contact.[15,16] The transmissibility of transient flora depends on the species present, the number of microorganisms on the surface, and the skin moisture.[17,18] The hands of some HCWs may become persistently colonized by pathogenic flora such as *S. aureus*, Gram-negative bacilli, or yeast.[19]

Normal human skin is colonized by bacteria, with total aerobic bacterial counts ranging from more than 1×10^6 colony-forming units (CFU)/cm^2 on the scalp, 5×10^5 CFU/cm^2 in the axilla, and 4×10^4 CFU/cm^2 on the abdomen to 1×10^4 CFU/cm^2 on the forearm.[20] Total bacterial counts on the hands of HCWs generally range from 3.9×10^4 to 4.6×10^6 CFU/cm^2.[14,21–23] Fingertip contamination ranged from 0 to 300 CFU when sampled by agar contact methods.[15] Price and subsequent investigators documented that although the count of transient and resident flora varies considerably among individuals, it is often relatively constant for any given individual.[6,24]

The skin is composed of three layers of different thickness: the thin outer layer called epidermis (50–100 μm), the thick inner layer called dermis (1–2 mm), and the subcutaneous tissue or hypodermis (1–2 mm) containing adipocyte lobules and interlobular septa (Figure 3.1). The epidermis is composed of 10–20 layers of

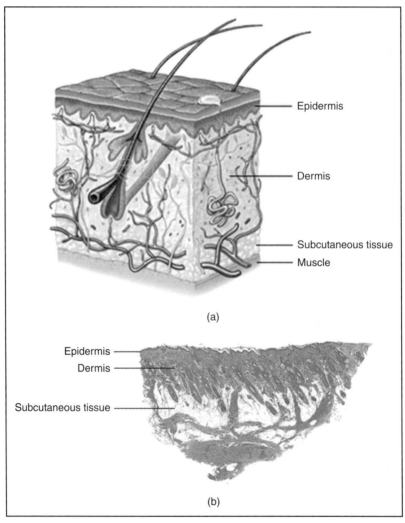

(a)

Epidermis

Dermis

Subcutaneous tissue

(b)

Figure 3.1   The anatomical layers of the skin *Source*: Shier 2004. Reproduced with permission from McGraw-Hill. *See plate section for color representation of this figure.*

keratinocytes and has four layers (from inside to outside): *stratum basale, stratum spinosum, stratum granulosum,* and *stratum corneum.* Keratinocytes of the *stratum basale* migrate towards the surface by differentiating through different layers of the epidermis. The entire epidermis is replaced every four weeks. It is estimated that an individual will lose about 500 grams of skin every year by shedding. The epidermis also contains melanocytes involved in skin pigmentation, and Langerhans' cells, involved in antigen presentation and immune responses.

The barrier to percutaneous absorption is the *stratum corneum,* the most superficial layer of the epidermis. The function of the *stratum corneum* is to reduce water loss, provide protection against abrasive action, and prevent penetration of infectious agents and chemicals. *Stratum corneum* is about 10–20 μm thick, and consists of a multilayered stratum of flat, polyhedral-shaped, 2–3 μm thick non-nucleated cells named corneocytes. Corneocytes are composed primarily of insoluble bundled keratins surrounded by a cell envelope stabilized by cross-linked proteins and covalently bound lipids. Corneodesmosomes are membrane junctions interconnecting *corneocytes* and contributing to the cohesion of the *stratum corneum.* The intercellular space between corneocytes is composed of lipids primarily generated from the exocytosis of lamellar bodies during the terminal differentiation of the keratinocytes. These lipids are required for an effective skin barrier function.

The epidermis is a dynamic structure, and the renewal of the *stratum corneum* is controlled by complex regulatory systems of cellular differentiation. Current knowledge of the function of the *stratum corneum* has come from studies of the epidermal responses to perturbation of the skin barrier such as (i) extraction of skin lipids with apolar solvents; (ii) physical stripping of the *stratum corneum* using adhesive tape; and (iii) chemically induced irritation. All of these experimental manipulations lead to a transient decrease of the skin barrier efficacy, as determined by transepidermal water loss. These alterations of the *stratum corneum* generate an increase of keratinocyte proliferation and differentiation in response to this "aggression" in order to restore the skin barrier. This increase in the keratinocyte proliferation rate could directly influence the integrity of the skin barrier by perturbing (i) the uptake of nutrients, such as essential fatty acids; (ii) the synthesis of proteins and lipids; or (iii) the processing of precursor molecules required for skin barrier function.

Cystine disulfide bonds play an important role in the solidity and resistance of the *stratum corneum* and are inert to a majority of reactive chemicals. They are vulnerable, however, to strong antioxidants and to a direct cleavage by chemical substances such as cyanide ion.[25]

RESEARCH AGENDA

- Explore the impact of sample collection method, DNA extraction techniques and sequencing modalities on the dynamics of hand microbial community structure.

- Explore the role of the skin microbiome and the differential impact of soap and water handwashing, alcohol-based handrubbing, as well as other hand hygiene agents and lotions on the skin microbiome.

REFERENCES

1. Chen YE, Tsao H, *J Am Acad Dermatol* 2013;**69**:143–155.
2. Dethlefsen L, McFall-Ngai M, Relman DA, An ecological and evolutionary perspective on human-microbe mutualism and disease. *Nature* 2007;**449**:811–818.
3. Turnbaugh PJ, Ley RE, Hamady M, et al., The human microbiome project. *Nature* 2007;**449**:804–810.
4. Grice EA, Kong HH, Renaud G, et al., A diversity profile of the human skin microbiota. *Genome Res* 2008;**18**:1043–1050.
5. Fierer N, Hamady M, Lauber CL, et al., The influence of sex, handedness, and washing on the diversity of hand surface bacteria. *Proc Natl Acad Sci USA* 2008;**105**: 17994–17999.
6. Price PB, The bacteriology of normal skin: a new quantitative test applied to a study of the bacterial flora and the disinfectant action of mechanical cleansing. *J Infect Dis* 1938;**63**:301–318.
7. Montes LF, Wilborn WH, Location of bacterial skin flora. *Br J Dermatol* 1969;**81** (Suppl. 1):23–26.
8. Wilson M, *Microbial inhabitants of humans: their ecology and role in health and disease.* New York: Cambridge University Press, 2005.
9. Rayan GM, Flournoy DJ, Microbiologic flora of human fingernails. *J Hand Surg Am* 1987;**12**:605–607.
10. Lee YL, Cesario T, Lee R, et al., Colonization by Staphylococcus species resistant to methicillin or quinolone on hands of medical personnel in a skilled-nursing facility. *Am J Infect Control* 1994; **22**:346–351.
11. Evans CA, Smith WM, Johnston EA, et al., Bacterial flora of the normal human skin. *J Invest Dermatol* 1950;**15**:305–324.
12. Hay RJ, Fungi and fungal infections of the skin. In: Noble WC, ed. *The skin microflora and microbial skin disease.* Cambridge: Cambridge University Press, 1993:232–263.
13. Kampf G, Kramer A, Epidemiologic background of hand hygiene and evaluation of the most important agents for scrubs and rubs. *Clin Microbiol Rev* 2004;**17**:863–893.
14. Lark RL, VanderHyde K, Deeb GM, et al., An outbreak of coagulase-negative staphylococcal surgical-site infections following aortic valve replacement. *Infect Control Hosp Epidemiol* 2001; **22**:618–623.
15. Pittet D, Dharan S, Touveneau S, et al., Bacterial contamination of the hands of hospital staff during routine patient care. *Arch Int Med* 1999;**159**:821–826.
16. Pessoa-Silva CL, Dharan S, Hugonnet S, et al. Dynamics of bacterial hand contamination during routine neonatal care. *Infect Control Hosp Epidemiol* 2004;**25**:192–197.
17. Marples RR, Towers AG, A laboratory model for the investigation of contact transfer of micro-organisms. *J Hyg (London)* 1979;**82**:237–248.
18. Patrick DR, Findon G, Miller TE, Residual moisture determines the level of touch-contact-associated bacterial transfer following hand washing. *Epidemiol Infect* 1997;**119**:319–325.
19. Adams BG, Marrie TJ, Hand carriage of aerobic gram-negative rods may not be transient. *J Hyg (London)* 1982;**89**:33–46.

20. Selwyn S, Microbiology and ecology of human skin. *Practitioner* 1980;**224**:1059–1062.
21. Larson E, Effects of handwashing agent, handwashing frequency, and clinical area on hand flora. *Am J Infect Control* 1984;**12**:76–82.
22. Larson EL, Hughes CA, Pyrek JD, et al., Changes in bacterial flora associated with skin damage on hands of health care personnel. *Am J Infect Control* 1998;**26**:513–521.
23. Maki D, Control of colonization and transmission of pathogenic bacteria in the hospital. *Ann Intern Med* 1978;**89**(Suppl. 5 Pt 2):777–780.
24. Sprunt K, Redman W, Leidy G, Antibacterial effectiveness of routine hand washing. *Pediatrics* 1973;**52**:264–271.
25. Magee PS, Percutaneous absorbtion: Critical factors in transdermal transport. In: Marzulli FN, Maibach HI, eds. *Dermatotoxicology* 4th edn. New York: Hemisphere Publishing, 1991:1–35.

Chapter 4

Dynamics of Hand Transmission

Andrew J. Stewardson,[1,2] **Benedetta Allegranzi,**[3] **and Didier Pittet**[2]

[1] *Infectious Diseases Department, Austin Health and Hand Hygiene Australia, Melbourne, Australia*
[2] *Infection Control Program and WHO Collaborating Centre on Patient Safety, University of Geneva Hospitals and Faculty of Medicine, Geneva, Switzerland*
[3] *Infection Prevention and Control Global Unit, Department of Service Delivery and Safety, World Health Organization, and Faculty of Medicine, University of Geneva, Geneva, Switzerland*

KEY MESSAGES

- Healthcare workers' (HCWs') hands are considered a key vector in the transmission of pathogenic organisms and antimicrobial resistance determinants in the healthcare setting.

- Contact with intact skin and contaminated environmental surfaces is sufficient to result in transmission of organisms from patients or the environment to HCWs' hands; bacterial hand contamination increases with the duration of patient care.

- Appropriate hand hygiene behavior is critical in reducing organism transmission in the healthcare setting.

Healthcare workers' (HCWs') hands are frequently in contact with patients and inanimate surfaces and are highly mobile throughout the healthcare environment. As such, they are considered a key vector in the transmission of pathogenic organisms and antimicrobial resistance determinants in the healthcare setting. This chapter presents a summary of the relevant evidence in this domain. We will focus on studies that directly assess transmission events rather than epidemiologic or interventional studies. A discussion of mathematical models of transmission dynamics follows in Chapter 5.

Hand Hygiene: A Handbook for Medical Professionals, First Edition.
Edited by Didier Pittet, John M. Boyce and Benedetta Allegranzi.
© 2017 John Wiley & Sons, Inc. Published 2017 by John Wiley & Sons, Inc.

WHAT WE KNOW – THE EVIDENCE

A conceptual model of hand transmission has previously been proposed (Table 4.1).[1] This chapter will follow the same framework, addressing in turn each of the five steps required for transmission of organisms between patients.

Organisms Present on Patients' Skin or Immediate Environment

Human skin is colonized by a diverse range of organisms; their collective genetic material is referred to as the skin microbiome[2] (see Chapter 3). These include organisms that have a beneficial role in human health as well as those that are relevant in the healthcare setting, either as potential infectious agents or as vehicles of transmission for antimicrobial resistance determinants. Culture-independent (metagenomic) studies have provided recent insights into factors that contribute to variation in the skin microbiome, including host physiology (such as anatomic site) and genotype, environment and lifestyle, immune system, and pathophysiology.[2]

Variation by body site is of obvious importance when considering the dynamics of organism transfer in the hospital setting.[2] Sebaceous sites, including the face, chest, and back, are generally dominated by *Propionibacterium* species. Moist sites, including umbilicus, axillae, inguinal creases, and other folds and creases, are most abundantly colonized by *Staphylococcus* and *Corynebacterium* species. Finally, dry sites have the greatest microbial diversity, with organisms from the phyla Actinobacteria, Proteobacteria, Firmicutes and Bacteriodetes. Of potential significance, given the global threat of antimicrobial resistance amongst *Enterobacteriaceae*, these sites include an abundance of Gram-negative bacteria. The skin microbiome of hospitalized patients is likely to be altered for a number of reasons, including greater prevalence of systemic diseases (particularly diabetes), disrupted

Table 4.1 The Five Sequential Steps for Cross-Transmission of Microbial Pathogens

1. Organisms are present on the patient's skin or have been shed onto inanimate objects immediately surrounding the patient
2. Organisms must be transferred to the hands of healthcare workers
3. Organisms must be capable of surviving for at least several minutes on healthcare workers' hands
4. Handwashing or hand antisepsis by the healthcare worker must be inadequate or omitted entirely, or the agent used for hand hygiene inappropriate
5. The contaminated hand(s) of the caregiver must come into direct contact with another patient or with an inanimate object that will come into direct contact with the patient

Source: Pittet 2006. Reproduced with permission from Elsevier.

skin integrity due to skin conditions, wounds, or invasive devices, and the presence of dressings.

HCWs are accustomed to considering *Staphylococcus aureus* as part of skin flora. However, patients colonized by antimicrobial resistant bacteria traditionally considered gastrointestinal tract commensals may also have these organisms present on their skin. For example, extended-spectrum beta-lactamase (ESBL)-producing *Enterobacteriaceae* colonize the groin of 35% of patients with infections due to such organisms.[3] Vancomycin-resistant enterococci (VRE) could be found on the hands of 25–54% of fecally continent VRE-colonized patients.[4] Therefore it is important to bear in mind that contact with wounds, body fluids, secretions, or fecal material is not required to determine the risk of contamination with organisms of importance for healthcare-associated infections: most of such organisms can be found on intact patient skin.[1]

The immediate patient environment receives a steady influx of organisms via direct patient contact and squames shed from patient's skin.[1] Organisms that are resistant to desiccation, including staphylococci, enterococci, *Clostridium difficile* and *Acinetobacter baumannii*, exhibit high capacity to contaminate and persist in the patient zone. One study detected methicillin-resistant *S. aureus* (MRSA) environmental contamination in the rooms of approximately 70% of patients that were either infected or colonized with MRSA.[5] Commonly contaminated objects included floor surfaces, bed linen, patient gowns, over-bed tables, and blood pressure cuffs. In another study, 36–58% of patient chairs and 42–48% of patient couches were contaminated by VRE after mock outpatient, hemodialysis or radiology sessions involving VRE-colonized patients.[4] Fecal density of VRE appeared to correlate with risk of contamination.[4] Multi-drug-resistant *A. baumannii* can be detected in environmental samples from 78% of colonized patients' rooms.[6] Not surprisingly, we can expect a greater degree of environmental contamination by healthcare pathogens in the setting of diarrhea and fecal incontinence; however, this should certainly not be considered a requirement for environmental contamination.[7]

Less robust organisms can also survive for limited periods on inanimate surfaces. For example, at room temperature, live influenza A virus can be recovered from most environmental surfaces four hours after application, and up to nine hours on nonporous materials.[8]

Organism Transfer to Healthcare Workers' Hands

There are scarce data with which to stratify patient care activities according to risk for transmission of organisms to HCWs' hands.[1] However, there is sufficient evidence to conclude that – as suggested above – "clean activities" involving contact with patient skin provide ample opportunity for such transmissions and that a key determinant of HCWs' hand contamination is duration of patient care. Pittet et al. followed HCWs during routine patient care to determine risk factors for bacterial hand contamination.[9] This study estimated that ungloved hands accumulate

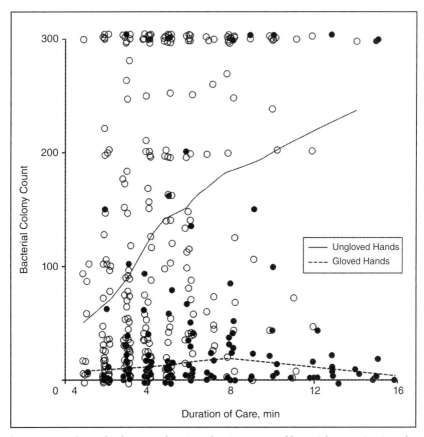

Figure 4.1 Relationship between duration of patient care and bacterial contamination of hands of hospital staff who wore gloves (solid circles and dashed line) and those who did not wear gloves (open circles and solid line) in 417 observations conducted at the University Hospitals of Geneva, Geneva, Switzerland, in 1996. Lines represent the average trend in each group, obtained using nonparametric regression (LOWESS). *Source*: Pittet 1999. Reproduced with permission from The American Medical Association.

bacteria at a rate of 16 colony-forming units per minute (Figure 4.1). Risk factors for contamination included patient contact, respiratory care, body fluid/secretion contact, and distractions from care flow (Table 4.2).[9] Pessoa-Silva et al. performed a similar study in a neonatal unit.[10] They demonstrated that HCWs' hands become progressively contaminated during patient care, and that skin contact, respiratory care, and diaper changes were independently associated with increased bacterial count.

A number of studies have examined the transmission risk associated with specific pathogens or specific activities. For example, Hamburger demonstrated that Group A streptococcus can be transferred between individuals during a

Table 4.2 Relationship Between the Time Spent in Various Patient Care Activities and
Bacterial Contamination of the Hands of Gloveless Hospital Staff (Multiple Linear
Regression Model)

Activity	Bacterial Colonies, CFU/min (95% Confidence Interval)	P
Direct patient contact	20 (14–26)	<0.001
Rupture in the sequence of care	19 (10–27)	<0.001
Respiratory care	21 (8–35)	0.002
Handling body fluid secrections	16 (3–29)	0.02
Blood sampling and intravenous injection or care	6 (–2–14)	0.14
Skin contact	4 (–5–13)	0.35
Housekeeping activities	–10 (–32–12)	0.38

CFU, colony-forming units.
Source: Pittet 1999. Reproduced with permission from The American Medical Association.

handshake.[11] In one study, 52% (95% CI, 42–62) of HCWs contaminated their
hands or gloves with VRE after contact with the patient environment only.[12]
Another small study suggested that HCW hands were most likely to become
colonized by VRE, and subsequently transmit this organism to inanimate surfaces,
after contact with patients' antecubital fossa or a blood pressure cuff.[13] In mock
clinical interactions, 16% of HCWs' gloved hands were contaminated by VRE
after collecting a rectal swab from a colonized patient.[4]

Several studies have examined contamination of HCWs' gloves. These studies
demonstrate the variation in risk of contamination according to organism. For
example, 17.7% (95% CI, 9.3–26.1) and 7.7% (95% CI, 2.2–13.2) of HCWs had
MRSA and VRE, respectively, on their gloves when exiting the room of a patient
colonized by those organisms.[14] The risk of transfer of MRSA to gloved-hands
while caring for a colonized patient is similar whether touching skin sites or
environmental surfaces (40% vs. 45%, $P=0.59$).[15] In another study, glove
contamination was detected more frequently when exiting the room of a patient
colonized by multi-drug-resistant *A. baumannii* (36.2% [95% CI, 29.5–42.9])
than multi-drug-resistant *Pseudomonas aeruginosa* (6.7% [95% CI, 2.5–11.0]).[16]
Independent risk factors for contamination of HCW gloves or gown with
multi-drug-resistant organisms include positive environmental cultures, duration
of time spent in the patient room, performance of a physical examination, and
contact with a ventilator.[6]

Under experimental conditions, influenza A (H1N1) and influenza B at physiological concentration can be transferred from nonporous material to human
hands.[17] There is also evidence to suggest that contact with infected patients and
contaminated environmental surfaces can result in respiratory syncytial virus and
rhinovirus acquisition.[18,19]

Organism Survival on Hands

Bacterial contamination of HCWs' hands increases with the duration of patient care (Figure 4.1). Based on a review including 24 studies, the prevalence of MRSA carriage on HCWs' hands was 6.4%.[20] Studies performed before the widespread introduction of alcohol-based handrubs found that Gram-negative bacilli were present on the hands of 20–30% of HCWs.[21–24] Predominant organisms included *Acinetobacter*, *Klebsiella*, *Enterobacter*, and *Serratia* species. These prevalence data demonstrate that such organisms are present on HCWs' hands, but there are fewer data regarding duration of persistence. Available studies suggest that while *Acinetobacter* spp., *P. aeruginosa*, *Shigella dysenteriae* and VRE may remain viable for 60 minutes, *E. coli* and *Klebsiella* spp. have a half life of approximately five minutes only.[1] Determinants of the skin microbiome composition discussed above are relevant here. For example, HCWs with hand dermatitis may be colonized by pathogens for longer periods.[1] In an experimental model, influenza A (H3N2) and A (H1N1)pdm09 remained viable on human fingertips for at least one minute after contamination.[25] Thereafter, there was a rapid reduction in viral recoverability, so that only a small minority of subjects had detectable virus after 30 minutes. Factors favoring prolonged survival included larger droplet size and higher viral concentration.

Defective Hand Cleansing Results in Hands Remaining Contaminated

Defective hand cleansing can take two forms: complete omission or suboptimal performance such that the reduction in organisms is affected. Evidently, the former will facilitate transmission of organisms by HCWs' hands. However, the latter – a suboptimal hand hygiene action – warrants further consideration. Parameters include the antimicrobial efficacy of the product, the quantity of product applied on hands, the presence of foreign materials such as rings or false nails, the duration of the hand hygiene action, and the steps (distinct movements) performed during it. These are discussed in detail in Chapters 8, 9, and 10.

Contaminated Hands Cross-Transmit Organisms

A mix of laboratory-based, epidemiologic, and outbreak investigation studies, summarized elsewhere,[1] demonstrate the role of HCWs' hands in transmitting organisms including *S. aureus*, norovirus, *Serratia* spp., *Acinetobacter* spp., and VRE. Factors determining the risk of transmission from HCWs' hands to patients or environmental surfaces include the organism involved, the nature of the destination surface, the duration of contact, moisture, and inoculum size.[1]

In a landmark early study by Mortimer et al.,[26] *S. aureus* colonization occurred in 92% (45/49) of neonates cared for by a nurse who had had contact with an index neonate known to be colonized by *S. aureus*. More recently, a review published in 2008 identified 27 studies reporting clear molecular and epidemiological evidence of MRSA transmission from HCWs to patients, with a further 52 studies categorizing such transmission as likely.[20] This review concluded that with regards to MRSA, HCWs "are likely to be important in the transmission of MRSA, most frequently acting as vectors and not as the main sources of MRSA transmission."

Transmission of organisms from patients to the environment via HCW hands was elegantly illustrated by Duckro et al.[13] By culturing HCW hands and clinical surfaces touched after touching a site known to be VRE positive, this study demonstrated that 10.6% (95% CI, 6.2–16.6) of contacts result in contamination of a previously culture-negative site by the same VRE strain found on HCWs' hands.

Impact of Hand Hygiene on Transmission

One can clearly expect, given the conceptual model of transmission outlined above when combined with an understanding of the efficacy of hand hygiene products (see Chapter 8), that hand hygiene will reduce the transmission of organisms in the healthcare setting. This applies to both interpatient transmission as well as intrapatient transmission.[1] In addition to numerous reports of healthcare outbreaks where hand hygiene is associated with epidemic control, a relatively small number of studies have described the impact of hand hygiene on organism transfer and colonization in the nonoutbreak healthcare setting.[1,27,28] Such studies have typically focused on *S. aureus*. Mortimer et al. demonstrated that handwashing after contact with a *S. aureus*-colonized neonate reduced *S. aureus* acquisition events amongst subsequently handled neonates from one event per 35 hours to one event per 135 hours of exposure.[26] The multimodal hand hygiene campaign implemented by Pittet et al. also resulted in a reduction in MRSA transmission events, from 2.16 to 0.93 events per 10,000 patient days (<0.001).[29] The ultimate indicator of this effect on organism transmission is the impact of hand hygiene on healthcare-associated infection rates. That topic is addressed in detail in Chapter 41.

WHAT WE DO NOT KNOW – THE UNCERTAIN

An understanding of the dynamics of microbial transmission in healthcare is of central importance in determining when hand hygiene should be performed. The central problem is that it is extremely challenging, if not unfeasible, to pinpoint exactly when a transmission event takes place during patient care. Each piece of evidence presented in this chapter provides a small snapshot of the steps that make up a conceptual model of microbial transmission.[1] This model identifies moments of risk for organism transmission and formed the basis for development of "My Five Moments for Hand Hygiene" (see Chapter 20).

Many questions remain open, and difficult to address. For example, while this chapter has focused on HCWs' hands as vectors for transmission of organisms between multiple patients or between patients and the environment, there is less evidence regarding their role in transferring organisms from one body site to another (for example, to a sterile body site) within an individual patient.

There are substantial gaps in our knowledge regarding "defective hand cleansing." There are few data regarding the relative importance, for example, of the different steps – or poses – recommended to be performed during each hand hygiene action. We do not know the impact on transmission risk of omitting each of these poses. For a detailed discussion of hand hygiene technique, please refer to Chapter 10.

We don't yet fully understand the role of the skin microbiome in colonization resistance: the action by commensal flora to prevent colonization by new – potentially harmful – organisms. The extent to which microbiome perturbation secondary to the use of antimicrobials, antiseptics, antivirals, or even other medications and conditions could affect this action is also unclear. These concepts have previously been difficult to study, but appropriate methods are becoming available.

RESEARCH AGENDA

As a general comment, given the significance of healthcare-associated infection and transmission of antimicrobial resistance determinants, there are surprisingly few studies that seek to directly describe and quantify the dynamics of transfer. There is therefore still a need for well conducted studies that address this topic. In particular, few studies quantify the impact of hand hygiene on organism acquisition events in the absence of concurrent interventions, particularly regarding organisms other than *S. aureus*.

Knowledge in the field of healthcare transmission dynamics can be expected to benefit greatly from the increasing feasibility of studies involving culture-independent microbiology techniques. Topics for further investigation include the role of commensal skin flora in resisting colonization by potential pathogens, and the extent to which this activity is perturbed among hospitalized patients.

There has been recent interest in the use of novel devices and surface materials to reduce organism transmission in the healthcare setting. These include use of copper surfaces, hydrogen peroxide vapor, and ultraviolet light to reduce the environmental burden of micro-organisms. These approaches would benefit from further study.

REFERENCES

1. Pittet D, Allegranzi B, Sax H, et al., Evidence-based model for hand transmission during patient care and the role of improved practices. *Lancet Infect Dis* 2006;**6**:641–652.

2. Grice EA, Segre JA, The skin microbiome. *Nat Rev Microbiol* 2011;**9**:244–253.

3. Tschudin-Sutter S, Frei R, Dangel M, et al., Sites of colonization with extended-spectrum beta-lactamases (ESBL)-producing enterobacteriaceae: the rationale for screening. *Infect Control Hosp Epidemiol* 2012;**33**:1170–1171.

4. Grabsch EA, Burrell LJ, Padiglione A, et al., Risk of environmental and healthcare worker contamination with vancomycin-resistant enterococci during outpatient procedures and hemodialysis. *Infect Control Hosp Epidemiol* 2006;**27**:287–293.

5. Boyce JM, Potter-Bynoe G, Chenevert C, et al., Environmental contamination due to methicillin-resistant *Staphylococcus aureus*: possible infection control implications. *Infect Control Hosp Epidemiol* 1997;**18**:622–627.

6. Morgan DJ, Rogawski E, Thom KA, et al., Transfer of multidrug-resistant bacteria to healthcare workers' gloves and gowns after patient contact increases with environmental contamination. *Crit Care Med* 2012;**40**:1045–1051.

7. Boyce JM, Havill NL, Otter JA, et al., Widespread environmental contamination associated with patients with diarrhea and methicillin-resistant *Staphylococcus aureus* colonization of the gastrointestinal tract. *Infect Control Hosp Epidemiol* 2007;**28**:1142–1147.

8. Greatorex JS, Digard P, Curran MD, et al., Survival of influenza A(H1N1) on materials found in households: implications for infection control. *PLoS One* 2011;**6**:e27932.

9. Pittet D, Dharan S, Touveneau S, et al., Bacterial contamination of the hands of hospital staff during routine patient care. *Arch Intern Med* 1999;**159**:821–826.

10. Pessoa-Silva CL, Dharan S, Hugonnet S, et al., Dynamics of bacterial hand contamination during routine neonatal care. *Infect Control Hosp Epidemiol* 2004;**25**:192–197.

11. Hamburger M, Jr., Transfer of beta hemolytic streptococci by shaking hands. *Am J Med* 1947;**2**:23–25.

12. Hayden MK, Blom DW, Lyle EA, et al., Risk of hand or glove contamination after contact with patients colonized with vancomycin-resistant enterococcus or the colonized patients' environment. *Infect Control Hosp Epidemiol* 2008;**29**:149–154.

13. Duckro AN, Blom DW, Lyle EA, et al., Transfer of vancomycin-resistant enterococci via health care worker hands. *Arch Intern Med* 2005;**165**:302–307.

14. Snyder GM, Thom KA, Furuno JP, et al., Detection of methicillin-resistant *Staphylococcus aureus* and vancomycin-resistant enterococci on the gowns and gloves of healthcare workers. *Infect Control Hosp Epidemiol* 2008;**29**:583–589.

15. Stiefel U, Cadnum JL, Eckstein BC, et al., Contamination of hands with methicillin-resistant *Staphylococcus aureus* after contact with environmental surfaces and after contact with the skin of colonized patients. *Infect Control Hosp Epidemiol* 2011;**32**:185–187.

16. Morgan DJ, Liang SY, Smith CL, et al., Frequent multidrug-resistant *Acinetobacter baumannii* contamination of gloves, gowns, and hands of healthcare workers. *Infect Control Hosp Epidemiol* 2010;**31**:716–721.

17. Bean B, Moore BM, Sterner B, et al., Survival of influenza viruses on environmental surfaces. *J Infect Dis* 1982;**146**:47–51.

18. Hall CB, Douglas RG, Jr, Modes of transmission of respiratory syncytial virus. *J Pediatr* 1981;**99**:100–103.

19. Winther B, McCue K, Ashe K, et al., Environmental contamination with rhinovirus and transfer to fingers of healthy individuals by daily life activity. *J Med Virol* 2007;**79**:1606–1610.

20. Albrich WC, Harbarth S, Health-care workers: source, vector, or victim of MRSA? *Lancet Infect Dis* 2008;**8**:289–301.

21. Knittle MA, Eitzman DV, Baer H, Role of hand contamination of personnel in the epidemiology of gram-negative nosocomial infections. *J Pediatr* 1975;**86**:433–437.

22. Casewell M, Phillips I, Hands as route of transmission for *Klebsiella* species. *Br Med J* 1977;**2**:1315–1317.

23. Larson EL, Persistent carriage of Gram-negative bacteria on hands. *Am J Infect Control* 1981;**9**:112–119.

24. Adams BG, Marrie TJ, Hand carriage of aerobic Gram-negative rods by health care personnel. *J Hyg (London)* 1982;**89**:23–31.

25. Thomas Y, Boquete-Suter P, Koch D, et al., Survival of influenza virus on human fingers. *Clin Microbiol Infect* 2013;**20**:58–64.

26. Mortimer EA, Jr., Lipsitz PJ, Wolinsky E, et al., Transmission of staphylococci between newborns. Importance of the hands of personnel. *Am J Dis Child* 1962;**104**:289–295.

27. Girou E, Legrand P, Soing-Altrach S, et al., Association between hand hygiene compliance and methicillin-resistant *Staphylococcus aureus* prevalence in a French rehabilitation hospital. *Infect Control Hosp Epidemiol* 2006;**27**:1128–1130.

28. Cromer AL, Latham SC, Bryant KG, et al., Monitoring and feedback of hand hygiene compliance and the impact on facility-acquired methicillin-resistant *Staphylococcus aureus*. *Am J Infect Control* 2008;**36**:672–677.

29. Pittet D, Hugonnet S, Harbarth S, et al., Effectiveness of a hospital-wide programme to improve compliance with hand hygiene. *Lancet* 2000;**356**:1307–1312.

Chapter 5

Mathematical Models of Handborne Transmission of Nosocomial Pathogens

Ben S. Cooper[1,2] and Nantasit Luangasanatip[1,3]

[1] Mahidol-Oxford Tropical Medicine Research Unit, Faculty of Tropical Medicine, Mahidol University, Bangkok, Thailand

[2] Centre for Tropical Medicine and Global Health, Nuffield Department of Clinical Medicine, University of Oxford, Oxford, UK

[3] School of Public Health, Queensland University of Technology, Brisbane, Australia

KEY MESSAGES

- The impact of improving hand hygiene on a hospital pathogen depends critically not only on the importance of the handborne route for patient-to-patient spread within the hospital, but also on the relative importance of hospital versus community transmission.

- Mathematical models explain why hand hygiene interventions are likely to have a disproportionate effect in reducing the incidence of infections that are adapted to hospital transmission. Changes in the incidence of infections due to (typically less resistant) bacteria more adapted to spread in the community are likely to be smaller.

- The full benefits of interventions to improve hand hygiene will in general not be felt immediately, but can take several years to accrue because of the long-term effects on the community reservoir.

Mathematical models have proved to be useful tools to better understand the control of infectious diseases, and are increasingly used to address problems relating to nosocomial pathogens.[1] In this chapter, we review the key insights such models

Hand Hygiene: A Handbook for Medical Professionals, First Edition.
Edited by Didier Pittet, John M. Boyce and Benedetta Allegranzi.
© 2017 John Wiley & Sons, Inc. Published 2017 by John Wiley & Sons, Inc.

have provided concerning the control of nosocomial pathogens with hand hygiene interventions. We present illustrative results from simple models to show how changing hand hygiene practice can have dramatically different effects on different nosocomial pathogens. Finally, we highlight some of the most important uncertainties and propose an agenda for future research.

WHAT WE KNOW – THE EVIDENCE

Healthcare workers can act as disease vectors, transmitting pathogens between patients during healthcare delivery. For some important bacterial pathogens, such as *Staphylococcus aureus*, this is likely to be the dominant mode of patient-to-patient spread. Hand hygiene can interrupt this transmission, reducing the number of patients who carry these pathogens asymptomatically. This in turn leads to reductions in the incidence of clinically important infections.

The modern use of mathematical models to study infectious diseases can be traced back to the seminal work of Ronald Ross, who developed dynamic transmission models to investigate the control of malaria.[2] The first models of hospital-acquired infections adapted Ross's malaria model, replacing mosquitoes with healthcare workers, and examined how changing levels of hand hygiene affected the carriage prevalence of nosocomial pathogens.[3–6] This work highlighted the nonlinear relationship between hand hygiene and the incidence of nosocomial infections, the importance of chance effects in determining the course of any single hospital epidemic, and the central importance of threshold effects in hospital epidemiology. To bring an epidemic under control, interventions do not need to stop all transmission-related events, but only to a degree associated with a reduction of less than one of the mean number of secondary cases linked to an index (primary) case.

Later work extended models to take into account the interactions between antibiotic-resistant and susceptible bacteria.[7] A key result is that nonspecific interventions that reduce transmission, such as hand hygiene, are likely to have a much greater effect on antibiotic-resistant pathogens (provided they are rare in the community) than on susceptible organisms.

Models were also used to consider how community reservoirs of important nosocomial pathogens, such as methicillin-resistant *S. aureus* (MRSA), affected the dynamics.[8,9] An important finding was that even though every battle against a nosocomial pathogen might be won in the hospital (and all local outbreaks successfully controlled), the war could still be lost. The slow buildup of carriers in the community (even in the absence of community transmission) causes a gradual increase in the rate patients bring resistant organisms into a hospital, and thus short outbreaks increase in frequency. Eventually, although successfully controlled, these outbreaks coalesce, and endemicity is established.[9] This work showed also that interventions may take several years before achieving their full effect. Again, this is a consequence of long-term changes to the community reservoir.

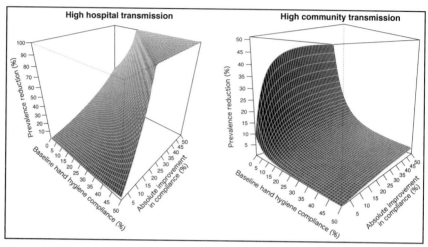

Figure 5.1   Results derived from a model combining vector-borne transmission of a nosocomial pathogen (assumed to be entirely mediated by the hands of healthcare workers), with transmission in the community reservoir. Results are shown for both a pathogen adapted to the hospital setting but assumed to transmit poorly in the community (left), and for a pathogen that transmits well in the community, but poorly in hospitals (right). The plots show how the equilibrium level of carriage prevalence (the percentage of hospital patients colonized or infected with the pathogen at any one time in the long term) changes in response to an intervention to improve hand hygiene compliance as a function of baseline (pre-intervention) compliance. See Table 5.1 for model assumptions.

The above themes are illustrated in Figure 5.1, which shows the results from a model that combines the assumptions of carer-mediated handborne transmission in the hospital setting with a community reservoir where transmission is not directly affected by hospital hand hygiene (see Table 5.1 for assumptions).[3–6,8,9] The impact of hand hygiene interventions can differ dramatically for organisms that have a high transmission in hospital settings with only limited community transmission compared to pathogens that spread mostly in the community. Typically, such hospital-adapted lineages have more antibiotic resistance determinants than those adapted to community transmission. In this example, once hand hygiene compliance (baseline + improvement) reaches about 70%, the hospital-adapted pathogen can be eliminated; that is, prevalence reduction is 100% (Figure 5.1, left panel). Whether such elimination is possible for a given pathogen depends on its transmission potential in the hospital and community and the degree to which hospital transmission can be interrupted by hand hygiene. If improving compliance is unable to eliminate the pathogen, substantial reductions in carriage prevalence are still possible. The percentage reduction becomes larger as compliance approaches the level needed for elimination.

For a pathogen that transmits poorly in the hospital, but well in the community, the potential impact of hospital-based hand hygiene interventions is far more limited. Even with 100% hand hygiene compliance, sustained community

Table 5.1   Model Parameter Values Used in Figures 5.1 and 5.2. These parameter values were chosen to illustrate model dynamics, and do not represent estimates from data. The models split the community population into two groups to account for the observation that recently hospitalized patients have an initially high rate of hospitalization that diminishes over time[9]

	Value(s)	
Model Parameter	Figure 5.1	Figure 5.2
Number of hospitalized patients	1000	1000
Number of healthcare workers (HCWs)	100	100
Number of people in the community	100,000	100,000
Ratio of hospital admission rate of the recently hospitalized to hospital admission rate for the general population	20	20
Number recently hospitalized having an elevated admission rate	10,000	5,000
Mean length of hospital stay (days)	10	10
Mean number of HCW contacts per patient day	10	10
Mean carriage duration in the community (days)	400	400
Ratio of probability of transmission from colonized patient to a susceptible HCW to the probability of transmission from colonized HCW to a susceptible patient	10	10
Baseline hand hygiene compliance	0–50%	40%
Reproduction number of pathogen A at 40% hand hygiene compliance*	3.0 (left) 6.5 (right)	1.5
As above, for pathogen B	–	1.5
Percentage of transmission events with pathogen A that occur in the hospital at 40% compliance (assuming an otherwise fully susceptible population, and that pathogen A is initially acquired in the hospital)	100% (left) 1% (right)	25%
As above, for pathogen B	–	2%
Bacterial interference: percentage reduction in risk of acquiring pathogen B (A) if carrying A (B) compared to risk in a non-carrier	–	100%

*Defined as the expected number of secondary cases in the hospital and community resulting from one typical initial case in an otherwise susceptible population, accounting for the possibility of repeated hospital admissions while still colonized.

Source: Adapted with permission from reference 9.

transmission means that elimination is not possible. In this case, the largest percentage reductions in prevalence occur when baseline compliance is low. There are rapidly diminishing returns as improvements in hand hygiene increase (Figure 5.1, right panel).

There has also been a lot of interest in how hospital-adapted bacterial lineages resistant to multiple antibiotics interact with less resistant community-adapted clones with which they may compete for host colonization sites.[7] Illustrative results using a model that extends the one used for Figure 5.1 to account for such interactions are shown in Figure 5.2. An intervention starting after one year in a hospital where nearly 10% of patients carry a hospital-adapted pathogen (Pathogen A) can have a large effect on the hospital prevalence of this organism. The full impact of the intervention is not felt for several years. This gradual reduction in hospital prevalence is a consequence of the long-term changes in the community prevalence (itself a consequence of fewer patients carrying the organisms when discharged and the long duration of carriage for typical nosocomial pathogens). The impact of the intervention on a competing, community-adapted organism (Pathogen B) is much less dramatic. In this example, although improving hand hygiene reduces transmission of both pathogen A and B in the hospital setting, there is a small increase in the prevalence of pathogen B. This occurs as a result of reduced competition with pathogen A. Results of simple models such as this can explain why major hand hygiene interventions have been followed by large reductions in the number of MRSA infections, but have had minimal impact on methicillin-sensitive *S. aureus*.[10]

A number of models have considered the effects of hand hygiene in the context of other infection control measures including antibiotic restriction, patient isolation, and ward cleaning.[4,6,11–14] These models have been applied to pathogens including vancomycin-resistant enterococci, MRSA, *Acinetobacter baumanii*, and extended-spectrum β-lactamase-producing Enterobacteriaceae. While these models have not reached consistent conclusions about the effectiveness of altering antibiotic prescribing, they have suggested important benefits associated with some forms of patient isolation and consistently found improving hand hygiene to be the most effective intervention.

A major criticism that could be levelled at many of the modelling studies discussed above is that, while assumptions may be plausible and qualitative insights are likely to be reasonably robust, key quantitative results depend critically on parameter values which are either guessed or plucked unsystematically from the literature, often with weak supporting evidence and poorly-quantified uncertainty. Researchers have addressed this problem by tackling what is known as the *inverse problem*: rather than just use models for forward simulations to evaluate what data would look like if the assumed parameter values and structural assumptions were correct, they aim to first use the model to work backwards from the data to learn about likely values of key parameters and to evaluate the support for different model assumptions. When models have been appropriately calibrated in this way they can be used to assess hypothetical interventions. This

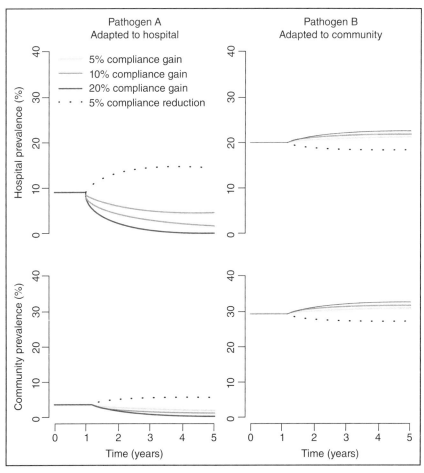

Figure 5.2   Results from a model combining hospital-based hand-borne transmission of a nosocomial pathogen with community transmission accounting for competitive interactions between a hospital-adapted clone (Pathogen A) and a community-adapted clone (Pathogen B). The plots show how the carriage prevalence (the percentage of people in the hospital or community who carry the pathogen at any one time) for both a pathogen adapted to the hospital setting (left) and a pathogen adapted to the community (right) changes over time in response to changes in hand hygiene compliance. Baseline compliance is 40%, and lines indicate trajectories resulting from absolute and immediate improvements in compliance after year 1 of 5, 10 and 20% and also from an immediate 5% absolute reduction. See Table 5.1 for model assumptions.

is much more computationally challenging than performing forward simulations alone (as most modelling studies do), but offers the potential for quantitative insights more firmly rooted in empirical data. Methods have been developed for this inverse problem for hospital infection data,[6,15] and successfully applied to estimate the effectiveness of isolation measures.[16] Data have so far been lacking to allow the effectiveness of hand hygiene in reducing transmission rates to be directly estimated using these methods, but these methodological developments make such an approach feasible. Moreover, recent developments in whole genome sequencing and extensions of transmission models to make use of such data for reconstructing transmission networks, promise to give us a more solid understanding of the relative importance of different transmission routes and more accurate estimates of the potential impact of hand hygiene interventions for different pathogens.[17]

WHAT WE DO NOT KNOW – THE UNCERTAIN

We currently have only a few good estimates of how much transmission of different pathogens occurs in hospitals (and how this is affected by interventions).[1,6] Corresponding estimates from the community are almost totally lacking. We also do not have reliable estimates for the amount of transmission that occurs via transiently colonized hands of healthcare workers for different pathogens, in particular for Gram-negative bacteria. For many important nosocomial pathogens, we do not know how long carriage typically persists and what dynamics are crucially involved in shifting the balance to infection.

We are only beginning to understand how the complex network of patient interactions with healthcare workers impacts on transmission dynamics. Finally, it is not clear to what extent improved carer hand hygiene practices can affect the risk of patients developing a clinical infection with an organism that they are carrying asymptomatically. A better understanding of all of these aspects is needed to develop more realistic models capable of use as predictive tools.

RESEARCH AGENDA

To better understand the dynamics of important nosocomial pathogens and the potential impact of interventions, we need to quantify the amount of transmission in different settings and through different means. In recent years, good-quality longitudinal data from hospitals have become available in some high-income countries, as have advanced statistical approaches for estimating key quantities from such data. There is a need for comparable high-quality longitudinal studies (and appropriate analysis) in healthcare settings other than the hospital, in community settings, and in low- and middle-income countries. This is particularly true for organisms such as community-associated clones of MRSA and resistant Gram-negative bacteria where a substantial component of transmission may be outside the hospital setting.

Another important research direction is to investigate the circumstances when further investment in hand hygiene promotion (alone or in combination with additional infection control interventions) is likely to be cost-effective. Such questions can be addressed by combining dynamic mathematical models with economic analysis (see also Chapter 39).

REFERENCES

1. van Kleef E, Robotham JV, Jit M, et al., Modelling the transmission of healthcare associated infections: a systematic review. *BMC Infect Dis* 2013;**13**:294.
2. Ross R, Some a priori pathometric equations. *Br Med J* 1915;**1**:546–547.
3. Sébille V, Chevret S, Valleron AJ, Modeling the spread of resistant nosocomial pathogens in an intensive-care unit. *Infect Control Hosp Epidemiol* 1997;**18**:84–92.
4. Austin DJ, Bonten MJ, Weinstein RA, et al., Vancomycin-resistant enterococci in intensive-care hospital settings: transmission dynamics, persistence, and the impact of infection control programs. *Proc Natl Acad Sci USA* 1999;**96**:6908–6913.
5. Cooper BS, Medley GF, Scott GM, Preliminary analysis of the transmission dynamics of nosocomial infections: stochastic and management effects. *J Hosp Infect* 1999;**43**:131–147.
6. McBryde ES, Pettitt AN, McElwain DL, A stochastic mathematical model of methicillin resistant *Staphylococcus aureus* transmission in an intensive care unit: predicting the impact of interventions. *J Theor Biol* 2007;**245**:470–481.
7. Lipsitch M, Bergstrom CT, Levin BR, The epidemiology of antibiotic resistance in hospitals: paradoxes and prescriptions. *Proc Natl Acad Sci USA* 2000;**97**:1938–1943.
8. Smith DL, Dushoff J, Perencevich EN, et al., Persistent colonization and the spread of antibiotic resistance in nosocomial pathogens: resistance is a regional problem. *Proc Natl Acad Sci USA* 2004;**101**:3709–3714.
9. Cooper BS, Medley GF, Stone SP, et al., Methicillin-resistant *Staphylococcus aureus* in hospitals and the community: stealth dynamics and control catastrophes. *Proc Natl Acad Sci USA* 2004;**101**:10223–10228.
10. Stone S, Fuller C, Savage J, et al., Evaluation of the national CleanYourHands campaign to reduce *Staphylococcus aureus* bacteraemia and *Clostridium difficile* infection in hospitals in England and Wales by improved hand hygiene: four year, prospective, ecological, interrupted time series study. *Br Med J* 2012;**344**:e3005.
11. D'Agata EM, Webb G, Horn M, A mathematical model quantifying the impact of antibiotic exposure and other interventions on the endemic prevalence of vancomycin-resistant enterococci. *J Infect Dis* 2005;**192**:2004–2011.
12. D'Agata EM, Horn MA, Ruan S, et al., Efficacy of infection control interventions in reducing the spread of multidrug-resistant organisms in the hospital setting. *PLoS One* 2012;**7**(2):e30170.
13. Doan TN, Kong DC, Marshall C, et al., Modeling the impact of interventions against Acinetobacter baumannii transmission in intensive care units. *Virulence* 2016;**7**:141–152.
14. Pelat C, Kardaś-Słoma L, Birgand G, et al., Hand hygiene, cohorting, or antibiotic restriction to control outbreaks of multidrug-resistant Enterobacteriaceae. *Infect Control Hosp Epidemiol* 2016;**37**:272–280.
15. Forrester ML, Pettitt AN, Gibson GJ, Bayesian inference of hospital-acquired infectious diseases and control measures given imperfect surveillance data. *Biostatistics* 2007;**8**:383–401.
16. Kypraios T, O'Neill PD, Huang SS, et al., Assessing the role of undetected colonization and isolation precautions in reducing methicillin-resistant *Staphylococcus aureus* transmission in intensive care units. *BMC Infect Dis* 2010;**10**:29.
17. Worby CJ, O'Neill PD, Kypraios T, et al., Reconstructing transmission trees for communicable diseases using densely sampled genetic data. *Ann Appl Stat* 2016;**10**:395–417.

Chapter 6

Methodological Issues in Hand Hygiene Science

Matthew Samore[1] and Stephan Harbarth[2]

[1] *Department of Epidemiology, University of Utah School of Medicine, Salt Lake City, USA*
[2] *Infection Control Program and WHO Collaborating Centre on Patient Safety, University of Geneva Hospitals and Faculty of Medicine, Geneva, Switzerland*

KEY MESSAGES

- Hand hygiene studies should clearly state the intended causal contrast.
- Confounding and contamination should be considered in hand hygiene studies.
- Hand hygiene studies should attempt to more fully address heterogeneity of adherence.
- New methods to estimate contact rates and characterize social networks are needed.

This chapter tackles the fundamental questions of how to advance knowledge and issue key recommendations for guiding future hand hygiene research. We focus on essential epidemiological concepts, which serve to guide study design and interpretation of results. A characteristic of the field of hand hygiene is that substantial obstacles exist that limit the application of these principles. As new technologies for measuring infection control practices emerge, the capability to meet these challenges will increase.

Hand Hygiene: A Handbook for Medical Professionals, First Edition.
Edited by Didier Pittet, John M. Boyce and Benedetta Allegranzi.
© 2017 John Wiley & Sons, Inc. Published 2017 by John Wiley & Sons, Inc.

METHODOLOGICAL CHALLENGES AND RECOMMENDATIONS

Recommendation 1: Studies Should Clearly State the Intended Causal Contrast

All studies designed to assess the impact of an intervention on hand hygiene should specify the causal question of interest. The question can be stated in terms of a hypothetical comparison: *what would have happened had the intervention been different from the one actually received?* The difference in outcome in a population exposed to alternative interventions (or treatments) represents the average causal effect. This contrast is called the "counterfactual" because it is not possible for a population to experience mutually exclusive conditions at the same time. In lieu of replaying history using a time machine, it is necessary to study distinct populations or examine the same population at different times.[1] When the intervention is randomly allocated, it is possible to derive an estimate of the unconfounded, average causal effect of the intervention. Unfortunately, only a few cluster-randomized trials have been performed in the field of healthcare workers' hand hygiene improvement.[2,3,4] In the absence of random allocation of the intervention, causal inference relies on plausible causal relationships and possible unmeasured confounders.[5]

Campaigns to affect hand hygiene are by their nature group-level interventions. In many hand hygiene studies the interventions that are being compared are incompletely delineated. Just labeling one group (or time period) the "control" is inadequate. To enhance interpretability and generalizability,[4] activities or policies regarding hand hygiene in the control arm should be defined. Conditions in both intervention and control groups/periods should be described in equivalent detail.[6]

Recommendation 2: Confounding and Contamination Should Be Considered in Hand Hygiene Studies but Generally Do Not "Explain" a Positive Result

Hand hygiene studies should address issues of confounding and bias. Confounding is produced when assignment of the intervention and occurrence of the outcome share a common cause. Factors that have the potential to confound group level interventions deserve particular attention. By design, time directly influences the intervention in before-and-after studies and other quasi-experimental designs.[7] Thus, time has the potential to be a particularly potent confounder if it affects other factors that alter hand hygiene practices. Unless these other factors decrease hand hygiene, the effect of confounding will be to attenuate the measured effect of the intervention.[4]

Contamination produces a different kind of bias because it means that the comparator group is partially receiving the intervention.[4] Contamination always reduces the observed differences in outcomes between groups.[4]

Information bias arises from systematic errors in measurement. It is potentially a very relevant problem because it may distort the association between intervention and outcome in either direction. Variation in methodology and performance of direct hand hygiene observation may engender information bias if there are nonrandom differences between groups or time periods.

Recommendation 3: Hand Hygiene Studies Should Characterize Their Target Populations of Healthcare Workers and Should Attempt to More Fully Address Heterogeneity of Compliance

Healthcare workers (HCWs) constitute the target population in hand hygiene studies. Typically, only a portion of HCWs exposed to the intervention are included in an analysis of hand hygiene adherence. Most hand hygiene studies do not enumerate the sizes of their HCW populations. Ideally, hand hygiene studies should describe the characteristics of the HCWs exposed to the intervention, analogous to what is done in patient-level research. Target populations of HCWs may vary across facilities with respect to position, experience, attitudes, and knowledge.

Furthermore, hand hygiene studies should attempt to more fully address heterogeneity of compliance. Reporting only average compliance may not represent the full picture, since low hand hygiene performers may contribute disproportionally to the risk of nosocomial cross-transmission. As suggested by an interesting agent-based simulation study, noncompliant HCWs may play a disproportionate role in disseminating pathogens (= superspreaders).[8,9] Thus, average compliance to hand hygiene is not a good indicator of nosocomial risk in real-life healthcare settings. We conclude that aggregate, average compliance data should be complemented by observational data about low performers and outliers using individual-level data. However, this complementary approach may encounter ethical and feasibility barriers.

Recommendation 4: Hand Hygiene Studies Should Explore New Approaches to Measuring Contact Rates Between Healthcare Workers and Patients

Most hand hygiene studies do not attempt to measure rates of contact between HCWs and patients. The usual calculation of compliance using the denominator of observed hand hygiene opportunities does not by itself support an analysis of contact rates. An ideal evaluation method would include an estimation of the frequency with which HCWs enter patient rooms and interact with the patient or touch the environment. The impact of a hand hygiene intervention on transmission of nosocomial pathogens is likely to be governed by these rates of contact. It is useful to recognize that HCWs and patients form a social network, identified by the patterns of their connections to each other. The nature of contacts in terms of timing, frequency, and duration defines the strengths of those links. A potential advantage of new technologies such as wireless sensor nodes (motes) is that they provide this additional capability.

Recommendation 5: Qualitative Research Methods Should be Developed to Better Understand Group-Level Components and Social Norms That Influence Hand Hygiene Behavior

Hand hygiene behavior is influenced by peers and opinion leaders. Several studies have shown that group pressure and adherence to social norms can increase adherence to hand hygiene recommendations.[10] However, few of them used a structured approach to investigate interactions between HCWs and role models, as suggested in behaviorial sciences. New models to measure the influence of peer pressure on hand hygiene compliance are therefore needed. In particular, qualitative studies could provide better understanding of the social and behavioral determinants including role models and peer groups that influence hand hygiene performance.

RESEARCH AGENDA

Future research related to methodological issues of hand hygiene improvement science should consequently focus on the following key questions:

- How much reduction in bias can be achieved by performing cluster-randomized trials compared to other interventional study designs?
- What are alternatives and better indicators of hand hygiene practices compared to data on average aggregate hand hygiene adherence?
- How can agent-based simulation studies contribute to further advances in this field?
- What are suitable methods to measure contact rates between healthcare workers and patients?
- Can qualitative research help in better understanding peer group influence on hand hygiene behaviour?

For future guidance of clinical hand hygiene studies, we list below a summary of the quality ranking of research designs in hand hygiene science, with a classification scheme of the evidence level (Table 6.1).

Table 6.1 Quality Ranking of Research Designs in Hand Hygiene Science, with a Classification Scheme of the Evidence Level

Type of Study Design	Quality of Evidence	Example & Reference
Uncontrolled before-after study	Low	Hand hygiene practices in a neonatal intensive care unit: a multimodal intervention and impact on nosocomial infection[11]
Controlled before-after study	Medium	Interventional study to evaluate the impact of an alcohol-based hand gel in improving hand hygiene compliance[2]
Interrupted time-series with step-wedge design	Medium	Interventions to reduce colonization and transmission of antimicrobial-resistant bacteria in ICUs: an interrupted time series study and cluster randomized trial[3]
Cluster-randomized clinical trial	High	Universal glove and gown use and acquisition of antibiotic-resistant bacteria in the ICUs: a randomized trial[12]
Meta-analysis of controlled clinical trials	High	Searching for an optimal hand hygiene bundle: a meta-analysis[13]

ICU, intensive care unit.

REFERENCES

1. Samore MH, Harbarth S, A methodologically focused review of the literature in hospital epidemiology and infection control. In: Mayhall CG, ed. *Hosp Epidemiol Infect Control*, 3rd edn. Philadelphia: Lippincott Williams & Wilkins, 2004:1645–1657.
2. Harbarth S, Pittet D, Grady L, et al., Interventional study to evaluate the impact of an alcohol-based hand gel in improving hand hygiene compliance. *Pediatr Infect Dis J* 2002;**21**:489–495.
3. Derde LP, Cooper BS, Goossens H, et al., Interventions to reduce colonisation and transmission of antimicrobial-resistant bacteria in intensive care units: an interrupted time series study and cluster randomised trial. *Lancet Infect Dis.* 2014;**14**:31–39.
4. Stewardson A, Sax H, Gayer-Ageron A, et al., Enhanced performance feedback and patient participation to improve hand hygiene compliance of health-care workers in the setting of established multimodal promotion: a single-centre cluster-randomised controlled trial. *Lancet Infect Dis.* 2016;**16**:1345–1355.
5. Maldonado G, Greenland S, Estimating causal effects. *Int J Epidemiol* 2002;**31**:422–429.
6. Mayer J, Mooney B, Gundlapalli A, et al., Dissemination and sustainability of a hospital-wide hand hygiene program emphasizing positive reinforcement. *Infect Control Hosp Epidemiol* 2011;**32**:59–66.
7. Harbarth S, Samore MH, Interventions to control MRSA: high time for time-series analysis? *J Antimicrob Chemother* 2008;**62**:431–433.
8. Temime L, Opatowski L, Pannet Y, et al., Peripatetic health-care workers as potential superspreaders. *Proc Natl Acad Sci USA* 2009; **106**:18420–18425.

9. Hornbeck T, Naylor D, Segre AM, et al., Using sensor networks to study the effect of peripatetic healthcare workers on the spread of hospital-associated infections. *J Infect Dis* 2012;**206**:1549–1557.

10. Pittet D, Simon A, Hugonnet S, et al., Hand hygiene among physicians: performance, beliefs, and perceptions. *Ann Intern Med* 2004;**141**:1–8.

11. Lam BC, Lee J, Lau YL, Hand hygiene practices in a neonatal intensive care unit: a multi-modal intervention and impact on nosocomial infection. *Pediatrics* 2004;**114**:e565–e571.

12. Harris AD, Pineles L, Belton B, et al., Universal glove and gown use and acquisition of antibiotic-resistant bacteria in the ICU: a randomized trial. *JAMA* 2013;**310**:1571–1580.

13. Schweizer ML, Reisinger HS, Ohl M, et al., Searching for an optimal hand hygiene bundle: a meta-analysis. *Clin Infect Dis* 2014;**58**:248–259.

Chapter 7

Statistical Issues: How to Overcome the Complexity of Data Analysis in Hand Hygiene Research?

Angèle Gayet-Ageron[1] and Eli Perencevich[2]

[1] Infection Control Program and WHO Collaborating Centre on Patient Safety, University of Geneva Hospitals and Faculty of Medicine, Geneva, Switzerland

[2] Department of Internal Medicine, University of Iowa, Carver College of Medicine, Iowa City, USA

KEY MESSAGES

- There are many factors explaining hand hygiene compliance; some are intercorrelated or have causal relationships between each other, leading to a complex causal model.

- There is no current single appropriate design to study the causal relationship between hand hygiene and healthcare-associated infections that allows for combined analysis of individual and group-level data.

- Before-and-after quasi-experimental studies are a widely used design. They are of interest, in particular if well designed with an appropriate control group and accompanied by adequate statistical regression models. The statistical analyses aiming to assess the association between various parameters and hand hygiene need to take into account the complexity of data and their intercorrelation; however, there is, as yet, no perfect statistical model.

Improving healthcare workers' (HCWs') attitudes and compliance towards hand hygiene is complex. Challenges are related to primary health education, cultural aspects, individual beliefs on risks and responsibility, and perception of their own role in the prevention and control of infection.[1,2] HCW perception of hand hygiene's importance depends upon the degree of support from the institution and health authorities.[3] Finally, infrastructures in the hospital and at the patient bedside (number of sinks available in the hospital room or in the ward, enough handrub dispensers, etc.) are obviously playing a role in the compliance with hand hygiene practices.[4–6] At the individual level, it has been shown that hand hygiene compliance is associated with professional category, workload, day of the week, and indications for hand hygiene (Tables 7.1 and 7.2). These and other predictors of compliance are potentially correlated (i.e., collinearity) with one another[7,8] (Figure 7.1).

This chapter outlines the complexity of the causative pathways between specific predictors of hand hygiene compliance including the existence of confounding and intercorrelation between the different variables. The aim is to describe optimal methods for analyzing epidemiological data in hand hygiene intervention studies in order to determine which components are optimal targets for future study with the ultimate goal of preventing healthcare-associated infections (HAIs).

Table 7.1 Parameters Associated with Successful Hand Hygiene Promotion

Education
Routine observation and feedback
Engineering controls
  Making hand hygiene possible, easy, and convenient
  Making alcohol-based handrub available (at least in high-demand situations)
Avoid overcrowding, understaffing, and excessive workload
Patient education, participation, empowerment
Reminders in the workplace
Administrative sanctions and rewards
Change in hand hygiene agent
Promote and facilitate healthcare worker hands' skin care
Obtain active participation at individual and institutional level
Drive and maintain an institutional safety climate around hand hygiene
Enhance individual and institutional self-efficacy
Consider important cultural issues/differences in promotion strategy
Imagine and implement innovative promotional initiatives to limit campaign fatigue

Source: Modified from Pittet 2000. Reproduced with permission from Cambridge University Press.

Table 7.2   Hand Hygiene: Distribution of Factors Associated with Noncompliance

Individual level
  Lack of education or experience
  Being a physician
  Male gender
  Lack of knowledge of guidelines
  Being a refractory noncomplier
Group level
  Lack of education or lack of performance feedback
  Working in critical care (high workload)
  Downsizing or understaffing
  Lack of encouragement or role model from key staffs
Institutional level
  Lack of written guidelines
  Lack of suitable hand hygiene agents
  Lack of skin-care promotion or agent
  Lack of hand hygiene facilities
  Lack of culture or tradition of compliance
  Lack of administrative leadership, sanction, rewards, or support
  Lack of innovative strategies to override campaign fatigue in long-term promotion

Source: Modified from Pittet 2000. Reproduced with permission from Cambridge University Press.

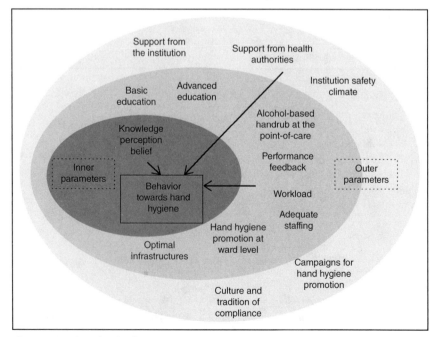

Figure 7.1   Three levels of parameters (from the most to the least influential) impacting healthcare workers' behavior towards hand hygiene.

WHAT WE KNOW – THE EVIDENCE

There is substantial evidence that hand antisepsis reduces the incidence of HAIs.[9] However, most studies of hand hygiene interventions have used observational designs,[10] including quasi-experimental studies.[11] Randomized or cluster-randomized trials are considered the gold standard study design, yet are rarely used in infection prevention research for logistical, ethical, and economic reasons.[12,13] First, in the case of hand hygiene evaluation, it would be unethical to use nothing or an alcohol-based handrub (ABHR) placebo as a controlled group in aiming to show the superiority of ABHR to reduce HAI rates. Second, all methods aiming to control information biases, such as blinding or concealment of allocation, would be difficult or impossible to implement. Finally, as hand hygiene is not a single intervention applied to one individual subject but is performed on multiple occasions by many HCWs who are taking care of multiple patients in single or multiple bedrooms, the implementation of individual randomized controlled trials is rarely feasible. It is possible that only mathematical modeling could ethically highlight the transmission of hospital pathogens in the healthcare setting,[12] as described in Chapter 5. Importantly, the study of pathogen transmission from hands to patient could be greatly enhanced through the emergence of new molecular-epidemiological methods including whole genome sequencing.[14,15]

Recently, cluster-randomized trials have emerged as a viable design, representing the method with the highest internal validity in evaluating the effectiveness of complex strategies randomly assigned to wards or hospitals (clusters) based on hand hygiene compliance improvement or specific HAI rates (see Chapter 6).[16,17] In regard to cluster-randomized trials, the assessment of the effectiveness of a program aiming to improve compliance, such as the World Health Organization (WHO) multimodal strategy[18] or a specific national campaign,[19] should also take into account data complexity and in particular clustering effects. The various levels of clustering (Figure 7.2) can be adjusted for through the use of appropriate regression models. Application of statistical analysis has improved along with the greater availability of statistical packages, most of which integrate generalized linear mixed models. The use of naïve regression methods (in the present case logistic regression with fixed effects only) that do not integrate random effects was shown to incorrectly estimate the standard errors around the intervention's effect.[20] Nonetheless, the use of mixed-effects regression models is not perfect, even when considering the integration of some variability in the outcome between the different clusters considered.

However, when randomized studies or cluster-randomized controlled trials are infeasible, the most appropriate design remains the before-and-after (or pre-post intervention) quasi-experimental study design.[21,22] In these studies, the intervention could be applied at the hospital level (e.g., educational intervention among anesthesiologists aiming to improve hand hygiene before versus after, and the effect on surgical site infections)[23] or at the individual level (e.g., semiautomatic treatment advice by email to improve compliance with the

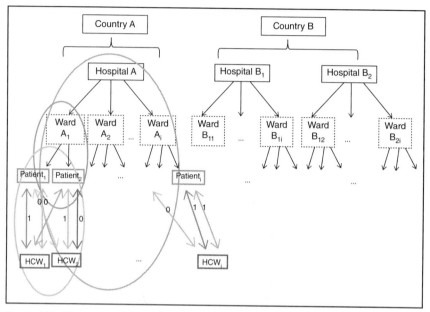

Figure 7.2 Illustration of the complexity in the data from a large observational study assessing the effectiveness of the WHO Multimodal Strategy in different pilot sites and countries.[6]
HCW, healthcare worker.

Infectious Diseases Society of America guidelines in the treatment of intravascular catheter-related infection)[24] and outcome data are collected before and after intervention at equally spaced time intervals (e.g., monthly). In these particular designs, nonrandomization of the intervention necessitates analytical control for potential confounders. Additionally, it is recommended that a control group unexposed to the intervention be included because regression to the mean and maturation effects are common pitfalls in these studies.[21] Depending on the format of the outcome (continuous, e.g., hospital length of stay; or count data, e.g., number of methicillin-resistant *Staphylococcus aureus* [MRSA] infections expressed as counts, proportions, or incidence rates) and on statistical assumptions, several statistical approaches could be used, from the simplest (two-group tests, such as Student's *t* tests, two-rates χ^2 test) to more sophisticated regression analyses: nonsegmented linear regression, which precludes the estimation of a change in a continuous outcome in time trend (i.e., slope) and presents two separate models (i.e., before and after intervention); segmented linear regression, which allows the slopes to differ before and after the intervention; nonsegmented or segmented Poisson regression for count outcomes and overdispersed Poisson regression if the assumption "mean equals variance" is violated. Finally, time-series analysis can be used to analyze quasi-experimental studies.[25] Those advanced techniques present the advantages to relax the independence assumption needed for the previous tests or regression models and to integrate the autocorrelation between observations collected at different times. Several approaches are available to integrate autocorrelation: autoregression if correlation between two observations gradually decreases as time between them increases; a moving-average model is more appropriate if autocorrelation between two observations is initially strong but abruptly decreases to 0; autoregressive moving-average (ARMA) models should be used if autocorrelation is strong for observations close in time and then sharply decreases to a nonzero level after some time threshold; lastly, when correlation between observations does not decrease with duration of time, autoregressive, integrated, moving-average (ARIMA or Box–Jenkins) models may be appropriate (e.g., incidence of hemorrhagic fever with renal syndrome).[26] In summary, the statistical validity of quasi-experimental studies depends on using well-designed studies with large (or adequately estimated) sample sizes and verifying modeling assumptions.[18,22]

WHAT WE DO NOT KNOW – THE UNCERTAIN

One of the barriers to proving causality is the use of data originating from at least two levels of observation without strict direct link between both entities: hand hygiene compliance by HCWs and HAIs at the patients' level. It is thus difficult or even impossible to implement an ideal clinical trial aiming to prove the causative association between increased hand hygiene compliance rates and a corresponding attributed decrease of HAIs. At the individual level, one ideal way of studying the causal relation would be to show that the lack of hand hygiene by one single HCW directly correlates with the subsequent acquisition of HAI in one identified patient. This can only be indirectly demonstrated by the use of an experimental or even quasi-experimental study showing the association between the intensity of bacterial contamination and the method of hand cleansing or the use of gloves during patient care.[27] As the association between specific pathogens and specific infections is clearly established, these experiments are critical in our quest to validate the link between inappropriate levels of hand hygiene and subsequent incident HAI.

Practical Example

Let's now use the example of a cluster-randomized controlled trial, which would aim to assess the efficacy of a new hand hygiene improvement intervention on HAI rates compared to baseline standard precaution recommendations. The intervention (new strategy versus standard precaution recommendations) will be randomly assigned to clusters (units of care). Here, we could distinguish two levels of observations with a certain degree of dependency: the HCW who will be observed regarding her/his compliance with hand hygiene in a selected session of care and the patient hospitalized in the ward where the intervention is implemented and who will be at risk of acquiring an HAI. In this example, two different outcomes are studied: (1) hand hygiene compliance and (2) HAIs. Due to the sources of information regarding data collected in the trial, two different kinds of analyses should be performed: (i) assess the association between the intervention (new strategy versus standard precautions) and hand hygiene compliance; and (ii) evaluate the association between the intervention and the subsequent decrease in HAI rates. In order to determine the association between hand hygiene compliance improvement and HAI rates, we could use mean compliance at the ward level to assess if above an arbitrary cut-off for compliance (e.g., >60%), HAI rate is demonstrated to be lower than below this cut-off. As one HCW could take care of several patients or one patient could be managed by several HCWs with different levels of hand hygiene compliance, it would be very difficult to combine these levels of data in the same analysis. It is likely that these two analyses would be best completed using two separate databases constructed at the unique level of observation, either HCW or patient.

Ideally, we would need to work on longitudinal data collected prospectively to show the link between hand hygiene improvement and subsequent decrease in HAI rates. But how could we implement such a study in practice? Due to the use of two levels of observations (HCWs and patients), it is difficult to have a simple method to study longitudinally the association between compliance and HAI. Thus, we must approach this level of complexity by using the currently imperfect yet ethical and feasible study designs available, namely the before-and-after quasi-experimental study.

RESEARCH AGENDA

Further research is needed regarding:

- A better understanding regarding what is driving HCWs' behaviors towards hand hygiene.
- More interventional studies focused on specific parameters explaining HCWs' attitudes towards hand hygiene.
- Development of new tools aiming to improve HCWs' compliance with hand hygiene.
- Reinforcing active and standardized surveillance for HAIs with the aim of describing their risk factors and directing future interventions.

REFERENCES

1. Pessoa-Silva CL, Posfay-Barbe K, Pfister R, et al., Attitudes and perceptions toward hand hygiene among healthcare workers caring for critically ill neonates. *Infect Control Hosp Epidemiol* 2005;**26**:305–311.

2. McAteer J, Stone S, Fuller C, et al., Using psychological theory to understand the challenges facing staff delivering a ward-led intervention to increase hand hygiene behavior: a qualitative study. *Am J Infect Control* 2014;**42**:495–499.

3. Pittet D, Simon A, Hugonnet S, et al., Hand hygiene among physicians: performance, beliefs, and perceptions. *Ann Intern Med* 2004;**141**:1–8.

4. Allegranzi B, Pittet D, Healthcare-associated infection in developing countries: simple solutions to meet complex challenges. *Infect Control Hosp Epidemiol* 2007;**28**:1323–1327.

5. Raka L, Lowbury Lecture 2008: infection control and limited resources – searching for the best solutions. *J Hosp Infect* 2009;**72**:292–298.

6. Shears P, Poverty and infection in the developing world: healthcare-related infections and infection control in the tropics. *J Hosp Infect* 2007;**67**:217–224.

7. Barahona-Guzman N, Rodriguez-Calderon ME, Rosenthal VD, et al., Impact of the International Nosocomial Infection Control Consortium (INICC) multidimensional hand hygiene approach in three cities of Colombia. *Int J Infect Dis* 2014;**19**:67–73.

8. Pittet D. Improving compliance with hand hygiene in hospitals. *Infect Control Hosp Epidemiol* 2000;**21**:381–386.

9. Larson E, A causal link between handwashing and risk of infection? Examination of the evidence. *Infect Control Hosp Epidemiol* 1988;**9**:28–36.

10. Schweizer ML, Reisinger HS, Ohl M, et al., Searching for an optimal hand hygiene bundle: a meta-analysis. *Clin Infect Dis* 2014;**58**:248–259.

11. Harris AD, Lautenbach E, Perencevich E, A systematic review of quasi-experimental study designs in the fields of infection control and antibiotic resistance. *Clin Infect Dis* 2005;**41**:77–82.

12. Perencevich EN, Lautenbach E, Infection prevention and comparative effectiveness research. *JAMA* 2011;**305**:1482–1483.

13. Saginur R, Research ethics and infection control. *Clin Infect Dis* 2009;**49**:1254–1258.

14. Price JR, Golubchik T, Cole K, et al., Whole-genome sequencing shows that patient-to-patient transmission rarely accounts for acquisition of Staphylococcus aureus in an intensive care unit. *Clin Infect Dis* 2014;**58**:609–618.

15. Snitkin ES, Zelazny AM, Thomas PJ, et al., Tracking a hospital outbreak of carbapenem-resistant Klebsiella pneumoniae with whole-genome sequencing. *Sci Transl Med* 2012;**4**.

16. Huang SS, Septimus E, Kleinman K, et al., Targeted versus universal decolonization to prevent ICU infection. *N Engl J Med* 2013;**368**:2255–2265.

17. Derde LP, Cooper BS, Goossens H, et al., Interventions to reduce colonisation and transmission of antimicrobial-resistant bacteria in intensive care units: an interrupted time series study and cluster randomised trial. *Lancet Infect Dis* 2014;**14**:31–39.

18. Allegranzi B, Gayet-Ageron A, Damani N, et al., Global implementation of WHO's multimodal strategy for improvement of hand hygiene: a quasi-experimental study. *Lancet Infect Dis* 2013;**13**:843–851.

19. Mathai E, Allegranzi B, Kilpatrick C, et al., Promoting hand hygiene in healthcare through national/subnational campaigns. *J Hosp Infect* 2011;**77**:294–298.

20. Moerbeek M, van Breukelen GJ, Berger MP, A comparison between traditional methods and multilevel regression for the analysis of multicenter intervention studies. *J Clin Epidemiol* 2003;**56**:341–350.

21. Harris AD, Bradham DD, Baumgarten M, et al., The use and interpretation of quasi-experimental studies in infectious diseases. *Clin Infect Dis* 2004;**38**:1586–1591.

22. Shardell M, Harris AD, El-Kamary SS, et al., Statistical analysis and application of quasi experiments to antimicrobial resistance intervention studies. *Clin Infect Dis* 2007;**45**:901–907.

23. Gastmeier P, Brauer H, Forster D, et al., A quality management project in 8 selected hospitals to reduce nosocomial infections: a prospective, controlled study. *Infect Control Hosp Epidemiol* 2002;**23**:91–97.

24. Rijnders BJ, Vandecasteele SJ, Van Wijngaerden E, et al., Use of semiautomatic treatment advice to improve compliance with Infectious Diseases Society of America guidelines for treatment of intravascular catheter-related infection: a before-after study. *Clin Infect Dis* 2003;**37**:980–983.

25. Fernández-Pérez C, Tejada J, Carrasco M, Multivariate time series analysis in nosocomial infection surveillance: a case study. *Int J Epidemiol* 1998;**27**:282–288.

26. Li Q, Guo NN, Han ZY, et al., Application of an autoregressive integrated moving average model for predicting the incidence of hemorrhagic fever with renal syndrome. *Am J Trop Med Hyg* 2012;**87**:364–370.

27. Pittet D, Dharan S, Touveneau S, et al., Bacterial contamination of the hands of hospital staff during routine patient care. *Arch Intern Med* 1999;**159**:821–826.

Chapter 8

Hand Hygiene Agents

Pascal Bonnabry[1] and Andreas Voss[2]

[1] University of Geneva Hospitals and Faculty of Medicine, and Univeristy of Lausanne, Geneva and Lausanne, Switzerland

[2] Radboud University Medical Centre and Canisius-Wilhelmina Hospital, Nijmegen, The Netherlands

KEY MESSAGES

- Hand hygiene products can be formulated with well-known and easy to find ingredients.

- Emollients and gelling agents can improve tolerability, but they can also negatively influence efficacy; each final formulation should be appropriately evaluated in terms of efficacy and acceptance.

- Manufacturing is easy and is possible in low-income countries, but a strict quality assurance system must be in place to guarantee the quality of the end product.

The objectives of hand hygiene can only be reached when the formulation has proven antimicrobial efficacy and when healthcare workers are compliant in using it at the right time and in the right way. This chapter focuses on the different agents that can be integrated in the composition of hand hygiene preparations, and will determine the activity of the product and possibly the acceptance by the users.

WHAT WE KNOW – THE EVIDENCE

The formulation of commercial hand hygiene preparations can be complex and expensive, but in fact, the process can be made relatively simple, as the basic ingredients commonly used are ubiquitous and inexpensive. For example, the World Health Organization (WHO) formulations contain alcohol (isopropanol

Hand Hygiene: A Handbook for Medical Professionals, First Edition.
Edited by Didier Pittet, John M. Boyce and Benedetta Allegranzi.
© 2017 John Wiley & Sons, Inc. Published 2017 by John Wiley & Sons, Inc.

or ethanol), hydrogen peroxide, glycerin and water,[1] all of which have been well-known and commonly used ingredients, for centuries. However, many different ingredients may be used in the preparation of hand hygiene products. Consequently, the number of different combinations and preparations is very high. The final objective of any product is to combine a high antimicrobial efficacy, high tolerability and optimal coverage to allow optimal compliance/use. The successful achievement of these three goals is associated with the ingredients, their concentrations and application form, and it must be demonstrated by standardized methods for each new combination.

All formulations are based on derivatives belonging to the following categories of products (Table 8.1):

- *Alcohol*:[1,2] the vast majority of alcohol-based handrubs contain isopropanol, ethanol or *n*-propanol, or a combination of two of these alcohols. The antimicrobial activity can be attributed to their ability to denature proteins. Solutions containing 60–95% alcohol are effective, and lower or higher concentrations are less potent; most of the time, concentrations between

Table 8.1   Examples of Ingredients Commonly Used in the Formulation of Hand Hygiene Preparations

Category	Products	Concentration	Objective
Alcohol	Ethanol Isopropanol *n*-Propanol	60–80%	Antimicrobial effect
Additional antiseptic	Chlorhexidine Chloroxylenol Hexachlorophene Iodine and iodophors Quaternary ammonium Triclosan	0.5–4% 0.5–4% 3% 1% iodine 0.1–2%	Antimicrobial effect Persistence of the activity
Sporicide	Hydrogen peroxide	0.125%	Spores elimination
Emollient	Glycerol Octoxyglycerine Isopropyl myristate Bisobolol	1–1.5% 1% 2% 0.1%	Improve tolerability
Gelling agent	Cellulose derivatives		Improve tolerability. Might decrease efficacy
Water	Quality for nonsterile pharmaceutical preparations	ad final volume	
Other additives	Colorant Fragrances		Not recommended

60 and 80% are selected for hand hygiene products. Alcohols effectively reduce bacterial counts on hands; they are rapidly germicidal when applied to the skin, but they have no appreciable persistent activity. They are also active against all enveloped and most non-enveloped viruses. The efficacy is affected by numerous factors including the type of alcohol used, the concentration, the contact time, the volume of solution used, and whether the hands are wet when the alcohol is applied (which reduces efficacy). The latter should never be done, since it furthermore increases the risk of skin irritation.

- *Additional antiseptic*:[1,2] antimicrobial agents can be added to the alcohol to increase efficacy and the duration of the effect (persistent or residual activity). Products dedicated to skin antisepsis are commonly included in hand hygiene formulations. The most frequently used antiseptics are chlorhexidine and quaternary ammonium derivatives. The additional activity and the persistent effect provided by chlorhexidine are well demonstrated in vitro,[3] but no robust in vivo data exist to definitively recommend the use of this agent in formulations.

- *Sporicide*: alcohols have a strong activity against many microorganisms, but their potential to eliminate spores is limited. In consequence, a risk of contamination by viable bacterial spores exists, with potential consequences during the use of the product.[4] To manage this risk, the solution should be either microbiologically filtered ($0.22 \mu m$) during the bottle-filling process or a spore-eliminating agent should be added to the formulation. Hydrogen peroxide (H_2O_2) at a low concentration (0.125% v/v) has demonstrated sporicidal activity in pharmaceutical alcohols[5] and was selected for the WHO formulations. At this concentration, H_2O_2 is not an active substance for hand antisepsis but is only useful during the first 72 hours post-production to eliminate any spore present in the alcohol. During this period of time, the bottles should be kept closed in quarantine.

- *Emollient*: although alcohols are less damaging for the skin than detergents, they can also cause dryness and irritation. Several studies have demonstrated that products including an emollient show improved tolerability and are associated with better skin condition.[6] The acceptance of the product is of utmost importance, as it will directly influence compliance and therefore the infection rate. Many different chemical products have been used as emollients, and this additive is often undeclared, as it can be the key element for the commercial success of a specific preparation. The impact of the emollient on tolerability should be evaluated, as well as its influence on the antimicrobial activity. Indeed, it was demonstrated that they can reduce the effect of alcohol,[7] and an adequate balance should be found between the antiseptics and the emollient to ensure both efficacy and acceptance.

- *Gelling agent*: gel formulations are more and more popular to reduce the drying effect of alcohol and potentially enhance compliance. A practical effect is also promoted as this type of formulation reduces the loss of solution onto the floor (and thus possible damage/discoloring of certain type of floors). Cellulose derivatives can be used for this purpose, by applying the formulation principles traditionally used for any external gel. However, like the emollients, the modification of the consistency of the product can potentially modify its efficacy[8] and tolerability, and these points should be strictly validated during the development of the product.

- *Water*: formulations always contain a certain amount of water, which is necessary to reach the expected titration of alcohol. The microbiological quality of the water should be appropriate to non-sterile pharmaceutical preparations, in accordance with the local pharmacopoeia or any local recommendation. When industrial sterile water is not available, distilled water or water that has been freshly boiled and cooled can be used.

- *Foams*: the foaming of formulations may allow for better coverage and spread of the products on hands. As current testing methods test the liquid solution (not the final product resulting from the foaming process), data on antimicrobial efficacy are missing; it can be assumed however that foams are equally effective as other application forms.

- *Other additives*: colorant and fragrances are sometimes added to the formulation, to differentiate the preparation from other fluids or to mask the odor of alcohol. These additives should be used with caution, as they increase the risk of allergic reaction. Fragrances can also have an unexpected negative impact on the acceptability by healthcare workers, as a pleasant odor can become disagreeable when the product has to be repeatedly applied throughout the day. As a result, it is recommended to limit the use of colorant and to carefully evaluate any fragrance that is being considered for addition to hand hygiene preparations.

In summary, the composition is crucial both to the efficacy and the tolerance of the hand hygiene product. It is possible to keep it simple and to use well-known active ingredients and additives. For example, the WHO proposes solutions with a final concentration of 80% v/v ethanol or 75% v/v isopropanol with 1.45% v/v glycerol and 0.125% v/v hydrogen peroxide. In any case, efficacy must be carefully evaluated as the formulation can greatly influence the overall antimicrobial activity.[9]

The quality of the final product is related not only to the selected ingredients, but also to the *manufacturing process*, which involves both production and quality control. Industrial manufacturing is the ideal way to provide large quantities of high-quality products, but in some situations local production in central hospital pharmacies or even dispensaries is necessary. This lower-scale production has been demonstrated to be feasible,[10] but requires the implementation of a facility working in accordance with good manufacturing practices (GMP). The level of GMP is regulated by the local rules in force and can vary according to the amount of solution produced. It concerns the facility, the operators, the documentation, the production process, and quality control. All these aspects should be strictly organized and described in the quality assurance system of the manufacturer.

The different ingredients of the preparation will only develop their expected action if their quality and quantity correspond to the specifications. For that reason, the *quality control* of both raw materials – especially active ingredients – and final products is essential to quality. In some countries, an adequate titration of alcohol is sometimes difficult to reach, and variation can exist between different purchased batches. It is therefore essential to measure the alcohol content before the first production, in order to avoid its use if the value is under the minimal concentration needed in the final preparation or to adapt the preparation protocol according to the effective titrate of alcohol. Although gas chromatography is the reference method to quantify alcohols, very simple procedures can also be used to rapidly verify the real content of a solution. The WHO Guidelines on Hand Hygiene in Health Care[1] recommend the use of an alcoholmeter.

If the formulation contains other active (additional antiseptic) or important (hydrogen peroxide) ingredients, they also have to be analyzed in the final preparation. Theoretically, even "inactive" additives – like emollients and gelling agents – should also be analyzed, as the efficacy of the final product can be influenced by their concentration. This can usually be done at an industrial level, but is very difficult to implement in small-scale production facilities, especially in developing countries. A simple e-learning module is freely available to help formulate an effective alcohol-based handrub, and to locally produce it with well-known and easy to find ingredients (pharmacie.g2hp.net/courses/hand-hygiene/).

WHAT WE DO NOT KNOW – THE UNCERTAIN

As was previously illustrated, even if the basic types of ingredients are limited, the number of different possible combinations is very high. Each formulation has to comply with efficacy testing (see Chapter 9), but only a few head-to-head studies exist, especially for commercial products. Each industrial company tries to keep as secret as possible the composition of its preparation – except for the ingredients that have to be declared – which is understandable from a commercial point of view but does not help to better understand the usefulness of specific antiseptics or additives. As a result, there is still no strong evidence on the need to add an antiseptic to alcohol, even if arguments related to the spectrum of activity or the persistence of the effect make sense. Chlorhexidine, which is probably the most discussed additional antiseptic, is frequently added to formulations without strict in vivo evidence of its superiority to alcohol-only formulations. In this condition, some may argue that the risks related to this substance surpass its potential benefit and that it is better not to use it. In the authors' view the question remains unsolved, with arguments for both sides but no conclusive scientific evidence. With regard to alcohol concentration, the sweet spot, hitting the broadest range of nosocomial pathogens, with the least chance of causing skin irritation and being accepted by healthcare workers is not well known, even so it might be in the 70–80% range.

As for antiseptics, there is an ongoing discussion on emollients and gelling agents, particularly regarding their impact on efficacy. No predictive model actually exists, and in vitro efficacy testing is the only way to demonstrate the suitability of a new formulation. However, even if this test is standardized, it is not uncommon to read contradictory conclusions between results obtained for the same product in different laboratories. This factor contributes to never-ending discussions about the real efficacy of products and the impact of additives on alcohol potency. In addition, any increase in acceptance of a product may outweigh any loss in in vitro efficacy. While foaming is usually achieved through the physical effect of the dispensing system, some foams may have additional ingredients to achieve foaming. They are frequently used in lower quantities than those used for the testing, according to European Norm (EN) standards, due to the fact that 3 mL solution as foam is too large in size and would take too long to dry. Future research still needs to demonstrate the ideal quantity of foam and gel products which cover the whole hand and are effective.

The quality of alcohol in developing countries is also a matter of uncertainty. As already mentioned, the concentration can vary, with important consequences on the production process. Moreover, purity cannot be verified in these facilities, and there is a risk of contamination by unexpected impurities. Even if the product is dedicated to an external use, one should avoid the presence of potentially toxic chemical entities.

Finally, the antimicrobial spectrum of hand hygiene preparations could be a challenge in the future, with the development of resistance and the emergence of new microbial agents, especially highly potent viruses. The efficacy of the actual preparations against these new pathogens is often unknown, which brings uncomfortable uncertainty when an outbreak or a pandemic situation with such a specific agent occurs.

RESEARCH AGENDA

To answer the above-mentioned uncertainties, the following research agenda should be addressed:

- The added-value of antiseptics should be demonstrated in real-life conditions, by conducting randomized controlled studies measuring the impact on infection rates as primary endpoint. Some of these endpoints may be pathogen-specific, such as rates of methicillin-resistant *Staphylococcus aureus* or Norovirus infections. This can be applied to chlorhexidine, but also to other antiseptic agents.

- A large in vitro study on the impact of emollients and gelling agents on the efficacy of alcohol should be designed, in order to get cartography between the ingredients, their concentration, their combination, and the final efficacy of the product. The final objective should be the development of a predictive model to help the formulation of new products.

- A large-scale analytical assessment of alcohols produced in developing countries should be proposed, with the use of technologies allowing for the determination of both concentration and purity. The inter-batch variability should also be measured, as well as the link between the quality and the source used to distil the alcohol. In the end, recommendations for distilleries should be established to help them produce alcohol answering to the pharmaceutical specifications.

- Knowledge on the efficacy of products on new microorganisms, especially viruses, should be increased by systematic studies. With the same objective of still having in the future potent antiseptics, the research and development of new active pharmaceutical ingredients suitable against a large spectrum of micro-organisms should be boosted.

REFERENCES

1. World Health Organization, *WHO Guidelines on Hand Hygiene in Health Care*. Geneva: WHO, 2009.
2. Centers for Disease Control and Prevention, *CDC Guidelines for Hand Hygiene in Healthcare Settings*. 2002. Available at www.cdc.gov/handhygiene/Guidelines.html. Accessed March 7, 2017.
3. Kühn S, Trends in hand disinfection. *Business briefing: global healthcare* 2003;**1–2**.
4. Baylac MG, Lebreton T, Darbord JC, Microbial contamination of alcohol solutions used in hospital pharmacies in antiseptic preparations manufacturing. *Eur J Hosp Pharm* 1998;**4**:74–78.
5. Lee MG, Hunt P, Weir PJ, The use of hydrogen peroxide as a sporicide in alcohol disinfectant solutions. *Eur J Hosp Pharm* 1996;**2**:203–206.
6. Larson E, Girard R, Pessoa-Silva CL, et al., Skin reactions related to hand hygiene and selection of hand hygiene products. *Am J Infect Control* 2006;**34**:627–635.
7. Suchomel M, Rotter M, Weinlich M, et al., Glycerol significantly decreases the three hour efficacy of alcohol-based surgical hand rubs. *J Hosp Infect* 2013;**83**:284–287.
8. Kramer A, Rudolph P, Kampf G, et al., Limited efficacy of alcohol-based hand gels. *Lancet* 2002;**359**:1489–1490.
9. Edmonds SL, Macinga DR, Mays-Suko P, et al., Comparative efficacy of commercially available alcohol-based hand rubs and World Health Organization-recommended hand rubs: formulation matters. *Am J Infect Control* 2012;**40**:521–525.
10. Allegranzi B, Sax H, Bengaly L, et al., Successful implementation of the World Health Organization hand hygiene improvement strategy in a referral hospital in Mali, Africa. *Infect Control Hosp Epidemiol* 2010;**31**:133–141.

Chapter 9

Methods to Evaluate the Antimicrobial Efficacy of Hand Hygiene Agents

Manfred L. Rotter,[1] Syed A. Sattar,[2] and Miranda Suchomel[1]

[1] *Institute of Hygiene and Applied Immunology, Medical University of Vienna, Vienna, Austria*

[2] *Department of Biochemistry, Microbiology and Immunology, Faculty of Medicine, University of Ottawa, Ottawa, Canada*

KEY MESSAGES

- Every new formulation for hand antisepsis should be tested for its antimicrobial efficacy together with all its ingredients to ensure that any excipients added for better skin tolerance do not compromise its activity.

- Economically affordable standardized in vivo laboratory tests on the hands of subjects are appropriate to ensure that a product meets an agreed-upon minimum performance in activity under simulated practical conditions, while also allowing for comparisons with other similar products.

- At present, the choice of *reference treatments* or *positive controls* requires further research. Firstly, because it is not known how their efficacy assessed by in vivo laboratory tests translates into clinical effectiveness. Secondly, because results from clinical trials with concomitant comparative in vivo laboratory testing of various hand hygiene treatments remain scarce.

Hand Hygiene: A Handbook for Medical Professionals, First Edition.
Edited by Didier Pittet, John M. Boyce and Benedetta Allegranzi.
© 2017 John Wiley & Sons, Inc. Published 2017 by John Wiley & Sons, Inc.

WHAT WE KNOW – THE EVIDENCE

Every new formulation for hand antisepsis should be tested for its antimicrobial efficacy together with all its ingredients to ensure that any excipients added for better skin tolerance do not compromise its activity.[1,2]

Possible ways to assess the antimicrobial activity of hand hygiene agents include in vitro tests, such as determinations of the minimal bactericidal concentration, kill-curves and quantitative suspension tests, or ex vivo protocols using explants of animal or human skin. Such testing, however, represents neither the inactivating potential of the tested formulation in vivo nor the conditions on live human skin under practical circumstances.[3] In contrast, properly designed and well controlled in vivo testing using the hands of human subjects or actual field testing are considered more appropriate to demonstrate the actual antimicrobial activity of antiseptics under field conditions. While in vitro testing is too artificial by its nature, in vivo protocols can be difficult to control for extraneous influences, and neither of them can provide information on a formulation's potential to reduce the spread of handborne pathogens.[1,3] Although clinical trials are the best way to demonstrate a candidate formulation's ability to prevent/reduce the spread of hand-borne pathogens, such studies are invariably difficult to design, expensive, time consuming, and labor intensive. It has been shown, for instance, by power calculations that the demonstration of a reduction in hand-transmitted infections from 2% to 1% by changing to a presumably better hand antiseptic presupposes the observation of almost 2500 subjects in each of two experimental arms at the statistical settings of α (unidirectional) = 0.05 and a power of $1 - \beta = 0.9$.[4] Therefore, the results of only a few clinical trials have been published.

Hence, economically affordable, standardized in vivo laboratory-based tests on the hands of subjects appear to be an appropriate choice to ensure that a product meets an agreed-upon minimum performance in activity under simulated practical conditions while also allowing for comparisons with other similar products.

Currently Available in Vivo Tests

The two major categories of products to be evaluated are (a) hand hygiene agents to eliminate transient pathogens from healthcare workers' (HCWs') hands by either a hygienic handrub or handwash, and (b) presurgical hand rubs or handwashes to reduce the release of resident microflora from the hands of the surgical team. In Europe, the only officially approved test methods are those of the Comité Européen de Normalisation (CEN). In the United States and Canada, the U.S. Food and Drug Administration (FDA) and Health Canada, respectively, regulate such formulations; both refer to the standards of American Society for Testing Methods (ASTM) International (www.astm.org/). See Table 9.1.

Table 9.1 Basic Experimental Design of Current Methods to Test the Efficacy of Hand Hygiene and Surgical Hand Preparation Formulations[*]

Method No.	Test Organism(s)	Basic Procedure
EN 1499 (Hygienic handwash)	*Escherichia coli* (K12)	Hands are washed with a soft soap, dried, contaminated by immersion in broth culture for 5 s, excess fluid is drained off, and hands are air-dried for 3 min. Bacteria are recovered for pretreatment values by kneading the fingertips of each hand separately for 60 s in 10 mL of broth without neutralizers. Hands of one half of the subjects are treated with the product following the manufacturer's instructions (allowed contact time between 30 and 60 s). Hands are then rinsed (10 s) and dried (5 s). The hands of the other half are washed in a standardized fashion for 60 s with the reference solution (a 20% solution of soft soap), rinsed (10 s) and dried (5 s). After thorough handwashing, the procedure is repeated by same subjects with reversed roles. Recovery of bacteria for post-treatment values (see EN 1500)
EN 1500 (Hygienic handrub)	*Escherichia coli* (K12)	Basic procedure for hand contamination and for pre-treatment recovery of test bacteria is the same as in EN 1499. For treatment with the test formulation, half of the subjects rub hands according to manufacturer's instructions (allowed contact time between 30 and 60 s). For reference treatment, the other half rub hands for 30 s with 3 mL of 2-propanol 60% v/v and repeat this operation with a total application time not exceeding 60 s. Fingertips of both hands are then rinsed in water for 5 s and excess water is drained off. For post-treatment sampling, fingertips of each hand are kneaded separately in 10 mL of broth with added neutralizers to obtain post-treatment values. After thorough handwashing, the same subjects repeat the procedure with reversed roles. Log_{10} dilutions of recovery medium containing neutralizer are prepared and plated out. Colony counts are obtained and log reductions calculated

ASTM E-1174 (Standard test method for evaluation of the effectiveness** of healthcare personnel handwash formulations)	*Serratia marcescens, Escherichia coli*	To test the efficacy of handwash agents for the reduction of transient microbial flora. Before baseline bacterial sampling and prior to each wash with the test material, 5 mL of a suspension of the test organism is applied to and rubbed over the hands. Test material is spread over hands and the lower third of forearms with lathering. Hands and forearms are then rinsed. Contamination and antisepsis are repeated consecutively 10 times. Elusions are performed after the 1st, 3rd, 7th, and 10th washes using 75 mL of eluent for each gloved hand. The eluates are tested for viable bacteria. (Alcohol-based handrubs and other leave-on formulations used without the aid of water may be tested using Test Method E-2755)
ASTM E-2755 (Standard test method for determining the bacteria-eliminating effectiveness of hand sanitizer formulations using hands of adults)	*Staphylococcus aureus, Serratia marcescens*	To test the efficacy of handwash or handrub agents on the reduction of high-density inoculum (10^{10} CFU/mL). This test method can be used to test any form of hand sanitizer, including gels, rubs, sprays, foams, and wipes according to label directions at typical "in-use" doses. It may be used as an alternative to test method E-2276, which limits the test bacteria to the fingerpads and does not incorporate actual use conditions such as friction during hand decontamination
ASTM E-1838 (Standard test method for determining the virus-eliminating effectiveness of hygienic handwash and handrub agents using the fingerpads of adults)	Adenovirus, Rotavirus, Rhinovirus, Hepatitis A virus, and Murine Norovirus	$10\,\mu$L of the test virus suspension in soil load is placed at the center of each thumb and fingerpad, the inoculum is left to dry, and exposed for 10–30 s to 1 mL of the test formulation or control. The fingerpads are then eluted and eluates are assayed for viable virus. Controls include an assessment of input titer, loss on drying of inoculum, and mechanical removal of virus. The method is applicable for testing of both handwash and handrub agents

(continued)

Table 9.1 (Continued)

Method No.	Test Organism(s)	Basic Procedure
ASTM E-2276 (Standard test method for determining the bacteria-eliminating effectiveness of hygienic handwash and handrub agents using the fingerpads of adults)	*Escherichia coli, Serratia marcescens, Acinetobacter baumannii, Staphylococcus aureus,* and *Staphylococcus epidermidis*	Similar to ASTM E-1838
ASTM E-2613 (Standard test method for determining the fungus-eliminating effectiveness of hygienic handwash and handrub agents using the fingerpads of adults)	*Candida albicans* and *Aspergillus niger*	Similar to ASTM E-1838
ASTM E-2011 (Whole hand method for viruses)	Rotavirus, Rhinovirus, Adenovirus, Feline Calicivirus, and Murine Norovirus	This method is designed to confirm the findings of the fingerpad method (E-1838), if necessary. Both hands are contaminated with the test virus, and the test formulation is used to wash or rub on them. The entire surface of both hands is eluted, and the eluates are assayed for infectious virus
ASTM E-2784 (Standard test method for evaluation of the effectiveness of handwash formulations using the paper towel (palmar) method of hand contamination)	*Serratia marcescens, Escherichia coli, Staphylococcus aureus, Shigella flexneri*	This method is designed to determine the effectiveness of antimicrobial handwashing agents for the reduction of transient microflora when using a handwashing procedure with the palmar surface only for experimental contamination

Method	Test organism(s)	Description
ASTM E-2870 (Standard test method for evaluating relative effectiveness of antimicrobial handwashing formulations using the palmar surface and mechanical sampling)	*Serratia marcescens, Escherichia coli*	This method is designed to determine the relative effectiveness of antimicrobial handwashing agents in reducing transient microflora using a controlled handwash The test method also uses a mechanical scrubbing machine in conjunction with the glove juice technique for more efficient recovery of viable test bacteria from the palms. The mechanical sampling results in greater recovery of bacteria from the palms than conventional recovery methods, such as massaging
EN 12791 (Test method for evaluation of surgical handrub or scrub)	Resident skin flora (no artificial contamination)	Same as for EN 1500 with the following exceptions: no artificial contamination, reference hand antisepsis 3-min rub with *n*-propanol 60% v/v, longest allowed treatment with product 5 min, 1 week between tests with reference and product. Test for sustained effect (3 h) with split hands model is optional (product shall be significantly superior to reference)
ASTM E-1115 (Standard test method for evaluation of surgical hand scrub formulations)	Resident skin flora (no artificial contamination)	The method is designed to assess immediate, sustained, and long-term persistent activity against the resident flora. Subjects perform simulated surgical scrub and hands are sampled by kneading them in loose-fitting gloves with an eluent. The eluates are assayed for viable bacteria

*Adapted from references 1 and 3, and amended.
**Effectiveness does not refer to "clinical effectiveness" but to antimicrobial efficacy.

TESTS FOR HYGIENIC HANDRUB OR HANDWASH AGENTS

These test methods use experimentally contaminated hands of adults to evaluate a formulation's ability to reduce the release of transient microorganisms from the hands without regard to the resident microflora. Products to be tested are intended for use by HCWs, except in the context of surgical hand preparation.

CEN STANDARDS. The respective tests evaluating the microbicidal efficacy of products for hygienic handrub or hygienic handwash are EN 1500 and EN 1499, respectively. The former, a recently revised standard, requires 18–22 subjects, the latter 12–15 subjects. To compensate for extraneous influences, the subjects are assigned at random to two groups, one applying the test product according to instructions provided by the manufacturer (between 30 and 60 s), and the other applying a standardized reference treatment instead. After a thorough decontamination of the hands, the same subjects reverse roles in a consecutive run (crossover design). To establish the microbicidal efficacy of the formulation, the fingertips of each contaminated hand are sampled before and after treatment.

For handrubs, the reduction in the release of test organism with the formulation under test shall be at least not inferior to that achieved by the reference treatment (= rubbing 2 × 3 mL of 2-propanol 60% v/v for twice 30 s). In contrast, the bactericidal efficacy assessed with an antiseptic soap shall be significantly stronger than that achieved with the reference treatment (= washing prewetted hands with 5 mL of dilute (20%) soft soap for 60 s).

For official approval, in vitro pretesting of a product is required in quantitative suspension tests with certain bacterial strains, yeasts, and viruses as described in EN 13727, EN 13624, and EN 14476, respectively.

ASTM STANDARDS. ASTM E-1174 (Efficacy of healthcare personnel handwash formulations). Currently, handwash agents are evaluated using this whole-hand method in North America. To establish the microbicidal efficacy of the formulations, contaminated hands are sampled before and after treatment. The efficacy criteria of FDA's Tentative Final Monograph (TFM) are a 2-$\log_{10}$ reduction of the test organism on each hand within 5 min after the first and a 3-$\log_{10}$ reduction after the tenth wash. (Alcohol-based handrubs and other leave-on formulations used without the aid of water may be tested using test method E-2755.)

ASTM E-2755 (Whole-hand method for bacteria-eliminating effectiveness of hand sanitizer formulations). This test method, which may use either *Staphylococcus aureus* or *Serratia marcescens* as the test organism, can be used to test any form of hand sanitizer, including gels, rubs, sprays, foams, and wipes according to label directions at typical "in-use" doses. It can be an alternative to E-1174 or in place of E-2276, which limits the test bacteria to the fingerpads and does not incorporate friction during hand decontamination.

ASTM E-1838 (Fingerpad method for viruses). This method can be applied to handrub or handwash agents. With handwashes, it can measure reductions of viable virus after exposure to the test formulation alone, after post-treatment water rinsing and postrinse drying of hands. In contrast to using whole-hand models, the infection risk to subjects is smaller with this method.

ASTM E-2276 (Fingerpad method for vegetative bacteria). The method can be applied to handrub and handwash agents. It is similar in design and application to ASTM E-1838.

ASTM E-2613 (Fingerpad method for fungi). The method can be applied to handrub and handwash agents. It is similar in design and application to ASTM E-1838.

ASTM E-2011 (Whole-hand method for viruses). This method requires a larger volume (0.5 mL) of test virus as the entire surface of both hands is contaminated. After treatment, the surface of both hands is eluted, and the eluates are assayed for viable virus. Though this method gives results similar to those with ASTM E-1838, it may be used for further confirmation of the findings. It may also serve as an alternative when the test formulation form is not amenable to testing by E-1838. In this method, the application of viruses on the entire surface of both hands entails a greater risk to the subjects than using fingerpads only (E-1838). Therefore, greater caution must be exercised to ensure the freedom of the hands from any apparent damage. Moreover, virus inocula must be thoroughly screened for freedom from extraneous or adventitious pathogens before use in such testing.

ASTM E-2784 (contamination of palmar surface only). This method is designed to determine the effectiveness of antimicrobial handwashing agents for the reduction of transient microflora when using a handwashing procedure with the palmar surface only for experimental contamination. It can be an alternative to E-1174.

ASTM E-2870 (contamination of palmar surface and with mechanical sampling). This method is designed to determine the relative effectiveness of antimicrobial handwashing agents in reducing transient microflora using a controlled handwash. In contrast to E-1174, E-2755, and E-2784, this method makes it possible to directly compare the performance of two different formulations on the same subject. The method also uses a mechanical scrubbing machine in conjunction with the glove juice technique for more efficient recovery of viable test bacteria from the palms.

TESTS FOR SURGICAL HANDRUB OR HANDWASH AGENTS
No experimental contamination of the hands is needed in these tests.

EN 12791 (surgical hand preparation). The protocol of the forthcoming amendment of this European Norm is comparable with that described in EN 1500 except that the bactericidal efficacy of a product is tested:

- on clean, artificial contamination-free hands of 23–26 subjects,
- using a split-hands model to assess the immediate effect on one hand and a possible 3-hour sustained effect on the other, otherwise gloved hand,

- using a crossover design, the two experimental runs are separated by one week to allow regrowth of the resident flora,
- with the reference antiseptic treatment using as many 3-mL portions of 1-propanol 60% v/v as are necessary to keep hands wet for 3 min,
- with the test formulation as applied according to manufacturer's instructions but with the contact time not to exceed 5 min,
- with the requirements that the immediate and 3-hours effects of a product shall not be significantly inferior to those of the reference hand antisepsis, and
- with the option to demonstrate sustained activity (3 hours) – if such a claim is being contemplated.

ASTM E-1115 (surgical hand scrub). The method measures the reduction in the release of bacterial skin flora from the hands. It is designed for determining immediate and sustained as well as long-term persistent microbial reductions, after single or repetitive treatments, or both. In addition, cumulative activity after repetitive treatments may be measured. In North America, a formulation must pass this test to be considered for registration.

The TFM requires that products:

- reduce the release of bacteria from the hands by $1\text{-}\log_{10}$ on each hand within 1 min,
- that, on day 1, the bacterial count on each hand does not subsequently exceed baseline within 6 hours,
- produce a $2\text{-}\log_{10}$ reduction in bacterial counts on each hand within 1 min by the end of the second day of the test period,
- accomplish a $3\text{-}\log_{10}$ reduction of bacterial counts on each hand within 1 min by the end of the fifth day when compared to the established baseline.

WHAT WE DO NOT KNOW – THE UNCERTAIN

With in vivo laboratory tests, serious uncertainty exists in the *choice of requirements concerning the necessary reduction of test organisms* from the hands. The three in vivo European methods, EN 1499, EN 1500, and EN 12791, compare the efficacy of a test product intra-individually – each subject representing its own control – with that of a reference treatment concurrently performed by the same subjects in a crossover fashion. Even more important is that this reference serves as the standard for performance. This standard is flexible and changes according to the performance of the actual test population of subjects. In contrast, the TFM methods use fixed $\log_{10}$ bacterial reductions as pass criteria without allowing for efficacy variation in the composition of the subjects. The efficacy of hand hygiene agents depends, however, very much upon the subjects using them.[5]

The TFM requires that a healthcare personnel handwash demonstrates an in vivo reduction of the indicator organism by ≥ 2 $\log_{10}$ within 5 min after the first experimental contamination and handwash or handrub, and by 3 $\log_{10}$ after the tenth treatment. This requirement is inappropriate for healthcare settings. First, a ≥ 2-$\log_{10}$ reduction within a maximum contact time of 5 min is quite lenient, as even unmedicated soap and water can achieve a minimum reduction of 3 $\log_{10}$ within 1 min.[5] Second, the necessity for cumulative and sustained action in non-surgical settings may be unnecessary.[1,3] What is really needed is a strong immediate effect against a broad spectrum of transient microflora in a short contact time after the first application of the antiseptic as, for ethical reasons, the first patient should be as safe as the tenth.

Another, often criticized uncertainty is the *duration of hand treatments* of 30 s or 60 s as stipulated in traditional test methods because in actual practice the average duration of contact may be less than 15 s. However, a possible justification for longer than field-relevant contact times is the fact that contact times as short as 15 s make determination of statistically valid differences between the performances of a test product as compared to the reference would require very large sample sizes, that is, number of subjects. Therefore, in a laboratory in vivo test the non-inferiority of a test product can much more easily and economically be demonstrated by using a reference treatment with longer skin contact than is usual in field practice.

The *volume of a hand hygiene agent* (handrub or soap) applied is crucial for its performance. Up to a volume of 3 mL the performance of hand hygiene agents increases significantly.[6] But that volume has been criticized as being too large compared to the output of most dispensers, shown to range between 0.6 and 1.3 mL.[7] Volumes such as these are, however, often too small to cover the entire surface of the hands and may, in some instances, fail to meet the efficacy requirements of the existing officially approved standards.[6–8]

Another point of criticism is frequently the choice of an *indicator organism*, such as *Escherichia coli*, which some regard as not representative enough for hand-transmitted pathogens. However, *S. aureus* and *S. marcescens* used in some ASTM test protocols may pose a higher infection risk to the subjects.

The overall *costs* of testing hand hygiene formulations to meet regulatory requirements can be a major impediment. This is especially true for the varied and extensive requirements as mandated in the TFM. This large expenditure could easily be reduced at the same statistical power by testing both formulations concurrently with the same subjects in a crossover fashion and comparing the results intra-individually, as described in the CEN test protocols.

Statistical comparisons of the results with test formulations and reference treatments or positive controls should be performed as in clinical drug trials by noninferiority tests rather than by comparative statistical models. This earlier point of criticism on EN 1500 and EN 12791 has now been addressed in the 2013 versions.

In addition to the *immediate effect*, the TFM model for surgical handrub and handwash requires verification of a *sustained* and *persistent effect* of the surgical scrub, whereas in EN 12791 testing for those effects is optional. The fast and strong bactericidal action of the applied concentrations of volatile agents such as ethanol, 2-propanol, and 1-propanol essentially generates a sustained effect by delaying the regrowth of the skin's resident microflora by several hours.[9] Better justification is also needed to show a long-term bactericidal effect increasing from the first to the fifth day, as mandated by the TFM model.

The argument of an extremely high *expenditure* with the TFM model for testing surgical handrubs and scrubs is even more applicable than with testing products for hygienic hand antisepsis as at least 64 subjects are required per arm. This means that no less than 130 subjects are necessary to test a product together with an active control. For some products, this number will even have to be multiplied for concomitant testing of the vehicle and possibly of a placebo to demonstrate efficacy. Hence, this can add up to 520 or even more subjects. This high number could easily be reduced if the tests were not performed with different populations of subjects for each arm, but if always the same individuals participated in each arm, being randomly allocated to the various components of a Latin Square design, the experiments of which could be carried out at weekly intervals. The results are then treated as related samples with intra-individual comparison as in the EN 12791 model.

RESEARCH AGENDA

At present, the choice of *reference treatments* or *positive controls* requires further research because it is not known how their efficacy assessed by in vivo laboratory tests translates into clinical efficiency and because results from clinical trials with concomitant comparative in vivo laboratory testing of various hand hygiene treatments remain scarce.

Furthermore, in contrast to existing methods used in North America, the virucidal activity of handrub or handwash agents is tested in Europe solely by in vitro suspension tests with polio- and adenovirus (EN 14476) because suitable tests under practical conditions are not yet available. The development of a European Norm with murine norovirus as a test organism is in progress, though.

REFERENCES

1. World Health Organization, *WHO Guidelines on Hand Hygiene in Health Care*. Part I, Section 10. Geneva: WHO, 2009.
2. Suchomel M, Rotter M, Weinlich M, et al., Glycerol significantly decreases the three hour efficacy of alcohol-based surgical hand rubs. *J Hosp Infect* 2013;**83**:284–287.
3. Rotter M, Sattar S, Dharan S, et al., Methods to evaluate the microbicidal activities of handrub and handwash agents. *J Hosp Infect* 2009;**73**:191–199.

4. Rotter ML, Are experimental handwashing models a substitute for clinical trials to assess the efficacy of hand disinfectants. *Infect Control Hosp Epidemiol* 1990;**11**:63–66.
5. Rotter M, Mittermeyer H, Kundi M, Investigations on the model of the artificially contaminated hand – proposal for a test method [in German]. *Zbl Bakt Hyg, I.Abt Orig B* 1974;**159**:560–581.
6. Goronczy-Bermes P, Koburger T, Meyer B, Impact of the amount of hand rub applied in hygienic hand disinfection on the reduction of microbial counts on hands. *J Hosp Infect* 2010;**74**:212–218.
7. Macinga DR, Edmonds SL, Campbell E, et al., Efficacy of novel alcohol-based hand rub products at typical in-use volumes. *Infect Control Hosp Epidemiol* 2013;**34**:299–300.
8. Kampf G, Ruselack S, Eggerstedt S, et al., Lesser and lesser – the impact of small volumes in hand disinfection on quality of hand coverage and antimicrobial efficacy. *BMC Infect Dis* 2013;**13**::472.
9. Rotter ML, Kampf G, Suchomel M, et al., Population kinetics of the skin flora on gloved hands following surgical hand disinfection with three propanol-based hand rubs – a prospective, randomized, double-blind trial. *Infect Control Hosp Epidemiol* 2007;**28**:346–350.

Chapter 10

Hand Hygiene Technique

Marie-Noëlle Chraïti[1] and Andreas F. Widmer[2]
[1] Infection Control Program and WHO Collaborating Centre on Patient Safety, University of Geneva Hospitals, Geneva, Switzerland
[2] Division of Infectious Diseases and Hospital Epidemiology, University Hospital of Basel, Basel, Switzerland

KEY MESSAGES

- Handrubbing with an alcohol-based handrub formulation is standard of care for routine hand hygiene in healthcare.

- The amount of product used must be large enough to meet the requirements of the procedure duration and favor the coverage of the whole hand surfaces. According to producers, 2 to 3 mL of alcohol-based handrub is commonly sufficient.

- A procedure by steps, or at least minimal instructions, must be taught and trained to achieve a systematic full coverage of hand surfaces.

Hand hygiene techniques will depend on ways to perform it, either by rubbing with an alcohol-based handrub (ABHR) or by washing with soap and water. Hand-rubbing has been recommended since 2006 by the World Health Organization (WHO)[1] as the standard to clean hands in healthcare daily practices. Some particular indications to routinely perform handwashing still remain relevant, when the mechanical rinsing is an asset over handrubbing. Only few studies focus on the technique: therefore, limited data are available to provide clinically validated evidence for a defined technique.[2]

WHAT WE KNOW – THE EVIDENCE

The antimicrobial efficacy of rubbing hands with an ABHR is usually higher than hand cleansing with plain and medicated soaps. The quality of formulations, their respective compounds and concentrations, are crucial to guarantee efficacy.[3,4] Hand hygiene agents should meet the American (ASTM) or European (EN) standards (see Chapter 9). For ensuring efficacy, WHO recommends following the steps of the modified techniques according to the EN 1500 (Figures 10.1 and 10.2). The technique for handrubbing in daily routine instructs the user to apply "a palmful of the product" likely to fit hand-size surfaces; the technique for handwashing suggests applying "enough soap to cover all surfaces". 2 to 3 mL of a compound is usually sufficient (in some cases even 1.5 mL), but the volume should be adapted to the size of the hands.[5] However, staff members should undergo training sessions, where the appropriate volume and technique are investigated.

The duration of rubbing and exposure to the product depends directly on the amount applied, but a 30-second application is usually sufficient.[6] Considering the procedural steps to rub and wash hands for routine hand hygiene, Widmer,[4,7] Tschudin,[8] and Reilly[9] showed that properly applying the WHO technique was associated with a significantly greater antibacterial efficacy of handrubs. In addition, improving hand hygiene technique correlated well with increased antimicrobial activity using the same product, but strictly applying the WHO technique. Fluorescent methods have been used to study different aspects of the hand hygiene technique, and Kampf and colleagues suggested that basic instructions regarding the amount of product used and whole hand coverage requirement are sufficient.[10] The authors recommended a "responsible application" that does not require the use of all steps of EN 1500 technique. In fact, the most important steps of the WHO hand hygiene protocol are probably listed as the two last steps, the *"rotational rubbing of left thumb clasped in tight palm and vice versa"*, and the *"rotational rubbing, backwards and forwards with clasped fingers of right hand in left palm and vice versa"* (Figure 10.1). It may be prudent to use these steps as the first ones, since they ensure proper moistening of fingertips and thumbs.[11] These areas of the hands are most likely to come into direct contact with the patient, and subsequently, are likely the most important.

Skin protection is one of the key advantages of the preferred use of ABHR over handwashing with soap and water. Handwashing is known to remove the fatty acids from the skin, leading to dryness and enhancing skin damage. The skin protection properties of ABHRs containing humectants make them effectively less aggressive and well perceived by users. This has been repeatedly reported, including recently by Asensio when introducing rub in a surgical unit.[12] Interestingly skin hydration might correlate with handrub effectiveness.[13]

As any technique, hand hygiene sequences should be reviewed repeatedly to assure that they are being properly performed. Often, all aspects of the technique are not performed entirely. Several observation studies reported the low adherence to the techniques of hand hygiene. Handrub and handwash steps were missed and duration was shortened as observed by Widmer and Paz Felix[4,14] in two different contexts and among different professional categories. Reduction in antimicrobial efficacy has been determined[3] using different approaches.[4,11,14]

Related to handwashing, the hand-dry step is crucial in order to both prevent hand recontamination and skin damage. A recent review of the efficacy of different hand-dry methods concluded in favor of the use of disposable paper towels over cloth towels and air-dryers.[15]

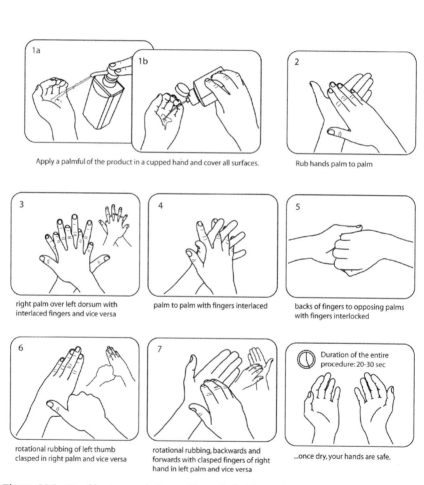

1a
1b
Apply a palmful of the product in a cupped hand and cover all surfaces.

2
Rub hands palm to palm

3
right palm over left dorsum with interlaced fingers and vice versa

4
palm to palm with fingers interlaced

5
backs of fingers to opposing palms with fingers interlocked

6
rotational rubbing of left thumb clasped in right palm and vice versa

7
rotational rubbing, backwards and forwards with clasped fingers of right hand in left palm and vice versa

Duration of the entire procedure: 20-30 sec

...once dry, your hands are safe.

Figure 10.1   Hand hygiene technique with an alcohol-based formulation. *Source: WHO Guidelines on Hand Hygiene in Health Care,* 2009 (Reproduced with permission from World Health Organization).

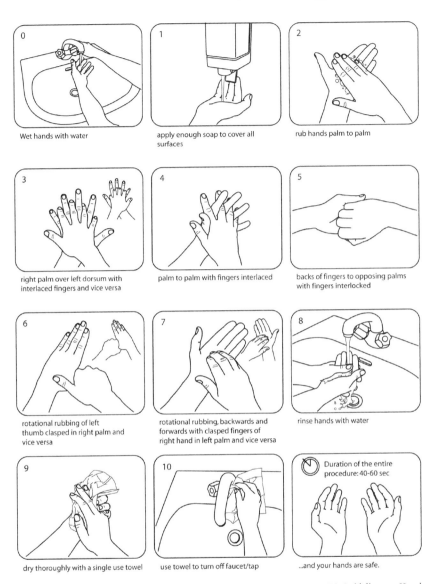

Figure 10.2   Hand hygiene technique with soap and water. *Source: WHO Guidelines on Hand Hygiene in Health Care*, 2009 (Reproduced with permission from World Health Organization).

WHAT WE DO NOT KNOW – THE UNCERTAIN

Studies have demonstrated that sequences to rub-in surfaces are key in antimicrobial efficacy of hand hygiene action. However the gain of one technique over another, provided the whole surfaces coverage, and the impact of the technique on the occurrence of healthcare-associated infection have not been quantified. In fact, the technique of EN 1500 was not developed for clinical use, but for evaluating minor differences between products in laboratory conditions following artificial contaminations (see Chapter 9). Although the antimicrobial efficacy of each step has not been studied so far, any technique that ensures proper moistening of the fingertips and the thumb is likely to be superior[11] and should be promoted, rather than leaving issues related to technique to the individual.

The amount of product applied seems critical to allow the coverage of all hand surfaces[5] and the minimal necessary duration of rubbing and exposure to active compounds. Although this component constitutes necessarily the first steps of either the handrub or handwash techniques to be applied for routine hand hygiene, there is no consensus on the minimal amount to be applied. Most of the European companies advise applying 2 to 3 mL of ABHR, and WHO recommends a "palmful" amount. Asensio has observed that the use of greater than 3 mL of product does not guarantee better coverage when handrubbing technique is suboptimal.[12]

RESEARCH AGENDA

Procedural steps for performing hand hygiene contribute to the antimicrobial efficacy of the action. Alternative simplified steps could be further explored.

However, we do not know how much compliance with the technique impacts on microbial transmission and healthcare-associated infection, and how it synergizes with compliance with indications for hand hygiene.

REFERENCES

1. World Health Organization, *WHO Guidelines for Hand Hygiene in Health Care*, Part II: **152**. Geneva: WHO, 2009. Available at whqlibdoc.who.int/publications/2009/9789241597906_eng.pdf. Accessed March 7, 2017.
2. Stewardson AJ, Iten A, Camus V, et al., Efficacy of a new educational tool to improve handrubbing technique amongst healthcare workers: a controlled, before-after study. *PLoS ONE* 2014;**9**:e105866.
3. Kampf G, How effective are hand antiseptics for the postcontamination treatment of hands when used as recommended? *Am J Infect Control* 2008;**35**:356–360.
4. Widmer AF, Dangel M, Alcohol-based handrub: evaluation of technique and microbiological efficacy with international infection control professionals. *Infect Control Hosp Epidemiol* 2004;**25**:207–209.
5. Bellissimo-Rodrigues F, Soule H, Gayet-Ageron A, et al., Should alcohol-based handrub use be customized to healthcare workers' hand size? *Infect Control Hosp Epidemiol* 2016;**37**:219–221.
6. Pires D, Soule H, Bellissimo-Rodrigues F, et al., Hand hygiene with alcohol-based handrub: how long is long enough? ICHE (in press).

7. Widmer AF, Conzelmann M, Tomic M, et al., Introducing alcohol-based hand rub for hand hygiene: the critical need for training. *Infect Control Hosp Epidemiol* 2007;**28**:50–54.

8. Tschudin Sutter S, Frei R, Dangel M, et al., Effect of teaching recommended World Health Organization technique on the use of alcohol-based hand rub by medical students. *Infect Control Hosp Epidemiol* 2010;**31**:1194–1195.

9. Reilly JS, Price L, Lang S, et al., A pragmatic randomized controlled trail of 6-step vs 3-step hand hygiene technique in acute hospital care in the United Kingdom. *Infect Control Hosp Epidemiol* 2016;**37**:661–666.

10. Kampf G, Reichel M, Feil Y, et al., Influence of rub-in technique on required application time hand coverage in hygienic hand disinfection. *BMC Infect Dis* 2008;**8**:149.

11. Pires D, Bellissimo-Rodrigues F, Soule H, et al., Revisiting the WHO "How to Handrub" hand hygiene technique: fingertips first? *Infect Control Hosp Epidemiol* 2017;**38**:230–233.

12. Asensio A, de Gregorio L, Practical experience in a surgical unit when changing from scrub to rub. *J Hosp Infect*, 2013;**83**:s40–s42.

13. Hautemanière A, Diguio N, Daval MC, et al., Short-term assessment of training of medical students in the use of alcohol-based hand rub using fluorescent-labeled hand rub and skin hydration measurements. *Am J Infect Control* 2009;**37**:338–340.

14. Paz Felix CC, Kaue Miyadahira AM, Evaluation of the hand washing technique held by students from the nursing graduation course. *Rev Esc Enferm USP* 2009;**43**:133–139.

15. Huang C, Ma W, Stack S, The hygienic efficacy of different hand-drying methods: a review of the evidence. *Mayo Clin Proc* 2012;**87**:791–798.

Chapter 11

Compliance with Hand Hygiene Best Practices

Benedetta Allegranzi,[1] Andrew J. Stewardson,[2,3] and Didier Pittet[3]

[1] *Infection Prevention and Control Global Unit, Department of Service Delivery and Safety, World Health Organization, and Faculty of Medicine, University of Geneva, Geneva, Switzerland*

[2] *Infectious Diseases Department, Austin Health and Hand Hygiene Australia, Melbourne, Australia*

[3] *Infection Control Program and WHO Collaborating Centre on Patient Safety, University of Geneva Hospitals and Faculty of Medicine, Geneva, Switzerland*

KEY MESSAGES

- Reports based on self-reported compliance systematically overestimate directly observed compliance.

- In the absence of promotional activities, healthcare workers' (HCWs') hand hygiene compliance with best practices is usually low, especially in developing countries. The quality of hand hygiene technique performance has also been found defective in most studies.

- Several objective and self-reported determinants of both low and good compliance have been identified, but additional research is still needed.

- Many interventions are effective in improving hand hygiene compliance, especially if aimed at addressing the determinants of defective practices.

Hand hygiene is a general term referring to any action of hand cleansing. Hand hygiene during healthcare delivery should be practiced either by handwashing or by handrubbing at specific moments when the risk of microbial transmission occurs. These moments have been identified by the World Health Organization (WHO) (see also Chapter 20) and other national and international agencies according to available scientific evidence, and are reflected in specific

Hand Hygiene: A Handbook for Medical Professionals, First Edition.
Edited by Didier Pittet, John M. Boyce and Benedetta Allegranzi.
© 2017 John Wiley & Sons, Inc. Published 2017 by John Wiley & Sons, Inc.

"opportunities" for hand hygiene.[1] The term "opportunity" for hand hygiene is defined as a "moment during healthcare activities when hand hygiene is necessary to interrupt germ transmission by hands."[1] This term is very close to the concept of hand hygiene "indication," which is the reason for a hand hygiene action. An opportunity is identified by the presence of one or more indications. Compliance or noncompliance with these indications has consequences for the transmission of pathogens and the development of healthcare-associated infections (HAIs). Technically, compliance with hand hygiene is calculated as the ratio of the number of performed actions to the number of opportunities.[1] In addition to compliance with recommended indications, it is important to consider the appropriateness of the technique used for handwashing or handrubbing. The WHO recommendations include the execution of specific movements to cover all hand surfaces while respecting recommended time duration of 20–30 s and 40–60 s for handrubbing and washing, respectively.[1] In this chapter, we focus mainly on findings from studies reporting hand hygiene compliance measured through direct observation. Other approaches to evaluate hand hygiene performance are discussed elsewhere in this book (see also Chapters 24 and 34).

WHAT WE KNOW – THE EVIDENCE

The issue of the *WHO Guidelines on Hand Hygiene in Health Care* in 2009 marked an important step in hand hygiene promotion worldwide because the recommendations were accompanied by an in-depth review of the scientific evidence and by a pilot-tested implementation strategy and tool package aimed at improving practices worldwide.[1,2] At the time of guideline publication, average compliance with hand hygiene best practices worldwide was estimated as being 38.7%, in the absence of hand hygiene promotion.[1] An additional systematic review, addressing the same time period, reported very similar results: an overall median compliance of 40%.[3] A multicenter European study conducted in 2009 in surgical wards showed marked interhospital variation in hand hygiene compliance (range, 14–76%)[4] and a study in 13 hospitals across Ontario, Canada, found a mean adherence of 31%.[5] Given that healthcare workers' (HCWs') hands are considered the main means of microbial transmission in healthcare, this compliance is unacceptably low.

Some national and subnational campaigns have published large-scale data on hand hygiene compliance. In Belgium, the average national compliance was 50% in 2005 before the launch of the first national campaign, and it progressively increased every year up to 73% after the fourth campaign in 2011.[6] Similarly, in Australia, compliance was 44% in hospitals that had recently joined the national campaign, and it increased to 68% after implementation.[7] Hand hygiene compliance was 47% in public hospitals in New South Wales (Australia) before a statewide campaign, and it increased to an average of 61% after.[8] A recently published large multicenter study conducted in intensive care units (ICUs) in a range of low- and middle-income countries documented that compliance before patient contact or an aseptic task was 48%. Lower compliance has been reported by other studies in poorly resourced settings (see also Chapter 43).

Unadjusted compliance estimates are usually lower in ICUs than in other settings (30–40% versus 50–60%), lower among physicians than among nurses (32% versus 48%), and before rather than after (21% versus 47%) patient contact.[3] These patterns are common in many single studies. Main predictors of poor adherence to recommended hand hygiene best practices have been summarized in the WHO Guidelines and include professional category, hospital ward, time of day/week, glove use (see also Chapter 23), and type and intensity of patient care, defined either as the number of opportunities for hand hygiene per hour of patient care or patient-to-nurse ratio. The average number of opportunities for hand hygiene per HCW varies markedly between hospital wards. For example, nurses in pediatric wards had an average of 8 opportunities per hour of patient care, compared with an average of 22 in ICUs.[1] The inverse relation between level of compliance and intensity of care was identified in a landmark study published in 1999 (Figure 11.1A).[9] Through multivariate analysis, the authors identified critical care units, procedures that carry a high risk of bacterial

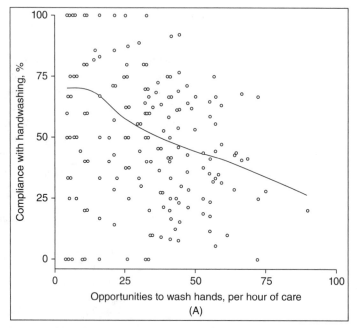

Figure 11.1A   Relation between level of hand hygiene compliance and opportunities per hour of patient care.*

* Opportunities per hour reflect the intensity of care. *Source*: Pittet 1999. Reproduced with permission from American College of Physicians.

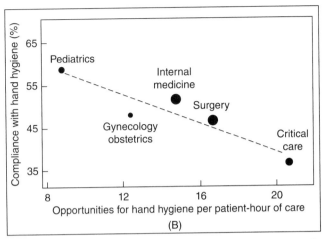

Figure 11.1B Relationship between opportunities for hand hygiene and compliance across hospital wards, University of Geneva Hospitals, 1994. Average compliance is indicated for handwashing and handrubbing. The size of the symbol is proportional to the number of opportunities observed in the different wards. *Source*: Pittet 2001. Reproduced with permission from Elsevier.

contamination, and high intensity of patient care as factors independently associated with low compliance. On average, compliance decreased by 5% per 10 opportunities per hour when the intensity of patient care exceeded 10 opportunities per hour. This inverse relation was also reflected in the type of ward (Figure 11.1B): the higher the average number of opportunities for hand hygiene per hour of patient care for a nurse, the lower the average compliance across hospital wards.

Hand hygiene compliance was found to be poorer before patient contact than after in most published studies.[3] In 2010, WHO conducted a global survey on Moment 1 (before patient contact), which showed an average compliance of 51%, ranging between 26% in the Americas and 64% in Europe (see Chapter 20).[10]

Poor compliance has been observed regardless of the national level of economic development and resources available at the local level. However, factors frequently identified as determinants of low compliance include inadequate infrastructures (lack of products or inconvenient location), high workload and understaffing, lack of understanding of hand hygiene recommendations, lack of recognition of the transmission risk, as well as of the impact of hand hygiene to reduce HAI.[1] Surgical subspecialty, professional category, type of care activity, and workload were independently associated with compliance in European surgical wards.[4] These factors and other barriers to hand hygiene compliance are discussed in detail in Chapter 12.

Predictors of good hand hygiene compliance or determinants for its improvement were also summarized in the WHO Guidelines and later confirmed in recent studies.[1] The most common were the introduction of widely accessible alcohol-based handrub (ABHR) or a multimodal improvement strategy, healthcare professionals other than physicians, care of patients under contact precautions or in isolation, activities perceived as having high risk of cross-contamination or infection for the HCW, and working in hemodialysis units or ICUs, in particular neonatal. In their large observational study in Ontario, Mertz and colleagues[5] confirmed that observations in ICUs, in single rooms, when contact precautions were indicated, when nurses rather than other HCWs were involved, and when ABHRs were accessible, were associated with a higher likelihood of good compliance.

Several studies investigated the level of hand hygiene compliance when self-reported by HCWs.[1,3] Interestingly, when asked about their own compliance with hand hygiene indications, HCWs demonstrate a perception at odds with the reality of defective compliance described above. Indeed, several studies showed that individuals of any professional category tend to overestimate their ability to clean their hands according to recommendations. This is illustrated by the absence of correlation between self-reported and observed hand hygiene compliance. Discrepancy between measured and self-reported compliance was also observed at baseline in the pilot study testing the WHO hand hygiene improvement strategy.[2] Despite differences in infrastructure, resource availability, and HCWs' knowledge across sites and countries, mean self-reported compliance was at least 80%, even in settings with very poor facilities for hand hygiene. In contrast, observed average compliance ranged between 8% and 55% (Figure 11.2).

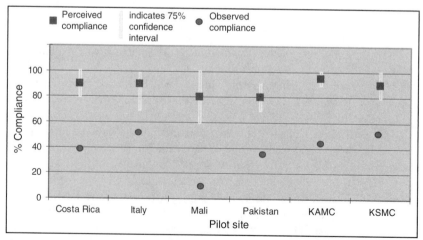

Figure 11.2   Self-reported vs. observed hand hygiene baseline compliance among healthcare workers in pilot sites testing the WHO Hand Hygiene Multimodal Improvement Strategy. KAMC/KSMC refer to hospitals in the Kingdom of Saudi Arabia.

Understanding the local determinants of and barriers to hand hygiene compliance, as well as any incorrect perceptions of self-performance, is of utmost importance in hand hygiene promotion strategies, and needs to be addressed with improved infrastructures, educational programs for HCWs, and performance feedback.

In addition to missed hand hygiene opportunities, defective behavior also concerns the technique used to perform hand hygiene. Indeed, the duration of hand hygiene actions is usually suboptimal (6.6 to 30 seconds in observational studies).[1] Furthermore, HCWs often fail to cover all surfaces of their hands and fingers.[11] Therefore, improvement strategies should also assess and, if necessary, address the appropriateness of hand hygiene technique (see Chapter 10).

WHAT WE DO NOT KNOW – THE UNCERTAIN

Despite the large number of studies published in the last 25 years about hand hygiene compliance in healthcare, methods used for direct observation have varied considerably. Therefore, estimates of average compliance are based on heterogeneous data, for instance, with regards to the type of opportunities detected, thus affecting reliability and benchmarking. Use of standardized methods, such as the WHO "My 5 Moments for Hand Hygiene" approach (see also Chapter 20),[1] would provide more generalizable estimates. For example, this would facilitate valid assessment of the extent of improvement achieved following campaigning and promotion efforts generated worldwide in recent years. Compliance calculated by recording all the "5 Moments for Hand Hygiene" according to the WHO observation method[1] are shown in the Table 11.1. Variability among studies remains evident, but it is very likely attributable to differences in settings and type of care.

Hand hygiene compliance has been measured at the level of single institutions in the great majority of studies. Although hand hygiene is regularly measured in several countries at the national level, a few publications have reported compliance on a large scale. Availability of hand hygiene compliance data at national or subnational level would allow more precise and generalizable analyses, including predictors and determinant factors, facilitated by a larger sample size. In particular, this would allow assessing the effect of national efforts and motivate their reinvigoration and long-term sustainment (see Chapter 36).

Although several insightful studies on hand hygiene behavior have been published over the last years (see Chapter 18), the understanding of social, cultural, and even religious factors influencing HCWs' attitude toward hand hygiene performance is still limited. We know much more about the external determinants and much less about intrinsic factors attributable to the individual or the social group. For instance, McLaws and colleagues recently demonstrated community-based handwashing practices in Iran, probably based on religious norms, exert a strong influence on HCWs' compliance in the hospital (see Chapter 18). If this interdependence between community and hospital hand hygiene practices would be

Table 11.1 Compliance with the Five Moments for Hand Hygiene Recommended by WHO (Measured Up to 2010)

Reference	Year of Measurement	Country	Scope	Setting	Baseline Compliance (%)
Mertz D et al.[5]	2005	Ontario, Canada	13 hospitals	Hospital-wide	31.2
Costers M et al.[6]	2005	Belgium	Nationwide	Hospital-wide	49.6
Allegranzi B et al.[2]	2006	Mali	One hospital	5 departments (internal medicine, surgery, emergency, intensive care, gynecology and obstetrics)	8.0
Allegranzi B et al.[2]	2006	Italy	38 hospitals	ICUs	55.2
Allegranzi B et al.[2]	2006	Costa Rica	One hospital	Medicine, surgery, paediatrics departments	39.7
Allegranzi B et al.[2]	2006	Pakistan	One hospital	3 ICUs	38.2
Allegranzi B et al.[2]	2006	Saudi Arabia	One hospital	6 departments (surgery, emergency, intensive care, gynecology and obstetrics, paediatrics, and others)	41.7
Allegranzi B et al.[2]	2006	Saudi Arabia	One hospital	2 departments (ICUs and surgical wards)	53.3
Caniza MA et al.[12]	2007	El Salvador	One pediatric hospital	5 high-risk wards	33.8
Abela N et al.[13]	2007	Malta	One hospital	3 wards	27.3
Tromp M et al.[14]	2008	The Netherlands	One hospital	Internal medicine department	27.0
Roberts SA et al.[15]	2009	New Zealand	One district	Hospital-wide	35.0
Marra AR et al.[16]	2009	Brazil	One hospital	ICU	62.3
Grayson L et al.[7]	2010	Australia	Nationwide	Hospital-wide	43.6
Scheithauer S et al.[17]	NA	Germany	One hospital	3 ICUs	61.3
Mathur P et al.[18]	2010	India	One hospital	2 ICUs	8.4

ICU, intensive care unit.

confirmed in other settings and on a larger scale, efforts to improve hand hygiene in the community could contribute to better behavior in healthcare.

Transmission models to identify specific indications for hand hygiene action in traditional medicine practices, home care, social care, and other types of care provided in the community are not yet available. As a consequence, the compliance levels of HCWs or carers working in these settings are unknown.

RESEARCH AGENDA

Further research is necessary regarding several unresolved issues concerning HCWs' hand hygiene compliance. Key research questions are:

- What are the determinants of HCWs' compliance in specific cultures and social environments?
- Based on identified barriers and predictors of hand hygiene compliance, what would be the most effective strategies to increase and sustain HCWs' compliance?
- Is measurement and reporting of hand hygiene compliance feasible on a large scale (national or international level), and would this contribute to improvement and sustainment of campaigning efforts around the world?
- What are the appropriate and essential indications for hand hygiene performance, and what is caregivers' compliance in traditional medicine, home care, and other types of care in the community?

REFERENCES

1. World Health Organization, *WHO Guidelines on Hand Hygiene in Health Care*. Geneva: WHO, 2009. Available at whqlibdoc.who.int/publications/2009/9789241597906_eng.pdf. Accessed March 7, 2017.
2. Allegranzi B, Gayet-Ageron A, Damani N, et al., Global implementation of WHO's multimodal strategy for improvement of hand hygiene: a quasi-experimental study. *Lancet Infect Dis* 2013;**13**:843–851.
3. Erasmus V, Daha TJ, Brug H, et al., Systematic review of studies on compliance with hand hygiene guidelines in hospital care. *Infect Control Hosp Epidemiol* 2010;**31**:283–294.
4. Lee A, Chalfine A, Daikos GL, et al., Hand hygiene practices and adherence determinants in surgical wards across Europe and Israel: a multicenter observational study. *Am J Infect Control* 2011;**39**:517–520.
5. Mertz D, Johnstone J, Krueger P, et al., Adherence to hand hygiene and risk factors for poor adherence in 13 Ontario acute care hospitals. *Am J Infect Control* 2011;**39**:693–696.
6. Costers M, Viseur N, Catry B, et al., Four multifaceted countrywide campaigns to promote hand hygiene in Belgian hospitals between 2005 and 2011: impact on compliance to hand hygiene. *Euro Surveill* 2012;**17**(18):pii=20161.
7. Grayson L, Russo P, Cruickshank M, et al., Outcomes from the first 2 years of the Australian National Hand Hygiene Initiative. *Med J Australia* 2011;**195**:615–619.

8. McLaws M-L, Pantle AC, Fitzpatrick KR, et al., Improvements in hand hygiene across New South Wales public hospitals: clean hands save lives, Part III. *Med J Australia* 2009;**191**:S18–S25.

9. Pittet D, Mourouga P, Perneger TV, et al., Compliance with handwashing in a teaching hospital. *Annals Intern Med* 1999;**130**:126–130.

10. World Health Organization, *WHOs, Hand hygiene moment 1 – global observation survey – summary report 2010.* Geneva: WHO, 2010. Available at www.who.int/gpsc/5may/news/ps_moment1_results_2010_en.pdf. Accessed March 7, 2017

11. Widmer AE, Dangel M, Alcohol-based handrub: evaluation of technique and microbiological efficacy with international infection control professionals. *Infect Control Hosp Epidemiol* 2004;**25**:207–209.

12. Caniza MA, Duenas L, Lopez B, et al., A practical guide to alcohol-based hand hygiene infrastructure in a resource-poor pediatric hospital. *Am J Infect Control* 2009;**37**:851–854.

13. Abela N, Borg MA, Impact on hand hygiene compliance following migration to a new hospital with improved resources and the sequential introduction of World Health Organization recommendations. *Am J Infect Control.* 2012;**40**:737–741.

14. Tromp M, Huis A, de Guchteneire I, et al., The short-term and long-term effectiveness of a multidisciplinary hand hygiene improvement program. *Am J Infect Control* 2012;**40**:732–736.

15. Roberts SA, Sieczkowski C, Campbell T, et al., On behalf of the Auckland District Health Board Hand Hygiene Steering and Working Groups, Implementing and sustaining a hand hygiene culture change programme at Auckland District Health Board. *New Zeal Med J* 2012;**125**:75–85.

16. Marra AR, Moura DF, Tavares Paes A, et al., Measuring rates of hand hygiene adherence in the intensive care setting: a comparative study of direct observation, product usage, and electronic counting devices. *Infect Control Hosp Epidemiol* 2010;**31**:796–801.

17. Scheithauer S, Haefner H, Schwanz T, et al., Compliance with hand hygiene on surgical, medical, and neurologic intensive care units: direct observation versus calculated disinfectant usage. *Am J Infect Control* 2009; **37**:835–841.

18. Mathur P, Jain N, Gupta A, et al., Hand hygiene in developing nations: experience at a busy level-1 trauma center in India. *Am J Infect Control* 2011;**39**:705–706.

Chapter 12

Barriers to Compliance

John M. Boyce,[1] Benedetta Allegranzi,[2] and Didier Pittet[3]

[1] *Hospital Epidemiology and Infection Control, Yale-New Haven Hospital, and Yale University School of Medicine, New Haven, USA*
[2] *Infection Prevention and Control Global Unit, Department of Service Delivery and Safety, World Health Organization, and Faculty of Medicine, University of Geneva, Geneva, Switzerland*
[3] *Infection Control Program and WHO Collaborating Centre on Patient Safety, University of Geneva Hospitals and Faculty of Medicine, Geneva, Switzerland*

KEY MESSAGES

- Providing healthcare personnel with readily accessible alcohol-based handrub dispensing systems and delivering products that result in minimal skin irritation should improve compliance.

- Developing patient empowerment strategies that are acceptable to both healthcare personnel and patients may lead to improved hand hygiene compliance.

- Electronic systems that provide reliable estimates of compliance and that are affordable and acceptable to caregivers should complement observational methods for measuring compliance.

WHAT WE KNOW – THE EVIDENCE

Studies conducted during the last 15 years have identified a number of factors (both observed and perceived) that result in poor hand hygiene compliance.[1] A number of investigators have observed that doctors, technicians, and a variety of other types of healthcare personnel usually have lower rates of hand hygiene compliance than nurses. Working in an intensive care unit, or in other specialty units where there is a high number of opportunities for hand hygiene per hour of patient care, has also been observed as a factor associated with poor hand

Hand Hygiene: A Handbook for Medical Professionals, First Edition.
Edited by Didier Pittet, John M. Boyce and Benedetta Allegranzi.
© 2017 John Wiley & Sons, Inc. Published 2017 by John Wiley & Sons, Inc.

hygiene compliance.[2] Understaffing and overcrowding can also adversely affect compliance rates. In several studies, wearing gowns and/or gloves has been associated with poor hand hygiene adherence.[1]

One of the most important self-reported barriers that prevents caregivers from frequently washing their hands with soap and water is the amount of time required. Voss et al. found that it took intensive care nurses an average of 62 seconds to go to a sink, apply soap to their hands, rinse and dry their hands, and return to patient care.[3] In contrast, the authors found that it only required about 15 seconds to use an alcohol-based handrub located at the patient's bedside. Nurses have often reported that they were too busy and did not have enough time to wash their hands as frequently as recommended. The routine use of alcohol-based handrubs when hands are not visibly soiled is less time-consuming than handwashing, and makes it possible for caregivers to perform hand hygiene many times during a shift. Other barriers to frequent handwashing include the fact that sinks are often inconveniently located and are not always accompanied by adequate supplies of soap and paper towels, which can discourage personnel from washing their hands when indicated. Skin irritation caused by frequent exposure to hand hygiene agents is another self-reported barrier affecting compliance. This was particularly a problem with frequent soap and water handwashing, which is more likely to cause skin irritation and dryness than frequent use of an alcohol-based handrub.[4] Multiple studies among healthcare personnel have shown that well-formulated alcohol-based handrubs cause less skin irritation and dryness than washing hands with soap and water.[5]

Other perceived factors associated with poor compliance rates include nurses' attitudes that patient care needs take priority over hand hygiene, and that hand hygiene interferes with the relationship that they have with patients.[1] Lack of knowledge of guidelines, inadequate education regarding the importance of hand hygiene, and lack of encouragement or rewards for good compliance have also been associated with poor adherence to hand hygiene policies.[1] Some caregivers continue to feel that there is insufficient evidence that improved compliance reduces healthcare-associated infections. Poor compliance rates have also been observed in settings lacking an institutional priority for hand hygiene or an institutional safety climate, and where no administrative actions promote a culture of personal accountability for performing hand hygiene.[6] Developing a culture of personal accountability for hand hygiene is also difficult to achieve in institutions where a hierarchical culture discourages younger or less experienced caregivers from speaking up when more senior members of the healthcare team have failed to clean their hands when indicated.[7]

Another barrier that can adversely affect efforts to improve hand hygiene is a reluctance on the part of some healthcare personnel to encourage patients to ask their caregivers if they have performed hand hygiene.[8] Attitudes voiced by such individuals include an unwillingness to be reminded by patients to perform hand hygiene, a belief that it is not part of the patient's responsibility to remind caregivers to clean their hands, and a feeling of guilt if patients discovered that they had failed to clean their hands when indicated.[8]

Reluctance of patients to remind caregivers to clean their hands is due to factors such as a belief that reminding caregivers is not part the patient's role, to avoid being perceived as disrespectful, being embarrassed, or fearing that their care may suffer.[9,10] In one recent study, some patients felt that it was not their role to remind physicians to clean their hands. Patients would also feel more comfortable discussing hand hygiene with their physician if the physician wore a button or light indicating that he or she had not cleaned their hands.[10] However, the willingness of healthcare personnel to wear personalized electronic devices (badges) that estimate their individual hand hygiene compliance has varied in different studies. Some healthcare workers who have worn electronic badges feel that they are useful reminders to perform hand hygiene and favor their use by all healthcare personnel, while others have refused to wear such badges for fear that the results may affect their annual performance evaluations.

WHAT WE DO NOT KNOW – THE UNCERTAIN

The most effective educational and motivational strategies for targeting physicians with poor hand hygiene compliance have yet to be defined. And despite several studies that have assessed the impact of wearing gloves on hand hygiene compliance rates, no clear answer has emerged. The ideal combination of ingredients (formulation) in handrub agents that results in little or no skin irritation among healthcare personnel who clean their hands many times per day has yet to be identified. The optimal placement (or combination of locations) of alcohol-based handrub dispensers in patient care settings, and the best design of wearable handrub dispensers have not been determined. The impact on hand hygiene compliance of emphasizing personal accountability, and the role of sanctions for lack of accountability for performing hand hygiene in various cultures and healthcare settings have not been well defined. Talbot and colleagues[11] implemented a multimodal initiative based on the WHO hand hygiene promotion strategy, that included leadership buy-in and goal setting, financial incentives linked to performance, and the use of an institution-wide accountability model. This initiative led to a significant and sustained improvement in hand hygiene compliance, and to a reduction of device-associated infections. Further research is needed to explore the role of institutional accountability in HCWs' behavioural change. We also need a better understanding of how to make healthcare personnel (especially physicians) more accepting of having patients remind them if they have not performed hand hygiene, and how to make patients feel more empowered to remind caregivers to clean their hands.[1, 8, 9, 12] Using a cluster-randomized controlled trial design[12] Stewardson and colleagues evaluated the potential effect of patient participation to improve hand hygiene compliance among HCWs. Both patient participation in hand hygiene promotion and enhanced performance feedback were compared to continuous (control) multimodal promotion. The authors observed an improvement in hand hygiene compliance during the intervention in all study arms, which was partly sustained during a 2-year follow-up. The impact of patient participation on HCWs' hand hygiene behaviour was difficult to estimate despite the use of a sophisticated study design; further research is needed to assess the impact of interventions on both HCWs' and patients' behaviour in infection control.

RESEARCH AGENDA

We need to identify more effective means of educating healthcare personnel regarding the need to perform hand hygiene in different clinical scenarios, and to establish methods to promote patient empowerment in a way that is acceptable to both caregivers and patients.[1] Manufacturers need to continue their efforts to formulate hand hygiene agents that are not only highly effective, but minimize skin irritation and dryness as well. Establishing with greater certainty the impact of glove and gown use on hand hygiene compliance is needed, and determining whether hand hygiene prior to donning nonsterile gloves reduces pathogen transmission is desirable.

REFERENCES

1. World Health Organization, *WHO Guidelines for Hand Hygiene in Health Care*. Geneva: WHO, 2009.
2. Pittet D, Mourouga P, Perneger TV, et al., Compliance with handwashing in a teaching hospital. *Ann Intern Med* 1999;**130**:126–130.
3. Voss A, Widmer AF, No time for handwashing!? Handwashing versus alcoholic rub: can we afford 100% compliance? *Infect Control Hosp Epidemiol* 1997;**18**:205–208.
4. Boyce JM, Kelliher S, Vallande N, Skin irritation and dryness associated with two hand hygiene regimens: soap and water handwashing versus hand antisepsis with an alcoholic hand gel. *Infect Control Hosp Epidemiol* 2000;**21**:442–448.
5. Larson E, Girard R, Pessoa-Silva CL, et al., Skin reactions related to hand hygiene and selection of hand hygiene products. *Am J Infect Control* 2006; **34**:627–635.
6. Pittet D, Improving compliance with hand hygiene in hospitals. *Infect Control Hosp Epidemiol* 2000;**21**:381–386.
7. Samuel R, Shuen A, Dendle C, et al., Hierarchy and hand hygiene: would medical students speak up to prevent hospital-acquired infection? *Infect Control Hosp Epidemiol* 2012;**33**:861–863.
8. Longtin Y, Farquet N, Gayet-Ageron A, et al., Caregivers' perceptions of patients as reminders to improve hand hygiene. *Arch Intern Med* 2012;**172**:1516–1517.
9. Longtin Y, Sax H, Allegranzi B, et al., Patients' beliefs and perceptions of their participation to increase healthcare worker compliance with hand hygiene. *Infect Control Hosp Epidemiol* 2009;**30**:830–839.
10. Michaelsen K, Sanders JL, Zimmer SM, et al., Overcoming patient barriers to discussing physician hand hygiene: do patients prefer electronic reminders to other methods? *Infect Control Hosp Epidemiol* 2013;**34**:929–934.
11. Talbot T, Johnson J, Fergus C, et al., Sustained improvement in hand hygiene adherence: utilizing shared accountability and financial incentives. *Infect Control Hosp Epidemiol* 2013;**34**:1129–1136.
12. Stewardson A, Sax H, Gayet-Ageron A, et al., Enhanced performance feedback and patient participation to improve hand hygiene compliance of health-care workers in the setting of established multimodal promotion: a single-centre, cluster-randomised controlled trial. *Lancet Infect Dis* 2016;**16**:1345–1355.

Chapter 13

Physicians and Hand Hygiene

Benedetta Allegranzi,[1] Andrew J. Stewardson,[2, 3] and Didier Pittet[3]

[1] *Infection Prevention and Control Global Unit, Department of Service Delivery and Safety, World Health Organization, and Faculty of Medicine, University of Geneva, Geneva, Switzerland*
[2] *Infectious Diseases Department, Austin Health and Hand Hygiene Australia, Melbourne, Australia*
[3] *Infection Control Program and WHO Collaborating Centre on Patient Safety, University of Geneva Hospitals and Faculty of Medicine, Geneva, Switzerland*

KEY MESSAGES

- Hand hygiene compliance is usually lower among physicians compared to other professionals, especially nurses. However, it was found to be higher in some studies conducted in developing countries.
- When exposed to hand hygiene promotion, physicians are usually more resistant to improvement than other professional categories.
- Several interventions and strategies have been shown to be effective to improve physicians' behavior but more targeted approaches are needed.

Healthcare worker (HCW) status has been repeatedly found to be a predictive factor for hand hygiene compliance. Most studies show that physicians have a worse performance than other professional categories, particularly nurses. As physicians often serve as role models for trainees, students, and other professionals, their poor performance may have an adverse effect on other HCWs' behavior. Therefore, it is important to understand physicians' behavior and perceptions towards hand hygiene and to identify successful strategies to induce behavioral change and improvement in this professional category.

Hand Hygiene: A Handbook for Medical Professionals, First Edition.
Edited by Didier Pittet, John M. Boyce and Benedetta Allegranzi.
© 2017 John Wiley & Sons, Inc. Published 2017 by John Wiley & Sons, Inc.

WHAT WE KNOW – THE EVIDENCE

A comprehensive review of the literature on hand hygiene in healthcare reported that the unadjusted average compliance rate among physicians was 32% versus 48% among nurses.[1] Repeated surveys conducted over several years in the context of national campaigns in Belgium and Australia showed that physicians' initial compliance, as well as their relative improvement, was significantly lower than that of nurses and other categories (see Chapter 11). By contrast, several studies conducted in developing countries reported that physicians had higher compliance than nurses (see Chapter 43). Observational studies also showed that physicians as a professional category represent an independent risk factor for missed hand hygiene actions.[2,3] Physicians have higher compliance after contact with patients' skin or body fluids than with other opportunities,[1,2] and they would appear to prioritize self-protection over patient safety. This phenomenon is common to all professional categories, but more pronounced among physicians (Table 13.1). Physician compliance with best practices may significantly vary between medical specialties. One study demonstrated that compliance is higher in neonatal and pediatric units,[4] while another showed that working in surgery, anesthesiology, and emergency and critical care medicine predicted missed hand hygiene actions among physicians (Table 13.1).[5] Defective behavior was observed also among medical students, including low levels of knowledge regarding hand hygiene indications, thus suggesting that hand hygiene should be given greater emphasis in their curriculum (Table 13.1).

Specific beliefs and perceptions have been found to influence physicians' lack of adherence to best practices. While other HCWs perceive physicians as role models, physicians frequently do not see themselves as such. In addition, physicians seem to be skeptical or less convinced than other professional categories about the effectiveness of hand hygiene to reduce healthcare-associated infection or to limit the spread of antimicrobial resistance and improve patient safety (Table 13.1).[6,7] Some researchers have suggested that physician resistance to hand hygiene promotion interventions may result from different personality traits or motivational frameworks compared with other categories.[8]

Physicians' poor compliance with best practices not only has direct consequences in terms of transmission and infection risk, but also influences junior colleagues' and other HCWs' behavior. A qualitative study reported that medical students explicitly mentioned that they follow the behavior of their superiors, which is often defective.[7] Furthermore, the behavior of attending physicians strongly influenced hand hygiene performance among team members following them in the patient encounter.[9] Finally, physicians' compliance was associated with awareness of being observed, the belief of being a role model for other colleagues, a positive attitude toward hand hygiene after patient contact, and easy access to handrub solution (Table 13.1).[5] High workload, activities associated with a high risk for cross-transmission, and working in some specific medical specialties were risk factors for lack of compliance (Table 13.1).[5]

Table 13.1   Main Determinants of Physicians' Hand Hygiene Behavior and Possible Specific Elements for Effective Targeted Improvement

	References
Determinants of Low Compliance	
Medical specialty (surgery, anesthesiology, emergency medicine, critical care)	5
High workload	2, 5
Activities associated with high cross-transmission risk	5
Low level of knowledge as medical students	11, 15
Lack of awareness about being role models	7
Skepticism about the effectiveness of hand hygiene to reduce healthcare-associated infection and antimicrobial resistance spread	6, 7, 14
Determinants of good compliance	
Medical specialty (neonatology and pediatrics)	4
Awareness of being observed	5
Belief of being role models	5
Self-protection prioritization (higher compliance with after contact with patients' skin or body fluids)	1, 2, 5, 10
Easy access to handrub solutions	5
Elements for promotion	
Education and practical training	2, 16
Focus groups	2, 12
Local data feedback and in-service presentations	13, 16
Medical champions	2, 16
Access to adequate hand hygiene supplies	16

Physicians have not only been found to be generally less compliant than other professional categories, they also usually show less improvement than other professions following hand hygiene promotion.[2] However, several interventions were shown to be effective to improve physicians' behavior. Better education, especially practical training, from the early stages of their curriculum is considered essential to improve practices.[2] In some settings where social pressure is high, separate training sessions for physicians only can be more effective. Focus groups were shown to be particularly useful to understand physicians' beliefs and attitudes towards hand hygiene and to tailor key educational messages to be promoted. Individual meetings with physicians to discuss observed hand hygiene compliance data and deliver in-service presentations were also very effective (Table 13.1). The identification and engagement of champions among physicians can facilitate behavioral change among their peers and others (Table 13.1).[2] An intervention targeting physicians based on improvement science methods was particularly effective and led to a significant compliance increase.

This intervention included an educational module, hand hygiene performance monitoring, daily display of compliance rates in the resident conference room, real-time identification and mitigation of failures by a hand hygiene champion, and access to adequate supplies (Table 13.1). Some studies assessing patients' intention to ask HCWs to perform hand hygiene showed that patients are more willing to ask nurses than physicians (see Chapter 30). Finally, the World Health Organization multimodal hand hygiene improvement strategy (see also Chapter 33) proved to be highly effective to increase compliance in all professional categories across a range of settings worldwide, although relative improvement was lower among physicians than among nurses in most sites.[2]

WHAT WE DO NOT KNOW – THE UNCERTAIN

Although several investigations and models have identified determinants of HCWs' hand hygiene behavior, further research is needed to understand physicians' attitudes and practices, especially as they are generally less compliant than other professionals. In addition, cultural, social, and religious factors may determine different hand hygiene behaviors in HCWs, particularly among physicians given their social role and position, and studies exploring this aspect should be encouraged. The reasons why physicians' compliance was observed to be higher than nurses in some studies from developing countries need to be better understood. Higher levels of knowledge and awareness of being role models may be factors, but confirmation through well-designed studies is needed.

Among the many strategies proposed to achieve hand hygiene improvement, only a few have specifically targeted physicians. Many healthcare facilities failed to observe a significant behavioral change initially among physicians, and in most cases improvement was achieved only later by implementing additional targeted actions. More evidence is needed to identify successful approaches targeting physicians and effectively integrate them in improvement strategies. In this context, it would be important to know whether physicians would be more responsive to improvement strategies focused on specific opportunities or procedures typically performed by medical staff.

RESEARCH AGENDA

Further research is necessary to understand more thoroughly hand hygiene behavior among physicians and the best strategies to improve performance.

Key research questions are:

- What are the specific determinants of physicians' hand hygiene behavior, and how do these vary in different cultures and social contexts?
- What are the best approaches to achieve sustained improvement of physicians' hand hygiene practices? In particular, how can physicians be

made more aware of their role as models for colleagues, students, and other professionals, and use this as a leverage for compliance improvement?

REFERENCES

1. Erasmus V, Daha TJ, Brug H, et al., Systematic review of studies on compliance with hand hygiene guidelines in hospital care. *Infect Control Hosp Epidemiol* 2010;**31**:283–294.
2. World Health Organization, *WHO Guidelines on Hand Hygiene in Health Care*. Geneva: WHO, 2009. Available at whqlibdoc.who.int/publications/2009/9789241597906_eng.pdf. Accessed March 7, 2017.
3. Alsubaie S, Maither AB, Alalmaei W, et al., Determinants of hand hygiene noncompliance in intensive care units. *Am J Infect Control* 2013;**41**:131–135.
4. Cantrell D, Shamriz O, Cohen MJ, et al., Hand hygiene compliance by physicians: Marked heterogeneity due to local culture? *Am J Infect Control* 2009;**37**:301–305.
5. Pittet D, Simon A, Hugonnet S, et al., Hand hygiene among physicians: performance, beliefs, and perceptions. *Ann Intern Med* 2004;**141**:1–8.
6. Tennant I, Nicholson A, Gordon-Strachan GM, et al., A survey of physicians' knowledge and attitudes regarding antimicrobial resistance and antibiotic prescribing practices at the University Hospital of the West Indies. *West Indian Med J* 2010;**59**:165–170.
7. Erasmus V, Brouwer W, van Beeck EF, et al., A qualitative exploration of reasons for poor hand hygiene among hospital workers: lack of positive role models and of convincing evidence that hand hygiene prevents cross-infection. *Infect Control Hosp Epidemiol* 2009;**30**:415–419.
8. Sladek RM, Bond MJ, Phillips PA, Why don't doctors wash their hands? A correlational study of thinking styles and hand hygiene. *Am J Infect Control* 2008;**36**:399–406.
9. Haessler S, Bhagavan A, Kleppel R, et al., Getting doctors to clean their hands: lead the followers. *BMJ Qual Saf* 2012;**21**:499–502.
10. Borg MA, Benbachir M, Cookson BD, et al., Self-protection as a driver for hand hygiene among healthcare workers. *Infect Control Hosp Epidemiol* 2009;**30**:578–580.
11. Graf K, Chaberny IF, Vonberg RP, Beliefs about hand hygiene: a survey in medical students in their first clinical year. *Am J Infect Control* 2011;**39**:885–888.
12. Jang JH, Focus group study of hand hygiene practice among healthcare workers in a teaching hospital in Toronto, Canada. *Infect Control Hosp Epidemiol* 2010;**31**:144–150.
13. Salemi C, Canola MT, Eck EK, Hand washing and physicians: how to get them together. *Infect Control Hosp Epidemiol* 2002;**23**:32–35.
14. Tai JW, Mok ESB, Ching PTY, et al., Nurses and physicians' perceptions of the importance and impact of healthcare-associated infections and hand hygiene: a multi-center exploratory study in Hong Kong. *Infection* 2009;**37**:320–333.
15. Van de Mortel TF, Apostolopoulou E, Petrikkos G, A comparison of the hand hygiene knowledge, beliefs, and practices of Greek nursing and medical students. *Am J Infect Control* 2010;**38**:75–77.
16. White CM, Statile AM, Conway PH, et al., Utilizing improvement science methods to improve physician compliance with proper hand hygiene. *Pediatrics* 2012;**129**:e1042–e1050.

Chapter 14

Surgical Hand Preparation

Andreas F. Widmer[1] and Joseph Solomkin[2]

[1] *Division of Infectious Diseases and Hospital Epidemiology, University Hospital of Basel, Basel, Switzerland*

[2] *University of Cincinnati College of Medicine, Cincinnati, USA*

KEY MESSAGES

- Surgical hand preparation is mandatory prior to surgery – either with antimicrobial soap or alcohol-based formulations. A 3-minute application is common, while some products allow shortening application to 1.5 minutes while still meeting European Standards (EN 12791).

- Alcohol-based handrubs work faster than medicated soap and water, are less irritating to skin, and avoid recontamination by contaminated water while rinsing hands. The addition of an agent that prevents regrowth of bacteria (such as chlorhexidine) is recommended. Chlorhexidine soap is an alternative for surgical hand preparation since it meets EN 12791.

- Alcohol-based handrubs should be applied using techniques recommended by the World Health Organization or national standards.

WHAT WE KNOW – THE EVIDENCE

Surgical hand preparation is the standard of care before any surgical procedure; either by surgical hand scrub with an antimicrobial soap or surgical handrub with an alcohol-based formulation. Joseph Lister was among the first to demonstrate the effect of skin antisepsis on the reduction of surgical site infections (SSI). At

Hand Hygiene: A Handbook for Medical Professionals, First Edition.
Edited by Didier Pittet, John M. Boyce and Benedetta Allegranzi.
© 2017 John Wiley & Sons, Inc. Published 2017 by John Wiley & Sons, Inc.

that time, surgical gloves were not yet available, thus making appropriate skin preparation of the surgical site and surgical hand preparation by the surgeon even more imperative. Surgical hand preparation with an antimicrobial soap and warm water was most common in the last century, frequently with the use of a brush. Today, 3-minute (to even 5 min) protocols are common and still suggested for surgical hand preparation when the World Health Organization (WHO) alcohol-based handrubs (ABHRs) formulations are recommended for use.[1] Despite this, a comparison of different countries showed almost as many protocols as listed countries.

The introduction of sterile and impermeable gloves does not render surgical hand preparation unnecessary. Pinholes in the gloves increase the risk for SSI by over fourfold if patients do not require antimicrobial prophylaxis, or routine surgical antimicrobial prophylaxis is not administered in a timely fashion.[4] In addition, pinholes occur in 4% of procedures even with double-gloving. Therefore, surgical hand preparation must be performed by all members of the surgical team prior to donning sterile gowns and gloves. Long fingernails or artificial fingernails are risk factors for pinholes in surgical gloves and might constitute microbial reservoirs, and thus are prohibited.

Surgical Handwash

Chlorhexidine or povidone-iodine-containing soaps result in similar initial reductions of bacterial counts (70% to 80%). Rapid regrowth occurs after the application of povidone-iodine, but not after the use of chlorhexidine. Povidone-iodine is still commonly used for surgical hand preparation, despite both in vitro and in vivo studies demonstrating that it is less efficacious in reducing bacterial counts on hands than chlorhexidine, induces more allergic reactions, and has a very limited residual effect. Skin irritation and dermatitis are more likely to be observed after surgical hand scrub with chlorhexidine than after surgical hand antisepsis with an ABHR formulation. Importantly, the epidermal water content decreases significantly during the handwash phase with soap and water compared to the ABHR phase.[5] Surgical handwash requires at least drinking water quality for rinsing and approximately 20 liters of water per HCW, per surgical procedure, which becomes an important problem in low-resource settings. Even drinking quality water commonly contains nonfermenting bacteria, such as *Pseudomonas aeruginosa*. Three- to five-minute applications are recommended by the manufacturers of antimicrobial soaps.

Alcohol-Based Handrubs

ABHRs are superior to other currently available surgical hand scrubs in both in vitro and in vivo studies.[6] Formulations containing 60–95% alcohol alone, or 50–95% when combined with small amounts of a quaternary ammonium compound, hexachlorophene, or chlorhexidine gluconate, lower bacterial counts on the skin immediately postscrub more effectively than other agents. The combination of alcohol and chlorhexidine fulfills most requirements for rapid killing and prolonged residual effect. While prior handwash may eliminate any risk of contamination with bacterial spores, experimental and epidemiological data fail to demonstrate an additional effect of washing hands before applying handrub in the overall reduction of the resident skin flora. Obviously, when hands and/or fingernails are visibly soiled, hand cleansing and/or nail shortening is mandatory.

Technique for the Application of Surgical Hand Preparation Using Alcohol-Based Handrubs

The application technique has not been standardized worldwide. The WHO approach for surgical hand preparation involves the same six basic steps as for hygienic hand antisepsis, but requires an additional step for rubbing the forearms (Figure 14.1).[7] During the whole procedure, the hands should remain wet from the ABHR, thus requiring approximately 9 to 15 mL, depending on the size of the hands. The procedure commonly requires 3 minutes, but a recent study with healthy volunteers under in vivo experimental conditions showed that even a 90-second rub was equivalent to a 3-minute rub with a product containing a mixture of iso- and n-propanol and mecetronium ethylsulfate. These results were corroborated in a similar study performed under clinical conditions with 32 surgeons.[8] However, further studies need to be conducted with other ABHRs to compare the usual 2–3 minute hand preparation with shorter times before such a recommendation can be generalized to other formulations.

Compliance with this recommendation remains a continuing problem. A recent study reported a mean handwashing time of 69.1 seconds, significantly lower than recommended by the manufacturer. Small differences in effectiveness between products become irrelevant if the surgical team does not follow the recommended application time.[9]

ABHRs are well tolerated,[10] better than surgical scrub with medicated soap (see also Chapter 15). Storing flammable fluids is of concern (see also Chapter 16), but fires are rarely, if ever, related to ABHRs.[10]

WHAT WE DO NOT KNOW – THE UNCERTAIN

The minimum antimicrobial activity of a formulation for surgical hand preparation is unknown. Both the European (EN 12791) and US standards (US Food and Drug Administration: Tentative final monograph for healthcare antiseptic drug products: Proposed rule. Federal Register. 1994;59:31441–31452) have been developed to provide a standard, primarily for clearing a product for the market. This uncertainty – not surprisingly – has led to different requirements from continent to

The handrubbing technique for surgical hand preparation must be performed on perfectly clean, dry hands. On arrival in the operating theatre and after having donned theatre clothing (cap/hat/bonnet and mask), hands must be washed with soap and water.
After the operation when removing gloves, hands must be rubbed with an alcohol-based formulation or washed with soap and water if any residual talc or biological fluids are present (e.g.the glove is punctured).

Surgical procedures may be carried out one after the other without the need for handwashing, provided that the handrubbing technique for surgical hand preparation is followed (images 1 to 17).

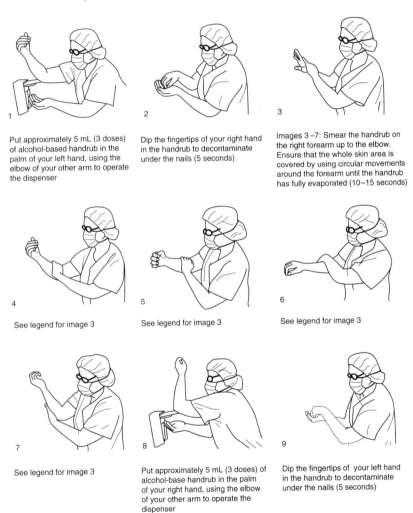

1 Put approximately 5 mL (3 doses) of alcohol-based handrub in the palm of your left hand, using the elbow of your other arm to operate the dispenser

2 Dip the fingertips of your right hand in the handrub to decontaminate under the nails (5 seconds)

3 Images 3 –7: Smear the handrub on the right forearm up to the elbow. Ensure that the whole skin area is covered by using circular movements around the forearm until the handrub has fully evaporated (10–15 seconds)

4 See legend for image 3

5 See legend for image 3

6 See legend for image 3

7 See legend for image 3

8 Put approximately 5 mL (3 doses) of alcohol-base handrub in the palm of your right hand, using the elbow of your other arm to operate the dispenser

9 Dip the fingertips of your left hand in the handrub to decontaminate under the nails (5 seconds)

Figure 14.1   Surgical hand preparation with an alcohol-based handrub. The first two steps of the surgical handrub ensure complete moistening of the forearms, starting from the elbow (see 1 to 10), then the forearms, and followed by a handrub for 1.5–3 minutes. *Source*: Reproduced with permission from the World Health Organization.

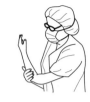

10

Smear the handrub on the left
forearm up to the elbow. Ensure
that the whole skin area is covered
by using circular movements around
the forearm until the handrub has
fully evaporated (10–15 seconds)

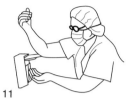

11

Put approximately 5 mL (3 doses) of
alcohol-based handrub in the palm of
your left hand, using the elbow of your
other arm to operate the distributor.
Rub both hands in the same time up to
the wrists, and ensure that all the steps
represented in images 12–17 are followed
(20–30 seconds)

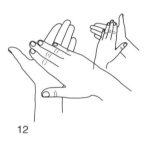

12

Cover the whole surface of the
hands up to the wrist with alcohol-
based handrub, rubbing palm
against palm with a rotating
movement

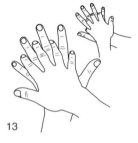

13

Rub the back of the left hand,
including the wrist, moving the
right palm back and forth, and
vice-versa

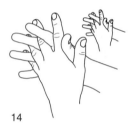

14

Rub palm against palm back and
forth with fingers interlinked

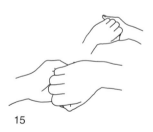

15

Rub the back of the fingers by
holding them in the palm of the
other hand with a sideways back
and forth movement

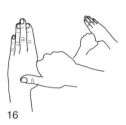

16

Rub the thumb of the left hand by
rotating it in the clasped palm of
the right hand and vice versa

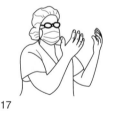

17

When the hands are dry, sterile
surgical clothing and gloves can
be donned

Repeat the above-illustrated sequence (average duration, 60 s) according to the number of times
corresponding to the total duration recommended by the manufacturer for surgical hand preparation
with an alcohol-based handrub.

Figure 14.1   (*Continued*)

continent, such as the ones from Europe and the United States listed above. The pathogenesis of SSI is multifactorial, and the impact of insufficiently cleaned hands as a predictive variable to prevent infections remains unclear.

RESEARCH AGENDA

The minimum antimicrobial activity for decreasing bacterial load on surgeons' hands has not yet been determined; such an estimate is needed to support or adapt current requirements by regulatory agencies.

The issue of spores on surgeons' hands is an unresolved issue if alcohol-based formulations are used. *Clostridium* spp, in particular *C. perfringens* and *C. difficile,* may raise concerns since spores are not destroyed by alcohol. However, postoperative clostridial wound sepsis is very rare.

There are few data on the interaction between emollients and hand hygiene agents, but healthy skin is important, since several outbreaks have been traced to colonization of skin injuries by the hands of surgeons and operating room nurses. In randomized studies, surgical hand preparation using ABHR has been shown to be at least as effective as antimicrobial/nonantimicrobial soap both in high-[11] and low-resource settings.[12] In the latter, the use of ABHR resolved the issue of poor quality/absence of water. Finally, replacing surgical hand preparation with an antiseptic handscrub with an alcohol-based handrub, is associated with a very significant reduction in the use of water estimated to an average of 18.5 liters per surgical procedure per individual in a recent study (i.e an average of 55.5 liters per procedure when three HCWs are involved).[13] Additional randomized clinical trials are needed to evaluate the cost-effectiveness of different strategies worldwide.[14,15,16]

The optimal hand hygiene technique has not been well established, but proper hand hygiene technique leads to improved antimicrobial killing. However, the issue has not been addressed for surgical hand preparation. Surgical hand preparation is part of the series of elements that participate to prevent surgical site infection, as recently summarized in the WHO Global Guidelines on the Prevention of Surgical Site Infection.[17,18,19]

REFERENCES

1. Suchomel M, Kundi M, Allegranzi B, et al., Testing of the World Health Organization-recommended formulations for surgical hand preparation and proposals for increased efficacy. *J Hosp Infect* 2011;**79**:115–118.
2. Widmer AF, Rotter M, Voss A, et al., Surgical hand preparation: state-of-the-art. *J Hosp Infect* 2010;**74**:112–122.
3. Widmer AF, Surgical hand hygiene: scrub or rub? *J Hosp Infect* 2013;**83**(Suppl. 1): S35–S39.

4. Misteli H, Weber WP, Reck S, et al., Surgical glove perforation and the risk of surgical site infection. *Arch Surg* 2009;**144**:553–558; discussion 558.

5. Boyce JM, Kelliher S, Vallande N, Skin irritation and dryness associated with two hand-hygiene regimens: soap-and-water handwashing versus hand antisepsis with an alcoholic hand gel. *Infect Control Hosp Epidemiol* 2000;**21**:442–448.

6. Rotter M, Sattar S, Dharan S, et al., Methods to evaluate the microbicidal activities of hand-rub and hand-wash agents. *J Hosp Infect* 2009;**73**(3):191–199.

7. Pittet D, Allegranzi B, Boyce J, et al., The World Health Organization Guidelines on Hand Hygiene in Health Care and their consensus recommendations. *Infect Control Hosp Epidemiol* 2009;**30**:611–622.

8. Weber WP, Reck S, Neff U, et al., Surgical hand antisepsis with alcohol-based handrub: comparison of effectiveness after 1.5 and 3 minutes of application. *Infect Control Hosp Epidemiol* 2009;**30**:420–426.

9. Umit UM, Sina M, Ferhat Y, et al., Surgeon behavior and knowledge on hand scrub and skin antisepsis in the operating room. *J Surg Educ* 2014;**71**:241–245.

10. Kramer A, Kampf G, Handrub-associated fire incidents during 25,038 hospital-years in Germany. *Infect Control Hosp Epidemiol* 2007;**28**:745–746.

11. Parienti JJ, Thibon P, Heller R, et al., Hand-rubbing with an aqueous alcoholic solution vs traditional surgical hand-scrubbing and 30-day surgical site infection rates: a randomized equivalence study. *JAMA* 2002;**288**:722–727.

12. Nthumba PM, Stepita-Poenaru E, Poenaru D, et al., Cluster randomized, crossover trial of the efficacy of plain soap and water versus alcohol-based rub for surgical hand preparation in a rural hospital in Kenya. *Br J Surg* 2010;**97**:1621–1628.

13. Graf ME, Machado A, Lopes Mensor L, et al., Surgical hand antisepsis with alcohol-based preparations: cost-effectiveness, compliance of professionals and ecological benefits in the Brazilian healthcare senario [Portuguese original]. *J Bras Econ Saúde* 2014;**6**:71–80.

14. Tschudin-Sutter S, Sepulcri D, Dangel M, et al., Compliance with the World Health Organization hand hygiene technique: a prospective observational study. *Infect Control Hosp Epidemiol* 2015;**36**:482–483.

15. Larson E, Aiello AE, Heilman JM, et al., Comparison of different regimens for surgical hand preparation. *AORN Journal* 2001;**73**:412–432.

16. Weight CJ, Lee MC, Palmer JS, Avagard hand antisepsis vs. traditional scrub in 3600 pediatric urologic procedures. *Urology* 2010;**76**:15–17.

17. World Health Organization, *Global guidelines on the prevention of surgical site infection*. Geneva: WHO, 2016. www.who.int/gpsc/ssi-prevention-guidelines/en/. Accessed March 7, 2017.

18. Allegranzi B, Bischoff P, de Jonge S, et al., New WHO recommendations on preoperative measures for surgical site infection prevention: an evidence-based global perspective. *Lancet Infect Dis* 2016;**16**:276–287.

19. Allegranzi B, Zayed B, Bischoff P, et al., New WHO recommendations on intraoperative and postoperative measures for surgical site infection prevention: an evidence-based global perspective. *Lancet Infect Dis* 2016;**16**:288–303.

Chapter 15

Skin Reaction to Hand Hygiene

Elaine Larson
Columbia University School of Nursing, New York, USA

KEY MESSAGES

- Irritant contact dermatitis and skin damage are prevalent among healthcare professionals, difficult to treat, and require consistent, long-term preventive care.
- The method used for hand hygiene is as important as the product.
- A regimen to minimize irritant contact dermatitis includes careful selection of products, use of alcohol-based handrubs whenever possible, and use of appropriate emollients or humectants.

WHAT WE KNOW – THE EVIDENCE

A concise summary of skin reactions associated with hand hygiene has been published in Chapter 14 of the *WHO Guidelines on Hand Hygiene in Health Care*. The reader is referred to that chapter and to a review article on skin care[1,2] for background; this chapter updates information published since 2009. Although both irritant contact dermatitis and allergic contact dermatitis can occur, this chapter focuses on irritant contact dermatitis because it is much more prevalent and potentially preventable. Allergic contact dermatitis can be associated with a variety of products (lotions, preservatives, fragrances, active ingredients), but is relatively

Hand Hygiene: A Handbook for Medical Professionals, First Edition.
Edited by Didier Pittet, John M. Boyce and Benedetta Allegranzi.
© 2017 John Wiley & Sons, Inc. Published 2017 by John Wiley & Sons, Inc.

uncommon and should be diagnosed and treated under the supervision of a dermatologist.

Hand hygiene has profound effects on the skin because products used for cleaning and drying hands cause reduced skin lipids, corneocytes, and proteins as well as increased transepidermal water loss in the *stratum corneum* (see also Chapter 3). Hence, healthcare professionals, because of their need for frequent hand hygiene, have higher rates of irritant contact dermatitis than the general population. Hand hygiene results in long-term, chronic structural changes in the *stratum corneum*, and there is insufficient time for recovery between work periods.[3] In fact, a majority of healthcare professionals report current or past skin problems.

A number of environmental factors over which one has no control can increase the risk of skin irritation: cold and excessively dry weather, increasing age, lighter skin color. It is therefore important to identify modifiable practices that can minimize skin irritation, including the product used and the method of hand hygiene. Choice of product clearly has an impact on risk of dermatitis. Although healthcare professionals often perceive that rubbing hands with an alcohol-based handrub (ABHR) is more damaging to hands than washing, numerous studies over the past several decades have confirmed that such products are considerably less damaging than detergent-based soaps and antiseptics. This misconception may lead to lower rates of adherence and, ironically, higher rates of dermatitis because staff continue with traditional handwashing.[4] While alcohol, as with any hand hygiene product, can cause skin dryness, this effect can be greatly minimized by using an ABHR containing emollients and humectants. The increased skin damage associated with other handwashing products is likely a combination of the effects of the product, the longer time required for washing, exposure to hot water, and the friction needed to dry hands with paper towels.

There are a number of strategies that healthcare professionals can use to reduce the risk of irritant contact dermatitis, summarized in Table 15.1.[1] First there

Table 15.1 Methods to Minimize Skin Irritation Associated with Hand Hygiene

- Use alcohol-based handrubs with emollients rather than detergent-based soaps
- Select products with the least potential for irritation
- Avoid unnecessary, prolonged glove use
- For handwashing
  - Avoid excessively hot water
  - Dry hands completely after washing and prior to gloving
  - Avoid rough paper towels; pat rather than rub dry
  - Do not wash hands after applying alcohol

- Develop a regular routine of applying emollients/lotions/humectants
  - Do not use soaps, detergents, or aqueous creams or lotions containing sodium lauryl sulfate

are specific practices with regard to hand hygiene that can help to minimize skin damage. When possible, ABHRs are recommended over detergent-based soaps. When soap and water are used, excessively hot water and rubbing with harsh paper towels should be avoided. In particular, soaps, detergents, or lotions that contain sodium lauryl sulfate have detrimental effects on normal skin lipids and should not be used in settings where frequent hand hygiene is needed.[5] Frequent gloving, particularly when hands are not completely dry, increases skin irritation and should also be avoided when possible.

Because of past problems with contamination of hand lotions or incompatibility of petroleum-based moisturizers with latex gloves and anionic (negatively charged) moisturizers with chlorhexidine gluconate, healthcare professionals may be wary of using emollients and moisturizers. A safe regimen to keep the *stratum corneum* intact (see Chapter 3), however, is essential to skin health. Emollients may be an important component to maintain the barrier properties of the hands to reduce cracking, inflammation, pruritus, and potential microbial colonization.[6] In fact, two consensus statements regarding management of dry skin and hand eczema both recommend a skin education program along with use of emollients and humectants as the primary methods to avoid and treat skin irritation.[5,7]

Emollients help to reduce water loss and drying of the hands by forming a protective layer on the skin. There is a variety of emollient formulations, some of which may contain other lipids, humectants (hold water in the *stratum corneum*), or anti-itching products. Because these products vary considerably in formulation and individuals respond differently to products, healthcare professionals must carefully select a product that is compatible with work requirements and most effective for them. Most importantly, moisturizers should be used consistently and frequently because irritant contact dermatitis is generally a chronic problem requiring constant monitoring and attention. Because many products are subject to potential microbial contamination, however, they should not be shared or be used from large open containers.

WHAT WE DO NOT KNOW – THE UNCERTAIN

Despite the important role of emollients and lotions in the treatment of skin problems, there is still a paucity of evidence comparing effectiveness of various products. The interaction of various components of hand hygiene practices (sanitizer or soap, emollient or moisturizer, drying and gloving), environmental conditions, skin type, and relative risk of irritant contact dermatitis needs further study.

A Cochrane systematic review to assess clinical trials of the effectiveness of barrier creams, moisturizers, gloves, complex educational interventions, and other strategies for the prevention of occupational hand dermatitis was published in 2010.[8] In four randomized clinical trials, which included almost 900 individuals from several occupations (print and dye workers, hairdressers, metal and kitchen workers, but not healthcare professionals), results were overall positive, but not statistically significant. The authors concluded that larger, well-designed studies are needed across a number of occupations.

RESEARCH AGENDA

Collaborative studies between dermatology and other cosmetic scientists with infection prevention and clinical staff to conduct realistic field trials of the impact of hand hygiene regimens on skin health are needed.

REFERENCES

1. Bissett, L, Skin care: an essential component of hand hygiene and infection control. *Br J Nurs* 2007;**16**:976–981.
2. World Health Organization, *WHO Guidelines for Hand Hygiene in Health Care*. Geneva: WHO, 2009. Available at whqlibdoc.who.int/publications/2009/9789241597906_eng.pdf. Accessed March 7, 2017.
3. Visscher MO, Said D, Wickett R, Stratum corneum cytokines, structural proteins, and transepidermal water loss: effect of hand hygiene. *Skin Res Technol* 2010;**16**:229–236.
4. Stutz N, Becker D, Jappe U, et al., Nurses' perceptions of the benefits and adverse effects of hand disinfection: alcohol-based hand rubs vs. hygienic handwashing: a multicentre questionnaire study with additional patch testing by the German Contact Dermatitis Research Group. *Br J Dermatol* 2009;**160**:565–572.
5. Moncrieff G, Cork M, Lawton S, et al., Use of emollients in dry-skin conditions: consensus statement. *Clin Exp Dermatol* 2013;**38**:231–238.
6. Voegeli D, The vital role of emollients in the treatment of eczema. *Br J Nurs* 2011;**20**:74–80.
7. English J, Aldridge R, Gawkrodger DJ, et al., Consensus statement on the management of chronic hand eczema. *Clin Exp Dermatol* 2009;**34**:761–769.
8. Bauer A, Schmitt J, Bennett C, et al., Interventions for preventing occupational irritant hand dermatitis. *Cochrane Database Syst Rev* 2010;**16**:CD004414.

Chapter 16

Alcohol-Based Handrub Safety

John M. Boyce[1] and M. Lindsay Grayson[2]

[1] *Hospital Epidemiology and Infection Control, Yale-New Haven Hospital, and Yale University School of Medicine, New Haven, USA*

[2] *Infectious Diseases Department, Austin Hospital and University of Melbourne, Melbourne, Australia*

KEY MESSAGES

- The risk of fires related to alcohol-based handrubs (ABHRs) is extremely low – if not negligible – when these products are used and stored properly.
- When performing hand hygiene with ABHRs, it is important to rub hands together until all the alcohol has evaporated and hands feel dry.
- The minimal absorption of alcohol through the skin or by inhalation of vapors that occurs with normal use of ABHRs does not pose a health risk to healthcare workers.

WHAT WE KNOW – THE EVIDENCE

Alcohol-based handrubs (ABHRs) are flammable, with flash points of products ranging from 17.5°C to 24.5°C.[1] The flash point of any given product depends on the concentration and type(s) of alcohol present. Despite this, the risk of fires related to the use or storage of ABHRs is very low. A questionnaire completed by infection preventionists in Switzerland did not reveal any ABHR-related fires over a period of five years.[2] Of 766 hospitals in the United States that had accrued 1430 hospital-years of use of ABHRs, none reported a fire related to a handrub

Hand Hygiene: A Handbook for Medical Professionals, First Edition.
Edited by Didier Pittet, John M. Boyce and Benedetta Allegranzi.
© 2017 John Wiley & Sons, Inc. Published 2017 by John Wiley & Sons, Inc.

dispenser.[3] A large German study reported that 788 hospitals had used a combined total of 35 million liters of ABHRs during 25,038 hospital-years.[4] Overall, seven nonsevere fire incidents were reported by 0.9% of hospitals, for a rate of 0.00028 incidents per hospital year. Two nurses and a construction worker lit cigarettes before handrub had fully evaporated and one nurse lit a candle before alcohol had evaporated. One incident was related to a suicide attempt by a psychiatry patient, and two cases were related to vandalism.[4] None of the fire incidents were attributed to storage of products or to fire caused by static electricity. One report of a healthcare worker (HCW) sustaining burns on her hands occurred following a complex sequence of events in which she removed a polyester over-gown immediately after applying ABHR to her hands. In removing the gown, she created significant static electricity, such that when she then pulled on a metal door, there was an audible discharge of static electricity and a spontaneous flame on her palm, causing erythema.[5] This rare event and several of those reported by Kramer et al., emphasize the need to rub hands together until all the alcohol has evaporated.[1,4]

Shortly after use of ABHRs became widespread in the United States, some fire safety personnel became concerned that the flammability of such products might pose a possible fire hazard in hospitals. As a result, the US National Fire Protection Agency (NFPA) amended their Life Safety Code, and prohibited the placement of ABHR dispensers in egress corridors.[1] However, the NFPA subsequently revised their recommendations in 2004. The US Medicare and Medicaid Services adopted the revision in 2005 and finalized its guidelines in 2006 stating that ABHR dispensers can be placed in egress corridors. To minimize the risk of fires, dispensers should not be installed over, or directly adjacent to, an ignition source (e.g., electrical outlet); nor should they be stored near high temperature sources or flames.[1]

Widespread adoption of ABHRs as the preferred method for hand hygiene performance in healthcare facilities caused some investigators to question whether or not significant absorption of alcohol through the skin or via the respiratory tract occurs following repeated applications of handrubs during hygienic hand hygiene or surgical hand preparation. Miller et al. had five volunteers apply 5 mL of an ABHR to their hands 50 times over a period of 4 hours, and found that all had blood ethanol concentrations of <5 mg/dL.[6] Kramer et al. studied 12 volunteers who applied 4 mL of handrubs varying in ethanol content from 55% to 95% 20 times for 30 s, with a 1-min break between applications.[7] The highest median blood acetaldehyde concentration was 0.57 mg/L after use of the 55% ethanol preparation. Blood ethanol levels ranged from 11.5 mg/L to 21 mg/L following hygienic handrub, and 8.8 mg/L to 30 mg/L following surgical hand preparation.[7] These levels were considered safe, since diminished fine motor coordination due to ethanol usually occurs with blood ethanol levels >200 mg/L. Other studies that had volunteers use an ABHR 50 times over 4 hours found that blood ethanol levels in the five volunteers were all <5 mg/dL. Another study involving 26 HCWs measured ethanol vapors in exhaled breath and ethanol, acetaldehyde, and acetate levels in blood and urine samples of volunteers.[8] None of the volunteers had detectable levels of ethanol or its metabolites in the blood or urine. Low concentrations (0.08 ± 0.07 mg/L) of ethanol were detected in exhaled breath of

10 HCWs 1–2 minutes after exposure. Since these HCWs used ABHR at a frequency commonly expected during a 4-hour work shift, the authors suggested that the study provided additional evidence that ABHRs are safe for routine use by healthcare personnel. Similarly, a group in Australia evaluated cutaneous ethanol and isopropanol absorption among 20 HCWs who applied the product to their hands 30 times in one hour.[9] Although ethanol was detected in the breath of 30% of the individuals 1 to 2 min after application, and in the serum at miniscule levels (i.e., below the detectable limit of a police breathalyzer) in 10% of individuals 5 to 7 min after application, this was thought to be related to inhalation of ethanol fumes since the study was conducted in a closed room. However, isopropanol levels in the blood were undetectable. For this reason, the authors concluded that both ethanol- and isopropanol-based products were safe for use, but that isopropanol-based products may be preferred by some religious groups who could be concerned about ethanol (see Chapter 31). A recent study that involved 33 HCWs during routine clinical work revealed measurable urinary ethanol and ethyl glucuronide levels that were negligible, and were 61 times lower than those observed when the HCWs were allowed to consume alcohol-containing beverages, food or cosmetic products.[10] There was no statistically significant correlation between urinary levels and the frequency of hand antisepsis. An accompanying editorial that reviewed the study and other literature dealing with the use of ethanol-based ABHRs concluded that ABHRs are safe for HCWs and patients.[11]

Although cutaneous absorption of alcohol-based products appears to be minimal, absorption following oral ingestion has been well documented.[12–16] For this reason, careful product placement is required in areas where young children or confused adults are managed. These include pediatric wards, outpatient clinics, geriatric/dementia wards, and psychiatric facilities.[12–16] A single report of eye irritation due to ABHR accidentally falling from a dispenser into a child's eye, causing pain and redness, suggests that equipping dispensers with drip trays might avoid this rare occurrence.[17] Additional case reports of accidental exposure have been published.[18–20]

WHAT WE DO NOT KNOW – THE UNCERTAIN

Most studies dealing with dermal or respiratory absorption of alcohol following use of ABHRs have been of relatively short duration. Few data are available on levels of alcohol absorption among HCWs who use ABHRs 40 to 100 times per day over long time periods. However, based on current information, longterm use appears to be safe.

RESEARCH AGENDA

Additional studies of HCWs who are chronically exposed to ABHRs on a very frequent basis are warranted. Further research on how to keep flash points as low as possible in handrub formulations with relatively high concentrations of alcohol is desirable. Development of effective non-alcohol-containing handrub formulations that can be made readily available in clinical areas where pediatric and psychiatric patients and those with dementia are managed would be helpful.

REFERENCES

1. World Health Organization, *WHO Guidelines for Hand Hygiene in Health Care*. Geneva: WHO, 2009.
2. Widmer AF, Replace hand washing with use of a waterless alcohol hand rub? *Clin Infect Dis* 2000;**31**:136–143.
3. Boyce JM, Pearson ML, Low frequency of fires from alcohol-based hand rub dispensers in healthcare facilities. *Infect Control Hosp Epidemiol* 2003;**24**:618–619.
4. Kramer A, Kampf G, Hand rub-associated fire incidents during 25,038 hospital-years in Germany. *Infect Control Hosp Epidemiol* 2007;**28**:745–746.
5. Bryant KA, Pearce J, Stover B, Flash fire associated with the use of alcohol-based antiseptic agent. *Am J Infect Control* 2002;**30**:256–257.
6. Miller MA, Rosin A, Levsky ME, et al., Does the clinical use of ethanol-based hand sanitizer elevate blood alcohol levels? A prospective study. *Am J Emerg Med* 2006;**24**:815–817.
7. Kramer A, Below H, Bieber N, et al., Quantity of ethanol absorption after excessive hand disinfection using three commercially available hand rubs is minimal and below toxic levels for humans. *BMC Infect Dis* 2007;**7**:117.
8. Hautemaniere A, Ahmed-Lecheheb D, Cunat L, et al., Assessment of transpulmonary absorption of ethanol from alcohol-based hand rub. *Am J Infect Control* 2013;**41**:e15–e19.
9. Brown TL, Gamon S, Tester P, et al., Can alcohol-based hand-rub solutions cause you to lose your driver's license? Comparative cutaneous absorption of various alcohols. *Antimicrob Agents Chemother* 2007;**51**:1107–1108.
10. Gessner S, Below E, Diedrich S, et al., Ethanol and ethyl glucuronide urine concentrations after ethanol-based hand antisepsis with and without permitted alcohol consumption. *Am J Infect Control* 2016;**44**:999–1003.
11. Pires D, Bellissimo-Rodrigues F, Pittet D, Ethanol-based handrubs: Safe for patients and health care workers. *Am J Infect Control* 2016;**44**:858–859.
12. Willmon HJS, Re: alcohol hand-rub in psychiatric units – A risk to patients? *Burns* 2009;**35**:610.
13. Gormley NJ, Bronstein AC, Rasimas JJ, et al., The rising incidence of intentional ingestion of ethanol-containing hand sanitizers. *Crit Care Med* 2012;**40**:290–294.
14. Tavolacci MP, Marini H, Vanheste S, et al., A voluntary ingestion of alcohol-based hand rub. *J Hosp Infect* 2007;**66**:86–87.
15. Schneir AB, Clark RF, Death caused by ingestion of an ethanol-based hand sanitizer. *J Emergency Med* 2013;**45**:358–360.
16. Batty LM, Brischetto AJ, Kevat AC, et al., Consumption of alcohol-based hand sanitisers by hospital inpatients. *Med J Aust* 2011;**194**:664.
17. Baylis O, Fraser S, When alcohol hand rub gets in your eyes. *J Hosp Infect* 2006;**64**:199–200.
18. Engel JS, Spiller HA, Acute ethanol poisoning in a 4-year-old as a result of ethanol-based hand-sanitizer ingestion. *Pediatr Emerg Care* 2010;**26**:508–509.
19. Henry-Lagarrigue M, Charbonnier M, Bruneel F, et al., Severe alcohol hand rub overdose inducing coma, watch after H1N1 pandemic. *Neurocrit Care* 2010;**12**:400–402.
20. May C, The risks to children of alcohol-based hand gels. *Paediatr Nurs* 2009;**21**:36–37.

Chapter 17

Rinse, Gel, Foam, Soap … Selecting an Agent

Andreas Voss

Radboud University Medical Centre and Canisius-Wilhelmina Hospital, Nijmegen, The Netherlands

KEY MESSAGES

- The agents chosen for hand hygiene in a healthcare settings should, where possible and when necessary, be targeted to fit specific patient populations and corresponding pathogens (e.g., choosing a product for a children's hospital with a better than average viral coverage). There is no "one-product-fits-all" in hand hygiene, which is why healthcare settings should offer at least two different rubs, when economics and availability allow.

- Despite (sometimes debatable) differences among various agents and formulations, the in vitro differences in efficacy are rendered insignificant if the compliance with use increases due to better acceptance of a rub, gel, or foam.

- Do not select a product you cannot afford or obtain. Only test products you selected and involve representatives from all major departments in testing (especially those with a high rate of use).

For most of history, handwashing with water and soap was the only method healthcare workers (HCWs) could use to clean their hands. In 1847, Semmelweis,[1] after understanding the role of HCWs' hands as a source of pathogen transmission, introduced an innovative way to perform hand hygiene based on the use of chlorinated lime solution (see Chapter 2). He thereby became the first to show the added value of antisepsis over cleaning with water and soap. Alcohol was used as skin antiseptic in the early 1900s prior to the availability of commercially

Hand Hygiene: A Handbook for Medical Professionals, First Edition.
Edited by Didier Pittet, John M. Boyce and Benedetta Allegranzi.
© 2017 John Wiley & Sons, Inc. Published 2017 by John Wiley & Sons, Inc.

produced agents.[2-4] Most agents at that time were "creams or jellies" containing hexachlorophene or chlorhexidine and were seen as far less effective than any hand rinse.[5] By whom and when alcohol-based handrubs (ABHRs) got introduced into clinical practice is far less clear. One of those scientists, who is mentioned to be associated with the first development of an alcohol-based product in 1965, is Peter Kalmar. Like Semmelweis, Kalmar was a Hungarian-born physician and worked in Hamburg, Germany.[6] In general it appears that much of the early development, commercialization, and clinical use of ABHRs originated from Germany in the early 1960s.[7] While Europe may have been an early adopter, in other parts of the world, including the United States, water and (medicated-)soap were the mainstay of hand hygiene until the early 2000s.

Today, ABHRs are the standard of care in many countries around the world, in large part due to the efforts of the WHO's global campaign on hand hygiene promotion (see also Chapter 38). Still, the system change reaches further than the mere introduction of a point-of-care ABHR, and it includes dispensing systems, monitoring of use, and – last but not least – availability of an adequate number of sinks continuously equipped with soap and disposable towels (see Chapter 21). Consequently, the complete set of hygienic hand products in the healthcare setting consists of a liquid soap and a skin care product that can be adequately dispensed. Any known interactions between products used to clean hands, skin care products, and the types of glove used in the institution should be determined and should not lead to side effects if combined. This chapter focuses on hand antiseptic products, with the exclusion of medicated soap. The latter is excluded, since it generally does not allow use at the point of care, its antimicrobial value is limited, and its dermal tolerance is frequently reduced compared to ABHRs.

WHAT WE KNOW – THE EVIDENCE

The first step in choosing a hygienic hand product is the selection of an effective, tolerated, affordable, and locally available product, with the "right feel." A team that broadly represents future users and professionals with specific knowledge such as infection control, occupational health, and pharmacology, should make a selection of one or several potential products. Factors that should be looked at during the selection procedure include efficacy (including considerations with regard to defined patient populations); dermal tolerance; cost; aesthetics such as color, fragrance, and texture; and use issues such as stickiness, drying time, ease of spreading the product, buildup, and mode of dispensing. In some settings, various products are made available as freedom of choice tends to improve hand hygiene compliance.

- *Dermal tolerance and skin reactions*
  Several studies have published methods to evaluate aspects of dermal tolerance such as dryness or irritation. Both self-assessment and expert clinical

evaluation correlate well with physiological measures that are not practical to use in clinical settings (see also Chapter 15).

- *Fragrance*
  While a lack of fragrance may render a product unappealing, a strong fragrance may cause side effects, including respiratory discomfort and allergic reactions among HCWs and patients. Consequently, a mild (or no) fragrance should be used.

- *Consistency*
  Handrubs are available as gels, rinses (solutions), or foams. Rinses generally have a consistency similar to water, dry faster than gels or foams, and may be less "sticky" after repeated use. On the other hand, they have a stronger smell and a higher chance of spillage, which may lead to damaged or slippery floors.[8] Foam is the type of handrub that came last to the market and some questions – related to drying time, optimal coverage, or amount to use – were only recently answered and may need further evaluation. Similar to gels, they decrease the chance of spillage and may lead to buildup after repeated use.

- *Antimicrobial efficacy*
  There is still some discussion with regard to efficacy, as some studies suggest that it depends on concentration and type of alcohol in the formulation, while other studies suggest that the volume applied may be the main factor influencing efficacy (see also Chapter 9).[9–11]

While all of these factors influence the choice of a product, dermal tolerance is one of the main parameters leading to product acceptability and, consequently, compliance with hand hygiene by HCWs. A decision-making tool for the selection of an appropriate product is available from the WHO website (www.who.int/gpsc/en/).

In addition to the above-mentioned criteria, "dispensing possibilities" of the selected product (e.g., within the patient zone, delivering appropriate volume) should be taken into account in the selection process. Manufacturers should also be questioned about the risk of product contamination, as well as any side effects that hand lotions, creams, (medicated) soap, or ABHRs may have.

The second step of choosing a hand hygiene product is pilot testing of the selected product(s). This should never happen in an *ad hoc* fashion (e.g., driven by internal or external players, such as a company-initiated "trial" to "test" a new product). Only "selected" products should be tested, which means that these must be locally available and affordable. Structured questionnaires should be used to assess HCWs' acceptability of hand hygiene products (available from the WHO website: www.who.int/gpsc/en/). While the above-mentioned selection factors should obviously be part of the evaluation or questionnaire, the main focus of the pilot study should be user acceptability issues. Where possible, multiple products should be tested and compared to the one currently used, and the product(s) with the highest user acceptability should be chosen, since this will have the largest influence on hand hygiene compliance.

WHAT WE DO NOT KNOW – THE UNCERTAIN

While it seems logical that high compliance and product use is more important than minimal differences related to in vitro efficacy of different hand hygiene products, little is known about the clinical impact (reduction of HAIs) of different antiseptic products, especially in a side-by-side comparison. Mere in vitro antimicrobial efficacy tests fail to predict the clinical performance of a hand antiseptic agent, which also depends on the above-mentioned selection criteria and characteristics such as the ease to cover the complete hand, or the drying time of the product.

In the past, ABHRs were made following the premise that "one solution fits all (purposes)." But actually, even those solutions geared at "virucidal activity" by increasing the alcohol content are not sufficiently active against all viruses. Specific products may be needed for specific circumstances, such as rotavirus spread in a neonatal intensive care, or a norovirus outbreak in a general adult ward.

As alcohols are flammable, storage and use of ABHRs may have to follow certain regulations, such as those of the US National Fire Protection Agency (see Chapter 16). Still, these regulations should not be in the way of appropriate use, namely at the point-of-care and with a suitable amount and placement of handrub dispensers in the patient room. In addition alcohol-based products may be a problem under specific conditions, such as during shipping for major rescue missions of "Médecins Sans Frontières" or comparable organizations. Nowadays, limited data are available on the efficacy and tolerability of alcohol-free handrubs. While the issue of the flammability of ABHRs is presently limited to certain states and rare situations, non-alcohol-based alternatives may become of interest in the future, due to discussions of dermal absorption after multiple handrubs. The Dutch Expert Committee on Occupational Safety suggested a "skin notification" for ethanol-based handrubs due to a possible carcinogenic effect after dermal absorption. This is a clear example of how regulations to increase human safety may actually increase patients' health risk; this statement contributes to deter hand hygiene compliance and a potential ban of ethanol would limit the number of available products. Hence, because of socio-cultural issues or other drivers, ABHRs – presently the best choice for hand hygiene – may not always be the undisputed alternative.

Most of the clinical and in vitro data on ABHRs originate from "developed" countries with a moderate climate, with some exceptions, however.[12] The differences in socio-cultural backgrounds, climate, environmental conditions, and clinical practices among users warrants more studies in countries with limited resources.

RESEARCH AGENDA

At present, most handrubs are tested and recommended for clinical use in accordance with the European Norms (EN), namely for at least 30 s and with a volume of 3 mL. In the daily routine, probably few of the handrubs are used for that "long" and the volume used differs significantly. Future studies should try to find a "sweet spot" that indicates, for each kind of agent (rinse, gel, foam), the optimal amount of product use that allows for full coverage of the hand in the shortest possible drying time. While not part of this chapter, one could furthermore evaluate if a "complete" coverage of the hands is even needed, since volume has a major impact on drying time, which in turn influences the willingness of HCWs to use a product (see Chapter 10).

Direct comparison of the clinical effects of different handrub formulations would be an ultimate research goal; but the vast amount of variables that might influence results and the expected low difference in outcomes (and thus the extremely large number of HCWs and patients) may impair getting these results.

In vitro and clinical effects of non-alcohol-based handrubs – in comparison to water and soap – is very well possible and should be encouraged in order to evaluate alternative point-of-care products for special situations, as described above.

With regard to particular circumstances, research into factors influencing the selection of a handrub in countries with limited resources is direly needed. Looking at the influence of temperature and humidity on characteristics such as drying time, ease of spread, and "stickiness" of different application forms of ABHRs would also be desirable.

REFERENCES

1. Semmelweis I, Die Aetiologie, der Begriff und die Prophylaxis des Kindbettfiebers. Pest, Wien und Leipzig: C.A.Hartleben's Verlag–Expedition, 1861.
2. Rotter ML, Alcohols for antisepsis of hands and skin. In Ascenzi JM (Ed). Handbook of disinfectants and antiseptics, Marcel Dekker, New York;1996:177–233.
3. Price PB, Ethyl alcohol as a germicide. *Arch Surg* 1939;**38**:528–542.
4. Birmingham DJ, Perone VB, Waterless hand cleaners. *Ind Med Surg* 1957;**26**: 361–368.
5. Banham TM, Hand hygiene. *Br Med J* 1965;**2**:315–316.
6. Peter Kalmar on Wikipedia. Available at https://de.wikipedia.org/wiki/Peter_Kalmár. Accessed March 7, 2017.
7. Mittermayer H, Rotter M, Comparative investigations on the efficacy of tap water, some detergents and ethanol on the transient flora of the hands. *Zentralbl Bakteriol Orig B* 1975;**160**:163–172.
8. Kramer A, Bernig T, Kampf G, Clinical double-blind trial on the dermal tolerance and user acceptability of six alcohol-based hand disinfectants for hygienic hand disinfection. *J Hosp Infect* 2002;**51**:114–120.

9. Barbut F, Maury E, Goldwirt L, et al., Comparison of the antibacterial efficacy and acceptability of an alcohol-based hand rinse with two alcohol-based hand gels during routine patient care. *J Hosp Infect* 2007;**66**:167–173.

10. Edmonds SL, Macinga DR, Mays-Suko P, et al., Comparative efficacy of commercially available alcohol-based hand rubs and World Health Organization-recommended hand rubs: formulation matters. *Am J Infect Control* 2012;**40**:521–525.

11. Macinga DR, Shumaker DJ, Werner HP, et al., The relative influences of product volume, delivery format and alcohol concentration on dry-time and efficacy of alcohol-based hand rubs. *BMC Infect Dis* 2014;**14**:511.

12. Allegranzi B, Sax H, Bengaly L, et al., Successful implementation of the World Health Organization hand hygiene improvement strategy in a referral hospital in Mali, Africa. *Infect Control Hosp Epidemiol* 2010;**31**:133–141.

Chapter 18

Behavior and Hand Hygiene

Mary-Louise McLaws[1] and Hugo Sax[2]

[1] Healthcare Infection and Infectious Diseases Control, University of New South Wales, Sydney, Australia

[2] Division of Infectious Diseases and Infection Control, University Hospital of Zurich, Zürich, Switzerland

KEY MESSAGES

- Hand hygiene in the healthcare setting is a practice for the benefit of others. Therefore, although interventions and education programs are based on a theoretical framework, the choice of theory may explain why improvements in hand hygiene have plateaued.

- Hand hygiene in the healthcare setting could be promoted as professionalism that is also altruistic.

- Promoting hand hygiene in messages of professionalism and altruism would benefit from using the elements in the marketing "hook cycle" to produce a "habit loop."

WHAT WE KNOW – THE EVIDENCE

"My Five Moments for Hand Hygiene" was designed as an extension of the before-after hand hygiene practice[1] on a multimodal platform (see Chapter 20). The literature is plentiful with healthcare facilities, singularly or country-wide, reporting baseline compliance rates, ranging from 13% to 51%, and improvements ranging from 10 to 20 percentage points (PP) with few reporting improvements of above 20 PP. Monitoring hand hygiene compliance is useful

Hand Hygiene: A Handbook for Medical Professionals, First Edition.
Edited by Didier Pittet, John M. Boyce and Benedetta Allegranzi.
© 2017 John Wiley & Sons, Inc. Published 2017 by John Wiley & Sons, Inc.

but only when it assists efforts to improve hand hygiene behavior. Interventions aimed at affecting behavior have the best likelihood of success when designed in the light of a behavioral theory.[2] Behavior theories consist of components that drive or inhibit behavior, and these components can be tested to identify which are the more influential on the targeted behavior. This can be difficult, however, given the myriad of theories. Behavioral theories that have been used to design hand hygiene interventions have included the Organizational Theory,[3] which aims to improve the behavior of the wider community, and the Control Theory, which utilizes feedback to goal-driven personalities. Other popular behavior change theories include the Health Belief Model, the Theory of Reasoned Action (TRA), the Social Cognitive Theory, and the Theory of Ecological Perspectives, which can include several of these models and theories.[3] In common to each of these theories is that the benefactor of the behavior change is the actor.

Social Marketing is a model rather than a theory, utilizing sequential strategic stages based on a commercial marketing technique–to understand the perceived needs of the audience, enhance and deliver perceived benefits associated with a product/idea to the audience, and reduce barriers to adopting or maintaining the product/idea. One benefit of application of this model is raising awareness in the actor (see Chapter 26). The Control Theory is effective when the targeted audience reacts well to goal-driven challenges. The very healthcare workers (HCWs) who are not goal driven may be the group needed to engage in the program if a targeted improvement of, say 20 PP, is needed to achieve an 80% compliance rate. Improvement by less than 20 PP is common, suggesting that an improvement of 20 PP or more may require a fundamental shift in efforts to change and sustain hand hygiene compliance rates greater than 80%.

The motivation to perform hand hygiene by the lay public and by HCWs is complex and has been hypothesized to have its basis in a childhood-learned behavior.[4] When HCWs practice hand hygiene in the healthcare setting, clinically prescribed behavior based on guidelines is in strong competition with childhood-learned behavior. Care situations that HCWs perceive as similar to those learned in childhood will trigger hand cleansing inherently; when patient contacts that require hand hygiene overlap a childhood-learned moment similar to toileting, HCWs will inherently comply. During childhood, hand hygiene was taught as self-protection, so when patient contacts are perceived as not posing a health risk to the HCWs, they will perceive hand cleansing as unnecessary self-protective behavior. As a consequence, in healthcare settings hand hygiene required before patient contact and before clean procedures is poor, while compliance will be inherently practiced after contact with ill patients and their body fluids.[4]

Knowledge of HCWs' translation of childhood-learned hand hygiene behavior was the result of a mixed-methods study using qualitative data from focus group discussions and quantitative data collected from a survey. This survey was structured according to the major components and wording of the Theory of Planned Behavior (TPB).[4] The TPB was chosen because the original theory, the Theory of

Reasoned Action, had successfully predicted several behavioral intentions beneficial to others as well as oneself, such as the intention to practice safe sex. For the purpose of the study, the theory was modified to include several potentially important components articulated by HCWs during qualitative interviews.

According to *World Health Organization (WHO) Guidelines on Hand Hygiene in Health Care*, the principal motivation for hand hygiene in healthcare is for the benefit of others – the patient. Professionalism presented within an altruistic frame may assist in reconfiguring childhood-learned behavior: "*You are a professional, and as a true professional your hand hygiene is for the benefit of your patient.*" The predictive model for HCWs' intention to practice hand hygiene associated with perceived *dirty* contacts,[4] termed "*inherent*" hand hygiene, explained 76% of variance for this behavior. Yet, the model to predict hand hygiene after perceived *clean* contacts, termed "*elective*" hand hygiene, explained only 64% of variance. The 36% of variance that was not explained for *electing* or not to comply may have been our omission of a component to test for the presence of empathy or altruism associated with performing hand hygiene for the benefit of the patient, in particular "before touching a patient." Empathy is said to evoke altruism where the benefit of the behavior is principally not oneself but *another*. Altruism is driven from a higher motivation that does not involve ego. By replacing the driver of self-protection with altruism, the HCW can start to practice hand hygiene in healthcare settings for its original intention – patient safety.

WHAT WE DO NOT KNOW – THE UNCERTAIN

So how can we replace the childhood-learned driver, self-protection, with professionalism presented as empathy and altruism to achieve habitual hand hygiene? We could look towards designers of software and Internet applications, such as Facebook, to help habitualize altruistic hand hygiene. Software designers understand that transforming occasional software use into habitual use requires a Hook ("a design that provides a solution to user's problem")[5] that produces the *habit loop.* This Hook must occur with sufficient frequency for the loop to develop into a circular behavior. There are four steps in designing a Hook. Step 1: the user is presented with a *trigger*; step 2: the user performs an *action* that is easy to carry out; step 3: the user gets a *reward* that humans are hardwired to look for; step 4: the user gives an *investment* or *commitment* to the software (Figure 18.1).[5]

Habit loops typically start with a cue that *triggers* repeat behavior. What makes behavior become habitual or ritual is how the human brain is programmed. The cue for the habit of community hand hygiene started with a parent reminding a child to handwash after toileting. This trigger moves children to undertaking hand hygiene for which they receive a reward, praise for their action from their role model or parent, which reinforces a message that handwashing associated with washing away assumed harmful germs is good. HCWs once had a role model in their childhood who acted as a cue to remember to perform hand

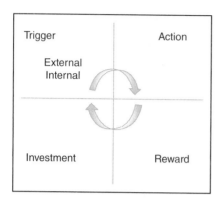

Figure 18.1 The Hook (modified) *Source*: Modified from Eyal. Reproduced with permission from Elsevier

hygiene. This role model rewarded the child until the habit loop of "toilet – verbal reminder – handwashing – praise" was established. By adulthood handwashing after toileting is a habit, where the act of toileting triggers memory to hand hygiene, referred to as an internal trigger.

Using the steps in *Hook* design for software such as Facebook we will now explore how well each *Hook* step can be utilized to improve hand hygiene performance, especially the altruistic moments 1 and 2 of the "My Five Moments for Hand Hygiene" (see Chapter 20) as a habitual or ritual practice based on altruism.

Step 1: the *trigger* that starts an action can be external or internal. External triggers should come in the form of "alarm" or "call to action" and simultaneously give the user a solution about "what to do next." There are several external *triggers* provided to HCWs in the form of May 5th "Hand Hygiene Day" worldwide, with activities and country campaign launches. These triggers are, however, too infrequent to establish a habit loop. Unlike the emotions of guilt or pleasure, mere knowledge about the indications for hand hygiene is a weak internal trigger.[5] An example of a good external trigger is the physical design of a surgical theater where the surgeon must enter the scrub room before entering the surgical theater. An even better trigger is the repeat request by a well-respected senior physician to use handrub before touching a patient. If repeated consistently, this trigger has a great chance of resulting in a higher internal engagement, intrinsic trigger, that now involves situation, place, and emotion.

Step 2: is an *action* that occurs when the trigger results in "doing." This step in the *habit loop* is a function of motivation and the ability or ease of performing the action.[6] "Ability" to perform the action includes physical effort, time, and money, and ability is affected when the action is nonroutine. There is an inverse relationship between motivation or ability and the size of the *trigger* required to achieve *action*: the stronger the motivation and ability to perform hand hygiene, the smaller the *trigger* needed to achieve the action (hand hygiene). Conversely, the less motivated, and hence the less ability the HCW has, then the more important the *trigger* has to become to achieve *action*. The *action* step to forming a *habit loop* should be the simplest behavioral requirement of the user. The requirement that the action must be easy is common to other theories and models. An example of an easy action has been designed in the "you have mail" icon, which is this same icon the user presses to access new email.

Hand hygiene action is now becoming easier than ever, ever since WHO instructed alcohol-based handrub (ABHR) to be placed at point-of-care. However, if hand hygiene compliance is low, motivation will most likely also be low, and hence the *trigger* to achieve hand hygiene will need to be big to obtain high compliance. An example of the size of a trigger required when motivation is low is the continued alarm from new wrist band technology to remind HCWs as they enter the patient's zone to perform hand hygiene, or the patient requesting the HCW to perform hand hygiene, or the continual presence of hand hygiene monitors who will speak up when they see that a HCW omits hand hygiene. Repeat hand hygiene (action) in HCWs will occur when they find more pleasure from complying (e.g., in the reward in the form of praise) than the perceived pain or emotional discomfort (e.g., from guilt or embarrassment for falling short in clinical professionalism) when they do not perform the action. This is when the *reward* part of the *Hook* is imperative.

Step 3: is providing the user with the *reward* (e.g., praise). When a strong internal *trigger* (e.g., emotion such as guilt or pleasure), *motivation*, and *ease of action* are present, the next step toward the final goal, *commitment* to a behavior, is the *reward*. Humans are hardwired to search for *rewards*.[7] *Rewards* can be grouped into reward given from the "tribe," reward obtained from the "hunt," and reward given to "oneself."[7] Anticipation of a *reward*, whether it is gained from the "tribe," the "hunt," or "oneself," stimulates dopamine in the brain, and dopamine is dampened when *reward* is withheld.[8] *Reward* given from the "tribe" includes receiving cooperation, competition, societal recognition, acceptance, sex, and empathetic joy. The custom of weddings provides the bridal couple with these "tribal" rewards. Facebook users posting photos on their Facebook page are *rewarded* from the *"tribe"* by being part of a wider social group. Money, food, and information are *rewards* gained through the *"hunt."* The *rewards* obtained by repeatedly searching apps or Facebook provides rewards for "oneself" in the forms of mastery, consistency, competency, and completion. When HCWs routinely practice altruistic hand hygiene, they should receive all three self-rewards.

Humans respond to variability in obtaining a *reward* by increasing their focus on finding more rewards.[8] If there is little *reward* from the *action*, hand hygiene, then the next step in the *habit loop – investment* towards habitual hand hygiene–will not occur. HCWs receive messages about the importance of complying and the association between compliance and low infection. Rewarding HCWs with messages incorporated into hand hygiene improvement interventions will need to be varied to prevent boredom and help HCWs move to the next step in the habit loop. Perhaps it's now time to invest in a *reward*-message that associates hand hygiene with their professionalism and altruism. When the human brain sees an image, it may relay a visual imagery message that may not be entirely correct.[9] The cause of this inaccuracy in visual imagery has been hypothesized as being of evolutionary advantage allowing us to swiftly respond to an image to increase our chances of survival.[9] We can use this visual imagery to increasingly link ABHR with professionalism and altruism; the emotional response when seeing ABHR for perceived "clean" patient contacts is to comply because it invokes a pleasurable sense of professionalism from helping others and engenders altruistic emotions rather than relying on a sense of obligation or demand.

Step 4: is *investment* and is the final step in the *hook*. This step in software design involves the user committing to the software action. *Investment* by users of, for instance, Facebook requires work or payment in terms of social capital, time, emotional commitment, and personal information. Personal investment is perceived by those who give something of themselves to the action as adding worth to that action.[10] Personal *investment* will increase the likelihood of a repeat passage through each step of the *hook* and stores value in all four steps. *Investment* by software users includes pressing the "Like" icon on Facebook or personalizing your Facebook home settings. This final step in the *hook* for hand hygiene would require HCWs to invest their emotion in the belief that their action is altruistic so that they add perceived value to their hand hygiene behavior as the penultimate patient safety action in their patient contact. This could be achieved by letting HCWs talk to patients about hand hygiene or involve them in defining the patient zone for their specific care setting.

RESEARCH AGENDA

> *People often say that motivation doesn't last. Well, neither does bathing – that's why we recommend it daily.*
>
> – Zig Ziglar (salesman and motivational speaker)

The first two steps (trigger and action) in the design of a *hook* for the habitual hand hygiene *loop* have been established without the motivation of fulfilling a sense of professionalism and altruism, while the importance of the innate human need for *reward* (such as praise by the hospital administration and auditors) has been undervalued in our previous attempts to improve hand hygiene. Our future strategy should be to develop programs that redirect HCWs' *motivation* to comply as fulfilling their sense of professionalism and engendering emotions of altruism that evoke a pleasurable desire to comply as we reward HCWs' compliance with praise.

REFERENCES

1. Sax H, Allegranzi B, Uckay I, et al., My five moments for hand hygiene: a user-centred design approach to understand, train, monitor and report hand hygiene. *J Hosp Infect* 2007;**67**:9–21.

2. French SD, Green SE, O'Connor DA, et al., Developing theory-informed behaviour change interventions to implement evidence into practice: a systematic approach using the Theoretical Domains Framework. *Implementation Sci* 2012;**7**:38.

3. Glanz K, Rimer BK, Viswanath K, eds, *Health Behavior and Health Education Theory, Research, and Practice*, 4th edn. San Francisco: Jossey-Bass, 2008.

4. Whitby M, McLaws ML, Ross MW, Why healthcare workers don't wash their hands: a behavioral explanation. *Infect Control Hosp Epidemiol* 2006; **27**:484–492.

5. Eyal N, Hooked: the psychology of how products engage us. Available at www.nirandfar.com. Accessed March 7, 2017.

6. Fogg BJ, A behavior model for persuasive design. Persuasive Technology Lab, Stanford University. Available at captology.stanford.edu and https://www.bjfogg.com.

7. Malone TW, Lepper MR, Making learning fun: a taxonomy of intrinsic motivations for learning. In: Snow RE, Farr MJ, eds. *Aptitude, Learning and Instruction III: Conative and Affective Process Analyses*. Hillsdale, NJ: Erlbaum Associates; 1987,223–253.

8. Knutson B, Peterson R, Neurally reconstructing expected utility. *Game Econ Behav* 2005;**52**:305–315.

9. Nairne JS, Pandeirada JNS, Adaptive memory: remembering with a stone-age brain. *Curr Dir Psychol Sci* 2008;**17**: 239–243.

10. Norton M, Mochon D, Ariely D, The IKEA effect: when labor leads to love. *J Consumer Psych* 2012;**22**:453–460.

ADDITIONAL REFERENCES

11. World Health Organization, Save Lives: Clean Your Hands – WHO's global annual campaign. Available at www.who.int/gpsc/5may/en/. Accessed March 7, 2017.

12. World Health Organization, *WHO Guidelines on Hand Hygiene in Health Care*, Geneva: WHO, 2009. Available at www.who.int/gpsc/5may/tools/en/. Accessed March 7, 2017.

13. Batson CD, Shaw LL, Evidence for altruism: towards a pluralism of prosocial motives. *Psychol Inq* 1991;**2**:107–122.

14. Whitby M, Pessoa-Silva CL, McLaws ML, et al., Behavioural considerations for hand hygiene practices: the basic building blocks. *J Hosp Infect* 2007;**65**:1–8.

15. Larson E, Monitoring hand hygiene: meaningless, harmful, or helpful? *Am J Infect Control* 2013;**41**(5 Suppl.):S42–S45.

16. Allegranzi B, Gayet-Ageron A, Bengaly L, et al., Global implementation of WHO's multi-modal strategy for improvement of hand hygiene: a quasi-experimental study. *Lancet Infect Dis* 2013;**13**:843–851.

17. McLaws ML, Pantle AC, Fitzpatrick KR, et al., Improvements in hand hygiene across New South Wales public hospitals: Clean hands save lives, Part III. *Med J Aust* 2009;**191** (8 Suppl.):S18–S24.

18. Grayson ML, Russo P, Cruickshank M, et al., Outcomes from the first 2 years of the Australian National Hand Hygiene Initiative. *Med J Aust* 2011;**195**:615–619.

19. Fakhry M, Hanna GB, Anderson O, et al., Effectiveness of an audible reminder on hand hygiene adherence. *Am J Infect Control* 2012;**40**:320–323.

20. Larson EL, Early E, Cloonan P, et al., An organizational climate intervention associated with increased handwashing and decreased nosocomial infection. *Behav Med* 2000;**26**: 14–22.

21. Pittet D, Hugonnet S, Harbarth S, et al., Effectiveness of a hospital-wide programme to improve compliance with hand hygiene. *Lancet* 2000;**356**:1307–1312.

22. Whitby M, McLaws ML, Slater K, et al., Three successful interventions in healthcare workers that improve compliance with hand hygiene: is sustained replication possible? *Am J Infect Control* 2008;**36**:349–355.

23. Fuller C, Michie S, Savage J, et al., The feedback intervention trial (FIT) – improving hand hygiene compliance in UK healthcare workers: a stepped wedge cluster randomized controlled trial. *PLOS One* 2012;**7**:e41617.

24. McLaws ML, Maharlouie N, Yousefi F, et al., Predicting hand hygiene among Iranian healthcare workers using the theory of planned behavior. *Am J Infect Control* 2012;**40**:336–339.

25. McLaws ML, Irwig LM, Oldenburg B, et al., Predicting intention to use condoms in homosexual men: an application and extension of the theory of reasoned action. *Psychol Health* 1996;**11**:745–755.

26. McLaws ML, The relationship between hand hygiene and healthcare associated infections: it's complicated. *Infect Drug Resist* 2015;**8**:7–18.

Chapter 19

Hand Hygiene Promotion Strategies

Benedetta Allegranzi[1] and Didier Pittet[2]

[1] Infection Prevention and Control Global Unit, Department of Service Delivery and Safety, World Health Organization, and Faculty of Medicine, University of Geneva, Geneva, Switzerland

[2] Infection Control Program and WHO Collaborating Centre on Patient Safety, University of Geneva Hospitals and Faculty of Medicine, Geneva, Switzerland

KEY MESSAGES

- A high burden of scientific evidence clearly shows that hand hygiene compliance can be significantly improved and that the most successful strategies are multimodal. The most important and commonly used key components of these strategies are system change, education, reminders, hand hygiene monitoring and feedback, and an institutional safety climate usually built through leadership, champions, and patient participation.

- Behavioral change theories have provided useful background and insights for the development of successful hand hygiene promotion strategies. Hand hygiene improvement requires strategies and efforts to be sustained in the long term.

- Further research is needed to establish the relative importance of specific components of multimodal hand hygiene improvement strategies to induce behavioral changes; to gather qualitative evidence on how institutions or teams succeed at improving hand hygiene; and to improve the quality and reliability of results in terms of impact of hand hygiene promotion to reduce healthcare-associated infections (HAIs).

Hand Hygiene: A Handbook for Medical Professionals, First Edition.
Edited by Didier Pittet, John M. Boyce and Benedetta Allegranzi.
© 2017 John Wiley & Sons, Inc. Published 2017 by John Wiley & Sons, Inc.

WHAT WE KNOW – THE EVIDENCE

Over the last three decades, many studies have investigated the best approaches to promote hand hygiene best practices and improve hand hygiene indicators, in particular healthcare workers' (HCWs') compliance. Early studies on hand hygiene improvement in healthcare were focused on single interventions promoting the importance of handwashing and introducing the use of antimicrobial soaps, and then focusing on the innovative role of alcohol-based handrubs (ABHRs), mostly accompanied by HCW education. However, understanding the factors influencing HCWs' behavior and resulting in poor hand hygiene practice is essential to identify the best improvement strategies. Determinants of HCWs' behavioral attitudes towards compliance with hand hygiene recommendations are extremely complex and multifactorial (see Chapters 11, 12, and 13). Indeed, factors negatively influencing adherence to hand hygiene best practices are not only related to individuals (e.g., lack of knowledge, professional category, and poor accountability) but also to the facility infrastructures (e.g., lack of ABHRs or soap and water), the institutional climate (lack of culture or tradition of compliance, no prioritization of patient safety), and more broadly governmental commitment (e.g., insufficient commitment to fight against HAIs, lack of hand hygiene national guidelines). Some of these factors (e.g., individual HCWs' or institutional factors) can be modified by applying behavioral change theories while developing hand hygiene improvement strategies; this approach has led to interesting results.[1–3]

Given the multifactorial determinants of hand hygiene compliance, improvement interventions need to tackle several of these factors, if not all, with different tailored strategies implemented in parallel or as a stepwise approach. This is in line with the current modern approach to infection control where evidence has shown that multidisciplinary and multifaceted strategies are the most successful to achieve practice improvement and patient harm prevention, mainly because they tackle the problem as a whole, addressing determinants from different sides and often in the context of a comprehensive patient safety approach. This concept has recently been demonstrated by the "Systematic review and evidence-based guidance on organization of hospital infection control programs" (SIGHT) study group through rigorous quantitative and qualitative work. The review paper, which also includes international experts' consensus, identified multimodal and multidisciplinary prevention programs taking into account principles of behavioral change among the 10 key components of effective hospital infection control programs.[4]

Based on this principle and on published evidence, in 2005, WHO developed the Hand Hygiene Multimodal Improvement Strategy (see Chapter 33) to support translation into practice of the recommendations on hand hygiene in healthcare.[5] This has represented one of the first ever multimodal strategies in the infection control field. It was built upon successful research on hand hygiene promotion conducted at the University of Geneva Hospitals and subsequently spread to several additional champion facilities in other countries.[6] The WHO strategy includes the following five key components with the "My Five Moments for Hand Hygiene" concept (see Chapter 20) at its core: system change; staff training and education; monitoring of hand hygiene indicators and performance feedback; reminders in the work place; and improvement of the institutional patient safety climate. Given that this strategy was based upon a vast review of available evidence and then has been used as the gold standard for hand hygiene promotion, we describe here the key components with reference to studies that implemented some or all these components, explored variations in the strategy implementation, or included additional elements. For details about the WHO strategy and associated toolkit, the definitions of the five key strategy components, the underlying scientific evidence, and subsequent studies to test or replicate it, the reading of Chapter 33 is recommended also. Various narrative or systematic reviews on hand hygiene improvement strategies have been published[1,7–15] with different objectives (e.g., either assessing effect on compliance or impact on HAIs) and different inclusion criteria (e.g., only randomized and/or controlled trials).[1,7,8] Therefore, the reviews' conclusions can be different. However, a very large number of papers reporting results of interventions to improve hand hygiene in healthcare exist nowadays. In Table 19.1, we indicate the most relevant studies[16–53] focusing on specific components of hand hygiene improvement strategies as well as those implementing multimodal strategies. The recent meta-analysis by Luangasanatip et al. demonstrates the key role of the WHO multimodal approach in successful hand hygiene promotion.[9] Importantly, the use of multimodal strategies is also the object of recommendations made by WHO to achieve effective implementation of infection prevention and control activities.[54,55]

Key Components of Effective Promotion Strategies

Actions aimed at making hand hygiene practices feasible during healthcare delivery by ensuring that the necessary infrastructure is in place are referred to as *system change* (see Chapter 21).[10] This is usually achieved by making ABHR readily accessible at the point of care, and in some settings around the world also ensuring access to safe, continuous water supply, as well as to soap and disposable towels. "Sufficient availability of and easy access to material and equipment and optimized ergonomics" were also identified as key components of effective hospital infection control programs by SIGHT.[4] Similarly, WHO strongly recommends that "materials and equipment to perform hand hygiene should be easily available at the point of care" as one of the core components for effective infection prevention and control programs.[54,55] System change is intended to overcome barriers to hand hygiene compliance, such as lack of time, lack of facilities, high workload, or the inconvenient location or malfunctioning of sinks and dispensers. It is a particularly important priority for healthcare facilities starting hand hygiene improvement activities. However, it is also essential to revisit the necessary infrastructure on a regular basis to detect emerging gaps. Commitment from key senior managers,

Table 19.1   Strategies for Hand Hygiene Promotion in Healthcare*

Strategy	Selected References**
1. System change	
• Make hand hygiene possible, easy, convenient	16–22
• Make alcohol-based handrub available	16
2. Education	16, 23–26
3. Routine observation and performance feedback	16, 27–29
4. Reminders in the workplace	16, 24, 30, 31
• Marketing and communication campaigns	32–34
5. Improvement of institutional safety climate	16, 35
• Patient education and participation	16, 36
• Champions, leadership, role models	16, 37–40
• Administrative sanction/rewarding	16
6. Avoid overcrowding, understaffing, excessive workload	16
7. Use of behavioral change theories and positive deviance	40–44
8. Combine several of above strategies	16, 32, 33, 34, 38, 45–53

*Adapted with permission from 16.
**Only selected references have been listed.

support through adequate budget allocation, and timely action planning are crucial. To facilitate system change, it is also essential to voice users' preferences and needs by involving key staff who rely upon adequate hand hygiene infrastructures and supplies. In settings with limited resources and/or where ABHRs are unavailable or too expensive, local production of the WHO formulations can promote and facilitate system change.[11] In addition to the continuous provision of ABHRs, optimizing the ergonomics (e.g., the location of the dispensers) is key.[4] Studies showed that ABHR dispensers directly in the view of HCWs and hand hygiene facilities at the point of care led to hand hygiene practices improvement (see Table 19.1). Easy-to-use pocket ABHR dispensers attached to scrubs or to the HCW's belt, or innovative dispensers, can also improve compliance. In some of these studies, research included the participation of frontline HCWs and users in the development of new innovative dispenser designs.[4]

Education of HCWs and managers is one of the pillars of any hand hygiene improvement strategy.[12] Many factors or beliefs associated with poor hand hygiene compliance can be targeted through staff education by providing solid evidence on hand transmission and the impact of HAIs, and by focusing on the importance of performing hand hygiene at the point of care (patient zone), at the right moment, and with the appropriate technique. In these regards, the concept of "My Five Moments for Hand Hygiene" promoted by WHO (see Chapter 20) proved very instrumental to gain HCWs' attention and make them understand, remember, and effectively focus on the essential moments when and why to clean hands at the bedside. Practical training on the correct technique and duration to achieve maximum hand decontamination is also of utmost importance because serious gaps in knowledge and practices are widespread. Educational objectives can be achieved with different methods; using regular presentations, e-learning modules, focus groups, reflective discussion, videos, self-learning modules, practical demonstrations, feedback from assessment, buddy systems, task-oriented in-service training, or combinations of different methods. However, qualitative studies have showed that, although formal training is effective, promotional strategies using traditional approaches based on logic and reasoning are less likely to improve hand hygiene.[4]

In association with feedback to HCWs, senior managers, and other key players, *monitoring* compliance and other hand hygiene indicators are very important and integral parts of improvement programs. Continuous monitoring is very helpful in measuring changes induced by the interventions (e.g., ABHR consumption trends following system change) and to assess their effectiveness in improving practices, perception, and knowledge among HCWs and in reducing infections. *Feedback* of local results to HCWs is a key element to make them feel part of the campaign, reward them for improvements, and highlight remaining gaps. Indeed, a systematic review on hand hygiene promotion in neonatal intensive care units, demonstrated that studies which specifically provided performance feedback at either the individual or group levels reported a more significant improvement in compliance compared to those that did not.[13] Therefore, provision of local tangible results to senior managers contributes to awareness-raising about the importance of hand hygiene and to motivate administrators to continue to support efforts. Details on approaches and methods for hand hygiene monitoring can be found in Chapter 24. Among the core components for effective infection prevention and control programs, WHO strongly recommends hand hygiene monitoring and feedback as a key performance indicator at national level.[54,55]

Posters as *reminders* to HCWs about hand hygiene are very commonly used in improvement strategies; they can include promotional messages as well as technical principles. Studies showed the usefulness of including front-line HCWs in the development of posters to be used in their settings (see Table 19.1). With the global spread of hand hygiene campaigning, creativity and original ideas respectful of the local culture have led to interesting variations of reminders. Other types of reminders are screen savers, pocket leaflets, stickers posted at the point of care, and special labels on ABHR dispensers and gadgets (e.g., mugs, badges, T-shirts, hats, pens, book notes with hand hygiene logos). Such reminders can be important for generating a sense of ownership of the campaign by HCWs. In some campaigns, reminders have been part of more comprehensive and thoughtful communication and marketing strategies (see Table 19.1).

Hand transmission of healthcare-associated pathogens should be seen as a patient safety issue, and therefore hand hygiene improvement should be embedded in efforts to establish or improve the *"safety climate"* within the institution. In many reported experiences, the implementation of hand hygiene promotion strategies worked as the entry door for addressing patient and HCWs' safety within the healthcare facility. Building a safety climate in this context means promoting all staff awareness-raising about the harm caused by HAIs, the system's and the HCWs' responsibilities leading to poor compliance, and to motivate all players (HCWs, senior managers, as well as patients) to achieve the shared objective of hand hygiene improvement as part of a strong institutional safety climate.

Hand hygiene is an easy example around which cohesion of healthcare community key players can be achieved. The creation and maintenance of this climate is not easy and requires leadership, together with high motivation and human and financial resources, to tackle patient safety from different angles and disseminate safety principles and spirit. Strategies to achieve this goal can be actions at the group level (e.g., ward) and may include efforts to prevent high workload (i.e., downsizing and understaffing), education and performance feedback on compliance, or buddy systems (i.e., HCWs addressing each other on desirable hand hygiene behavior at the point of care). The role of *leadership* (i.e., senior staff and leaders acting as excellence models in hand hygiene performance and holding other team members accountable for it) is crucial to establish a safety climate favorable to hand hygiene best practices (see Table 19.1). Identifying and supporting hand hygiene *champions* is also an effective approach. These individuals are more than role models because they not only act as examples but also are able to work around or through organizational barriers and activate dynamics driving teams towards behavior change. They demonstrate a strong motivation and enthusiasm about the practices they promote. At the institutional level, establishing mechanisms for *rewarding* individuals or units showing excellence in hand hygiene contributed to the safety climate in some settings; conversely, others established administrative and financial *sanctions* for individuals resistant to change, but this approach is not well documented and does not appear as a positive way to promote safety. Finally, many studies and campaigns have introduced *patient participation* in hand hygiene improvement as an interesting and challenging approach within strategies to establish or strengthen safety climate. Patient participation, also referred to as "patient empowerment," consists of educational initiatives emphasizing the importance of hand hygiene in preventing the spread of pathogens and encouraging patients to remind HCWs to perform hand hygiene (see Chapter 30). Based on the available evidence from most of these investigations and summarized in systematic reviews (see Table 19.1),[14] it appears that patient participation can contribute to compliance improvement; it is an important aspect to consider in multimodal improvement strategies. However, ideally this component should not be implemented in a setting where the culture of hand hygiene promotion has not yet been created, but rather at a more advanced stage and after considering local beliefs, and social and cultural features of the local environment.

WHAT WE DO NOT KNOW – THE UNCERTAIN

As explained in the previous section, most effective approaches to achieve hand hygiene improvement are multimodal, and indeed the vast majority of studies have introduced multifaceted interventions with some common key components. Some of these strategic elements may be unnecessary in certain settings, but may be helpful in others. To establish which strategy components contribute the most to determine HCWs' behavioral change towards best practices requires further research. This is in part also related to another limitation of hand hygiene research so far, which is the quality of the evidence produced given the limited number of randomized and/or controlled trials or clinical studies, interrupted time series analyses, and cluster-randomized, stepped wedge studies (see Chapter 6). The latter could help identify the effectiveness of different strategy components by gradually introducing them at different times and controlling for confounders. Stronger study designs could also provide more solid evidence about the impact of hand hygiene promotion on the ultimate outcomes of interest represented by reduction of pathogen transmission and HAIs (see Chapter 41).

A lot of debate has been recently generated about the most appropriate and efficient methods to monitor hand hygiene (see Chapter 24). Direct observation is considered the gold standard method for monitoring compliance; however, it is quite resource- and time-consuming; it also bears some limitations. Automatic electronic methods have been proposed and are being used recently. According to the results of systematic reviews,[15] although considered as innovative and promising, the reliability, impact, and cost-effectiveness of automatic methods require further investigations before they can be recommended.

Furthermore, not only do we not know what specific strategy components may be most effective in determining successful quantitative results in specific study settings, but also we don't know how institutions succeed at implementing complex multifaceted hand hygiene improvement strategies and what the facilitation and impediment factors are. Qualitative research and studies guided by implementation science are indeed very scarce and could help responses to both questions.

In addition, although multimodal strategies are comprehensive and usually effective in stimulating behavior change and improvement of hand hygiene indicators, their complexity may raise concerns regarding their long-term sustainability. Some recent studies have demonstrated maintenance of improvement and the possibility to overcome persistent barriers through positive deviance and continuous refreshment and reinforcement. However, other studies have documented difficulties in ensuring sustained effect and clear signs of "campaign fatigue" requiring further significant efforts. Further research is needed to identify best approaches to ensure sustainability of improvement with minimal efforts.

Finally, most studies implementing interventions to improve hand hygiene indicators have been conducted in hospital settings and in specific wards (e.g., intensive care units, anesthesiology, internal medicine, pediatrics). Additional research in some priority settings such as emergency, surgical, and gynecology and obstetrics departments is needed. Although over the last few years research and implementation in outpatient settings has increased, only limited information exists about the necessary adaptation of multimodal strategies in this different context while considering different practices, rapidity of patient turnover, type of health professionals involved, facility design, and other factors.

RESEARCH AGENDA

Further research is needed to:

- Establish the relative importance of the specific components of multimodal hand hygiene improvement strategies to induce HCWs' behavioral change and practices improvement.

- Gather more reliable results about the effectiveness of hand hygiene promotion to reduce HAIs through randomized and/or controlled studies interrupted time series analyses, and cluster-randomized, stepped wedge studies.

- Identify the best approaches to adapt and most successfully implement hand hygiene in nonhospital settings.

- Develop qualitative approaches to determine how institutions succeed at implementing complex multifaceted hand hygiene improvement strategies and what the barriers and facilitators are.

- Identify best approaches to ensure sustainability of hand hygiene improvements and overcome campaign fatigue.

- Evaluate the cost-effectiveness of hand hygiene promotion strategies in different settings.

REFERENCES

1. Huis A, van Achterberg T, de Bruin M, et al., A systematic review of hand hygiene improvement strategies: a behavioural approach. *Implement Sci* 2012;**7**:92.
2. Cumbler E, Castillo L, Satorie L, et al., Culture change in infection control: applying psychological principles to improve hand hygiene. *J Nurs Care Qual* 2013;**28**:304–311.
3. De Bono S, Heling G, Borg MA, Organizational culture and its implications for infection prevention and control in healthcare institutions. *J Hosp Infect* 2014;**86**:1–6.
4. Zingg W, Holmes A, Dettenkofer M, et al., Systematic review and evidence-based guidance on organization of hospital infection control programmes (SIGHT) study group. Hospital organisation, management, and structure for prevention of health-care-associated infection: a systematic review and expert consensus. *Lancet Infect Dis* 2015;**2**:212–224. Erratum in: *Lancet Infect Dis* 2015;**3**:263.
5. World Health Organization, *WHO Guidelines on Hand Hygiene in Health Care*. Geneva: WHO, 2009. Available at www.who.int/gpsc/5may/tools/en/. Accessed March 7, 2017.
6. Pittet D, Hugonnet S, Harbarth S, et al., Effectiveness of a hospital-wide programme to improve compliance with hand hygiene. *Lancet* 2000;**356**:1307–1312.
7. Allegranzi B, Pittet D, Role of hand hygiene in healthcare-associated infection prevention. *J Hosp Infect* 2009;**73**:305–315.
8. Gould DJ, Moralejo D, Drey N, Chudleigh JH, Interventions to improve hand hygiene compliance in patient care. *Cochrane Database Syst Rev.* 2010;**9**:CD005186.
9. Luangasanatip N, Hongsuwan M, Limmathurotsakul D, et al., Comparative efficacy of interventions to promote hand hygiene in hospital. Systematic review and network meta-analysis. *Br Med J* 2015;**315**:h37281.

10. Allegranzi B, Sax H, Pittet D, Hand hygiene and healthcare system change within multi-modal promotion: a narrative review. *J Hosp Infect*. 2013;**83**(Suppl. 1):S3–S10.
11. Guide to local production: WHO-recommended handrub formulations. World Health Organization, Geneva, Switzerland, 2009. Available at www.who.int/gpsc/5may/tools/en/. Accessed March 7, 2017.
12. Mathai E, Allegranzi B, Seto WH, et al., Educating healthcare workers to optimal hand hygiene practices: addressing the need. *Infection* 2010;**38**:349–356.
13. Ofek Shlomai N, Rao S, Patole S, Efficacy of interventions to improve hand hygiene compliance in neonatal units: a systematic review and meta-analysis. *Eur J Clin Microbiol Infect Dis* 2015;**34**:887–897.
14. McGuckin M, Govednik J, Patient empowerment and hand hygiene, 1997–2012. *J Hosp Infect* 2013;**84**:191–199.
15. Ward MA, Schweizer ML, Polgreen PM, et al., Automated and electronically assisted hand hygiene monitoring systems: a systematic review. *Am J Infect Control* 2014;**42**:472–478.
16. Pittet D, Allegranzi B, Sax H, Hand hygiene. In: Jarvis WR, ed. *Bennett and Brachmann's Hospital Infections*, 6th edn. Philadelphia: Lippincott Williams & Wilkins, 2013:26–40.
17. Birnbach DJ, Nevo I, Scheinman SR, et al., Patient safety begins with proper planning: a quantitative method to improve hospital design. *Qual Saf Health Care* 2010;**19**:462–465.
18. Melles M, Erasmus V, van Loon MPM, et al., Improving hand hygiene compliance in hospitals by design. *Infect Control Hosp Epidemiol* 2013;**34**:102–104.
19. Babiarz LS, Savoie B, McGuire M, et al., Hand sanitizer-dispensing door handles increase hand hygiene compliance: a pilot study. *Am J Infect Control* 2014;**42**:443–445.
20. Koff MD, Loftus RW, Burchman CC, et al., Reduction in intraoperative bacterial contamination of peripheral intravenous tubing through the use of a novel device. *Anesthesiology* 2009;**110**:978–985.
21. Thomas BW, Berg-Copas GM, Vasquez DG, et al., Conspicuous vs customary location of hand hygiene agent dispensers on alcohol-based hand hygiene product usage in an intensive care unit. *J Am Osteopath Assoc* 2009;**109**:263–267; quiz 280–281.
22. Whitby M, McLaws ML. Handwashing in healthcare workers: accessibility of sink location does not improve compliance. *J Hosp Infect* 2004;**58**:247–253.
23. Sladek RM, Bond MJ, Phillips PA, Why don't doctors wash their hands? A correlational study of thinking styles and hand hygiene. *Am J Infect Control* 2008;**36**:399–406.
24. Thomas M, Gillespie W, Krauss J, et al., Focus group data as a tool in assessing effectiveness of a hand hygiene campaign. *Am J Infect Control* 2005;**33**:368–373.
25. Scheithauer S, Kamerseder V, Petersen P, et al., Improving hand hygiene compliance in the emergency department: getting to the point. *BMC Infect Dis* 2013;**13**:367.
26. Scheithauer S, Eitner F, Mankartz J, et al., Improving hand hygiene compliance rates in the haemodialysis setting: more than just more hand rubs. *Nephrol Dial Transplant* 2012;**27**:766–770.
27. Fuller C, Michie S, Savage J, et al., The Feedback Intervention Trial (FIT) — improving hand-hygiene compliance in UK healthcare workers: a stepped wedge cluster randomised controlled trial. *PLoS One* 2012;**7**:e41617.
28. Moongtui W, Gauthier DK, Turner JG, Using peer feedback to improve handwashing and glove usage among Thai health care workers. *Am J Infect Control* 2000;**28**:365–369.
29. Lee L, Girish S, van den Berg E, et al., Random safety audits in the neonatal unit. *Arch Dis Child Fetal Neonatal Ed* 2009;**94**:F116–119.
30. Helder OK, Weggelaar AM, Waarsenburg DCJ, et al., Computer screen saver hand hygiene information curbs a negative trend in hand hygiene behaviour. *Am J Infect Control* 2012;**40**:951–954.

31. Helder OK, Brug J, van Goudoever JB, et al., Sequential hand hygiene promotion contributes to a reduced nosocomial bloodstream infection rate among very low-birth weight infants: an interrupted time series over a 10-year period. *Am J Infect Control* 2014;**42**:718–722.

32. Kirkland KB, Homa KA, Lasky RA, et al., Impact of a hospital-wide hand hygiene initiative on healthcare-associated infections: results of an interrupted time series. *BMJ Qual Saf* 2012;**21**:1019–1026.

33. Lederer JW, Jr, Best D, Hendrix V, A comprehensive hand hygiene approach to reducing MRSA health care-associated infections. *Jt Comm J Qual Patient Saf* 2009;**35**:180–185.

34. García-Vázquez E, Murcia-Payá J, Allegue JM, et al., Influence of a multiple intervention program for hand hygiene compliance in an ICU. *Med Intensiva* 2012;**36**:69–76.

35. Uneke CJ, Ndukwe CD, Oyibo PG, et al., Promotion of hand hygiene strengthening initiative in a Nigerian teaching hospital: implication for improved patient safety in low-income health facilities. *Braz J Infect Dis* 2014;**18**:21–27.

36. Davis R, Parand A, Pinto A, et al., Systematic review of the effectiveness of strategies to encourage patients to remind healthcare professionals about their hand hygiene. *J Hosp Infect.* 2015;**89**:141–162.

37. Lieber SR, Mantengoli E, Saint S, et al., The effect of leadership on hand hygiene: assessing hand hygiene adherence prior to patient contact in 2 infectious disease units in Tuscany. *Infect Control Hosp Epidemiol* 2014;**35**:313–316.

38. Tromp M, Huis A, de Guchteneire I, et al., The short-term and long-term effectiveness of a multidisciplinary hand hygiene improvement program. *Am J Infect Control* 2012;**40**:732–736.

39. Huis A, Schoonhoven L, Grol R, et al., Impact of a team and leaders-directed strategy to improve nurses' adherence to hand hygiene guidelines: a cluster randomised trial. *Int J Nurs Stud* 2013;**50**:464–474.

40. Huis A, Hulscher M, Adang E, et al., Cost-effectiveness of a team and leaders-directed strategy to improve nurses' adherence to hand hygiene guidelines: a cluster randomised trial. *Int J Nurs Stud* 2013;**50**:518–526.

41. Aboumatar H, Ristaino P, Davis RO, et al., Infection prevention promotion program based on the PRECEDE model: improving hand hygiene behaviors among healthcare personnel. *Infect Control Hosp Epidemiol* 2012;**33**:144–151.

42. Macedo Rde C, Jacob EM, Silva VP, et al., Positive deviance: using a nurse call system to evaluate hand hygiene practices. *Am J Infect Control* 2012;**40**:946–950.

43. White CM, Statile AM, Conway PH, et al., Utilizing improvement science methods to improve physician compliance with proper hand hygiene. *Pediatrics* 2012;**129**:e1042–e1050.

44. Marra AR, Noritomi DT, Westheimer Cavalcante AJ, et al., A multicenter study using positive deviance for improving hand hygiene compliance. *Am J Infect Control* 2013;**41**:984–988.

45. dos Santos RP, Konkewicz LR, Nagel FM, et al., Changes in hand hygiene compliance after a multimodal intervention and seasonality variation. *Am J Infect Control* 2013;**41**:1012–1016.

46. Lam BC, Lee J, Lau YL, Hand hygiene practices in a neonatal intensive care unit: a multimodal intervention and impact on nosocomial infection. *Pediatrics* 2004;**114**:e565–e571.

47. Schweon SJ, Edmonds SL, Kirk J, et al., Effectiveness of a comprehensive hand hygiene program for reduction of infection rates in a long-term care facility. *Am J Infect Control* 2013;**41**:39–44.

48. Scheithauer S, Rosarius A, Rex S, et al., Improving hand hygiene compliance in the anesthesia working room work area: more than just more hand rubs. *Am J Infect Control* 2013;**41**:1001–1006.

49. Rosenthal VD, Pawar M, Leblebicioglu H, et al., Impact of the International Nosocomial Infection Control Consortium (INICC) Multidimensional Hand Hygiene Approach over 13 years in 51 cities of 19 limited-resource countries from Latin America, Asia, the Middle East, and Europe. *Infect Control Hosp Epidemiol* 2013;**34**:415–423.

50. Roberts SA, Sieczkowski C, Campbell T, et al., Auckland District Health Board Hand Hygiene Steering and Working Groups, Implementing and sustaining a hand hygiene culture change programme at Auckland District Health Board. *N Z Med J* 2012;**125**;75–85.

51. Oh E, Mohd Hamzah HB, Chain Yan C, et al., Enhancing hand hygiene in a polyclinic in Singapore. *Int J Evid Based Healthc* 2012;**10**:204–210.

52. Martín-Madrazo C, Soto-Díaz S, Cañada-Dorado A, et al., Cluster randomized trial to evaluate the effect of a multimodal hand hygiene improvement strategy in primary care. *Infect Control Hosp Epidemiol* 2012;**33**:681–688.

53. Jamal A, O'Grady G, Harnett E, et al., Improving hand hygiene in a paediatric hospital: a multimodal quality improvement approach. *BMJ Qual Saf* 2012;**21**:171–176.

54. World Health Organization, *WHO Guidelines on core components of infection prevention and control programmes at the national and acute health care facility level.* Geneva: WHO, 2016. Available at www.who.int/entity/gpsc/ipc-components-guidelines/en/index.html. Accessed March 7, 2017.

55. Storr J, Twyman A, Zingg W, et al., and the WHO Guidelines Development Group, Core components for effective infection prevention and control programmes: new WHO evidence-based recommendations. *Antimicrob Resist Infect Control* 2017;**6**:6.

Chapter 20

My Five Moments for Hand Hygiene

Hugo Sax,[1] Benedetta Allegranzi,[2] and Didier Pittet[3]

[1] Division of Infectious Diseases and Infection Control, University Hospital of Zurich, Zürich, Switzerland

[2] Infection Prevention and Control Global Unit, Department of Service Delivery and Safety, World Health Organization, and Faculty of Medicine, University of Geneva, Geneva, Switzerland

[3] Infection Control Program and WHO Collaborating Centre on Patient Safety, University of Geneva Hospitals and Faculty of Medicine, Geneva, Switzerland

KEY MESSAGES

- The My Five Moments for Hand Hygiene concept is based on indications for hand hygiene and has been designed according to the human factors principles of simplicity. It serves to facilitate understanding, training, and monitoring gold-standard hand hygiene indications in healthcare.

- The concept targets the two infectious outcomes, microbial cross-transmission and healthcare-associated infections (HAIs).

- To advance the concept further, effectiveness research is warranted including behavioral and microbiological components.

WHAT WE KNOW – THE EVIDENCE

Design Requirements and Development

Homogenous recognition of indications for hand hygiene during patient care is a prerequisite to optimal staff education, monitoring, and performance feedback. A human factors approach (see Chapter 27) inspired an iterative process at the University of Geneva Hospitals with input from specialists from multiple countries and an international expert panel of the WHO First Global Patient Safety Challenge. It resulted in the innovative design of the "My Five Moments for Hand Hygiene" concept.[1] This approach was conceived for monitoring, training, and reporting hand hygiene in healthcare.[2] Specific methodological and design requirements had to be met (Table 20.1). Furthermore, it had to be applicable across a broad range of healthcare settings,[3,4] and to reduce the need for hand cleansing actions to the minimum necessary to be microbiologically effective.[5]

The Concept Explained: From Pathophysiology to Hand Hygiene Indications

Hands are considered the main vehicle of cross-transmission, while the main sources for transmission are the healthcare environment and colonized or infected patients. Two infectious patient outcomes are targeted for prevention by hand hygiene: microbial spread through cross-transmission and HAIs. Cross-transmission occurs when a vehicle (e.g., a hand) picks up bacteria from one surface and deposits them on another (see Chapter 4). Thus, to determine and describe relevant indications for hand hygiene, both surfaces need to be considered.

The Patient Zone and Critical Body Sites, Two Central Elements

Hand hygiene indications are closely related to the patient zone concept. The patient zone includes the patient, the area around the patient, and some surfaces and items (e.g., his/her bed, associated furniture and equipment) that are temporarily and exclusively dedicated to him/her.[1,2,4,5] These inanimate surfaces and items in direct physical contact with the patient and frequently touched by the patient and the healthcare worker (HCW) (for instance bed rails, bedside table, bed linen, medical equipment, monitors, knobs and buttons, etc.) become progressively colonized with the patient's own flora. The patient zone is the central element of the My Five Moments for Hand Hygiene concept. To establish the patient zone for each clinical setting is an important step in customizing the general concept to the specific local conditions. To foster a salient mental model, the patient zone may be imagined as a virtual "bubble" surrounding each patient and allowing only clean hands to cross its surface. The patient zone is not a static geographical area, but the area surrounding the patient and including him/her at any point in time. The model is not limited to a bedridden patient, but applies equally to patients sitting in a chair or being treated by physiotherapists in a common treatment location.[4] As a consequence, the concept of "My Five Moments" applies also to situations that define a "temporary" patient zone. The patient zone may also

Table 20.1 Design Requirements for a High-Usability Hand Hygiene Indication Concept

Issue	Explanation	Realization
High microbiological effect	The chosen indications for hand hygiene should prevent distinct infectious outcomes, i.e., microbial transmission including antibiotic-resistant pathogens, and HAI	In line with an evidence-based model for transmission;[5] consensus of a group of infection preventionists, epidemiologists, and microbiologists (WHO expert group; Swissnoso)
Minimal density	The chosen indications for hand hygiene should result in as few hand hygiene opportunities per time unit as possible	Bundling of indications in opportunities when the former overlap
Minimal effort for education	The concept should be easy to minimize expenditure for education and training	Simplicity and design of the concept helps to achieve this requirement (see further issues below)
Easy to understand	The concept should benefit from simplicity, from a reduced number of items to be remembered, helped by symmetry and chunking	The reduced number of items and symmetry helps understanding and remembering each indication for hand hygiene
Highly intuitive	The concept should take advantage of the intrinsic motivation for hand hygiene cleaning such as learned in early childhood, and general principles of hygiene and disgust	Intrinsic hand hygiene has an element of cleaning hands before performing a "clean" task (e.g., eating) and again after a dirty task (e.g., toileting). Fluids have a special place in the representation
Rich in cues to action	The concept should benefit from cues to action such as geographical dislocation	Especially indications 1, 4, and 5 benefit from geographical dislocation. Indications 2 and 3 are more challenging, since they have to be integrated in a complex workflow by anticipation of upcoming steps in the overall task
Meaningful for reporting	The data generated from observations should present enough detail to make sense for practical risk-analysis and to be meaningful for a performance improvement initiative	The concept distinguishes indications linked to transmission of multiresistant organisms and infection; it also distinguishes risk for the patient from risk for the healthcare worker

Table 20.1   (*Continued*)

Issue	Explanation	Realization
Patient centeredness	The concept should be centered on patient safety without ignoring HCW safety	This requirement was supported through the Five Moments pictogram
Stickiness	Based on insights from the realm of diffusion of innovation and social marketing, the concept should present itself in a way that sticks easily to memory	The My Five Moments name tag; the fact that the number corresponds to the five fingers of a hand certainly helped the successful global diffusion

vary considerably according to the setting, length of stay, and type of delivered care (see Chapters 42A,B,C,D,E, and F).

Once within the patient zone, hand hygiene should be performed only at critical moments. Identifying the patient's "critical body sites" is key to understanding when hand hygiene moments apply because they are associated with the risk of infection. "Critical sites" correspond to body sites or to medical devices that either have to be protected against microorganisms (*critical sites with infectious risk for the patient*), or potentially lead to hand exposure to body fluids and blood-borne pathogens (*critical sites with body fluid exposure risk*). Two of the five moments for hand hygiene occur before contact with the patient (Moment 1) and before a clean/aseptic procedure (Moment 2); the other three occur after body fluid exposure risk (Moment 3), contact with the patient (Moment 4), or the patient's surroundings (Moment 5) (Figure 20.1). Indications corresponding to the "before" moments prevent the risk of microbial transmission to the *patient*. The "after" indications prevent the risk of microbial transmission to the *healthcare worker* and the *healthcare area* (i.e., other patients, their surroundings, and the healthcare environment). More details on the five moments with their potential infectious outcomes and practical examples are provided in Table 20.2.

Moments during healthcare activities when hand hygiene is necessary to interrupt germ transmission by hands are defined as opportunities. Each opportunity requires one hand hygiene action. However, several indications for hand hygiene can arise at the same time (e.g., when walking directly from one patient to the next).[4]

The My Five Moments Image (Figures 20.1 and 20.2) has become a trademark for hand hygiene promotion and has undergone unprecedented viral spread worldwide. This image was designed according to human factors principles of intuitive understanding (see Chapter 27). In the Figure, the infusion and its vascular access represent a clean critical body site, whereas the urinary drainage represents the potential exposure to body fluids. Both point to breaks in skin and mucous membrane barriers. Both are associated with fluids, and appeal to basic

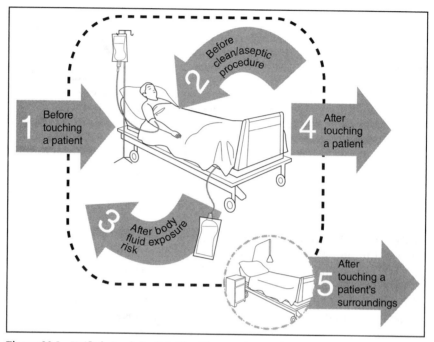

Figure 20.1 Unified visuals for "My Five Moments for Hand Hygiene". *Source*: Reproduced with permission from the World Health Organization. *See plate section for color representation of this figure.*

human notions of risk and inherent hand hygiene behavior (see Chapter 18): "clean" entering the patient's body, that is, a risk for the patient, and "dirty" coming from the patient's body, that is, a risk for the healthcare worker. The curved arrows within the patient zone underpin the need for hand hygiene within the patient zone when dealing with critical body sites.

The title "My Five Moments for Hand Hygiene," alluding to the five fingers of a hand and reinforcing the concept of ownership, was chosen for its "stickiness," a marketing feature (see Chapter 26) to facilitate its diffusion. Importantly, the central cartoon-like drawing has been adapted to specific settings and care situations (see Chapters 42C, 42D and 42E).

WHAT WE DO NOT KNOW – THE UNCERTAIN

My Five Moments for Hand Hygiene has been universally adopted without comparative effectiveness research. Hence, it remains unknown if alternative concepts would have a greater impact on patient safety. Yet, such effectiveness research would be very challenging.

Table 20.2 Five Moments Indications

Indication Term for Hand Hygiene	Donor Surface	Hand Transition and Microorganism Transmission Risk	Receptor Surface	Major Targeted Negative Infectious Outcome	Examples
(1) Before touching a patient	Surface outside the patient zone	Hand transmission of microorganisms from the healthcare environment to the patient	Patient's intact skin and other surfaces inside the patient zone	Colonization of the patient by hospital pathogens	Touching the door handle and then shaking hands with the patient
(2) Before aseptic/clean procedure	Any surface	Hand transmission of microorganisms from any surface (including the patient's skin) to a site that would facilitate invasion and infection	Critical site for infection in the patient	Endogenous or exogenous infection of the patient	Preparing the material and then giving an injection
(3) After body fluid exposure risk	Critical site for body fluid exposure in HCWs	Hand exposure to patient's body fluids potentially containing blood-borne or other pathogens	Any surface	Infection of the HCW by patient blood-borne pathogens	Drawing blood and then adjusting the infusion drop count
(4) After touching a patient	Patient's intact skin and other surfaces inside the patient zone	Hand transmission of microorganisms from the patient flora to other surfaces in the healthcare setting	Surface outside the patient zone	Dissemination of patient flora to the rest of the healthcare environment and infection of HCWs	Shaking hands with the patient, arranging the bedside table, and then touching the door handle
(5) After touching patient surroundings (without touching the patient during the same care sequence)	Surface inside the patient zone if the patient was not touched	Hand transmission of microorganisms from the patient flora to other surfaces in the healthcare setting	Surface outside the patient zone	Dissemination of patient flora to the rest of the healthcare environment and colonization of HCWs	Touching the bed rail (without touching the patient) and then touching the door handle

Source: Reproduced with permission from the World Health Organization.

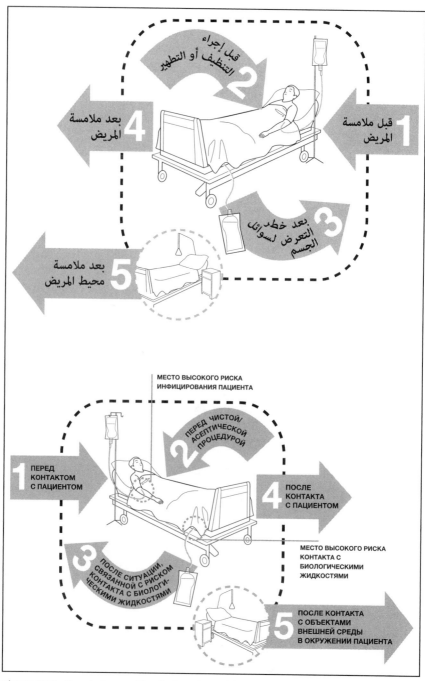

Figure 20.2 Translations and local adaptations of the "My Five Moments for Hand Hygiene" visual. *Source*: Reproduced with permission from the World Health Organization. *See plate section for color representation of this figure.*

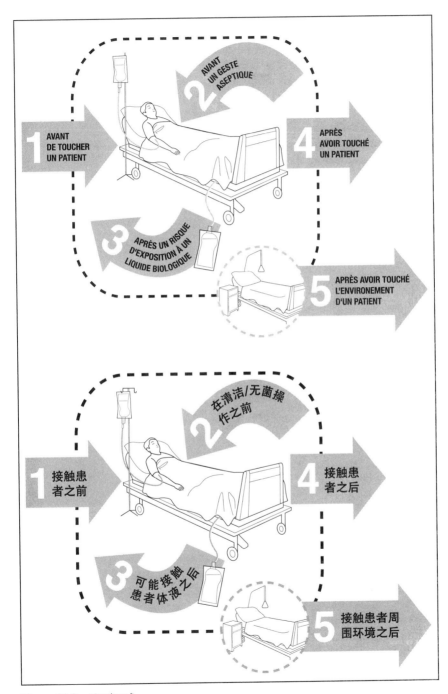

Figure 20.2   (*Continued*)

The large number of quasi-experimental studies published since 2000 (see Chapter 41) demonstrates the impact of improved hand hygiene following the implementation of the WHO multimodal strategy (including the use of the My Five Moments for Hand Hygiene).[6] It may well be that a simpler concept that would be less challenging to teach and survey and, consequently, to be adopted by HCWs, may increase overall patient safety, even if not fully covering all infectious risks. Furthermore, the transmission model on which the Five Moments are based[5] is not supported by research in every detail. Finally, the relative importance of each of the five moments to prevent microbial transmission and infection outcomes is unknown.

RESEARCH AGENDA

The following questions would add to the understanding and potential improvement of conceptualizing hand hygiene indications:

- To what extent is infectious risk harbored in specific steps in the care process, qualitatively and quantitatively, and how does this relate to hand hygiene?
- What is the contribution of each of the five moments to specific infectious outcomes and etiologies?
- Would any simplification of the My Five Moments concept be suitable?
- What alternative hand hygiene concepts could improve overall effectiveness on patient outcome?

Such research might be supported by and integrated in an overarching concept based on system level approach to infectious risks during patient care.[7]

REFERENCES

1. Sax H, Allegranzi B, Uckay I, et al., "My Five Moments for Hand Hygiene": a user-centred design approach to understand, train, monitor and report hand hygiene. *J Hosp Infect* 2007;**67**:9–21.
2. Sax H, Allegranzi B, Chraïti M-N, et al., The World Health Organization hand hygiene observation method. *Am J Infect Control* 2009;**37**:827–834.
3. Allegranzi B, Sax H, Bengaly L, et al., Successful implementation of the World Health Organization hand hygiene improvement strategy in a referral hospital in Mali, Africa. *Infect Control Hosp Epidemiol* 2010;**31**:133–141.
4. World Health Organization, *WHO Hand hygiene in outpatient and home-based care and long-term care facilities: a guide to the application of the WHO multimodal hand hygiene improvement strategy and the "My Five Moments for Hand Hygiene" approach.* Geneva: WHO, 2012.
5. Pittet D, Allegranzi B, Sax H, et al., Evidence-based model for hand transmission during patient care and the role of improved practices. *Lancet Infect Dis* 2006;**6**:641–652.

6. Allegranzi B, Gayet-Ageron A, Damani N, et al., Global implementation of WHO's multimodal strategy for improvement of hand hygiene: a quasi-experimental study. *Lancet* 2013;**13**:843–851.
7. Clack L, Schmutz J, Manser T, et al., Infectious risk moments – a novel, human factors-informed approach to infection prevention. *Infect Control Hosp Epidemiol* 2014;**35**:1051–1055.

Chapter 21

System Change

Benedetta Allegranzi,[1] Andreas Voss,[2] and Didier Pittet[3]

[1] *Infection Prevention and Control Global Unit, Department of Service Delivery and Safety, World Health Organization, and Faculty of Medicine, University of Geneva, Geneva, Switzerland*

[2] *Radboud University Medical Centre and Canisius-Wilhelmina Hospital, Nijmegen, The Netherlands*

[3] *Infection Control Program and WHO Collaborating Centre on Patient Safety, University of Geneva Hospitals and Faculty of Medicine, Geneva, Switzerland*

KEY MESSAGES

- System change, defined as a range of targeted actions aimed at making hand hygiene practices feasible by ensuring that the necessary infrastructure is in place, is essential to improve hand hygiene in healthcare. In particular, access to alcohol-based handrubs (ABHRs) enables appropriate and timely hand hygiene performance at the point of care.

- The feasibility and effect of system change within multimodal strategies to improve hand hygiene compliance and contribute to healthcare-associated infection (HAI) reduction have been demonstrated both at institutional level and at larger scale (nationwide).

- Implementation research and political actions to achieve broader availability of ABHRs are needed to overcome their limited access especially in developing countries. The local production of the World Health Organization (WHO) formulations is a feasible and low-cost alternative that yet requires improvements and more dissemination.

With regards to hand hygiene improvement strategies, "system change" refers to actions aimed at making hand hygiene practices feasible during healthcare delivery by ensuring that the necessary infrastructure is in place. This is achieved by making ABHRs readily accessible at the point of care, and in some settings around the world also ensuring access to safe, continuous water supply, as well as to soap and

Hand Hygiene: A Handbook for Medical Professionals, First Edition.
Edited by Didier Pittet, John M. Boyce and Benedetta Allegranzi.
© 2017 John Wiley & Sons, Inc. Published 2017 by John Wiley & Sons, Inc.

disposable towels.[1] However, the current use of the term "system change" usually focuses on the preferred recourse to ABHRs with subsequent implementation of actions to make it possible. Although this is one of the key elements enabling change within modern approaches to hand hygiene improvement, the recourse to a hand scrubbing solution was implemented for the first time by Semmelweiss back in the nineteenth century (see Chapter 2). Currently available ABHRs are the most efficacious and the best tolerated products for hand hygiene in healthcare, and system change leads to improvement of practices, especially when embedded within multimodal strategies.

WHAT WE KNOW – THE EVIDENCE

System change is one of the five key elements of the WHO multimodal hand hygiene improvement strategy and is based on the evidence of many studies.[1] At the basis of system change is the evidence that ABHRs have the following key advantages:[1]

1. Elimination of the large majority of germs (including viruses)
2. Short time required for action (15 to 30 seconds)
3. Availability and use at the point of care
4. Better skin tolerability
5. No need for any particular infrastructure

Most of these advantages overcome objective obstacles to hand hygiene performance as well as subjective reasons reported by healthcare workers (HCWs) that result in low hand hygiene compliance, such as lack of adequate agents for hand hygiene, lack of sinks and dispensers or their inconvenient location, lack of time, especially in settings with a high intensity of care, and skin damage caused by some hand hygiene products (see Chapters 11 and 12).

The results of in vivo efficacy studies have shown that ABHRs are more efficacious than antiseptic or plain soaps (see Chapter 8). Both the high- and broad-spectrum efficacy of ABHRs (see Chapter 8) justify system change and their preferred use as a key tool for system change.[1]

Based on the European Standard EN1500, efficacy of hand antisepsis is achieved by rubbing hands with an ABHR for 20–30 seconds; in contrast, the time to achieve efficacy with handwashing with soap and water increases to 40–60 seconds (see Chapter 10). The shorter duration of application together with the immediate availability at the point of care allow HCWs to minimize time dedicated to hand hygiene. Using ABHRs saves time by avoiding movements between the point of care and the sink. Indeed, key indications for hand hygiene performance, identified by WHO in five moments[1] (see Chapter 20) are typically actions to be performed in the patient zone or its surroundings. If ABHRs are available at the point of care through pocket bottles or dispensers placed on the cart or hung on the wall or the bed rail, they offer the advantage of avoiding the need for any particular infrastructure (clean water supply network, washbasin, plumbing, soap, hand towel). This can be a significant asset considering that sinks are often far from the point of care or that the infrastructure can be deficient at multiple levels (e.g., lack of running water supplies in remote areas in developing countries).

Although the frequent performance of hand hygiene actions may lead to some adverse events that need to be prevented, numerous reports confirm that ABHRs are associated with better acceptability and tolerance than other products (see Chapter 15), mainly because they contain humectants. The results of a recent multicenter investigation based on 1932 assessments showed that traditional handwashing is a risk factor for dryness and irritation.[2]

All these specific technical reasons why ABHRs should be preferred to soap and water are at the basis of the success of strategies that have led to hand hygiene performance improvement. System change represented by the introduction of ABHRs has revolutionized the approach to hand hygiene promotion. Some early studies demonstrated an immediate significant effect of simply introducing ABHRs can achieve an increase of hand hygiene compliance and reduction of HAIs (see Chapter 41).

More recently, it became evident that satisfactory and sustainable behavioral change is better achieved by multimodal strategies that integrate system change in a broader approach mainly including HCWs' education, hand hygiene indicators, monitoring and performance feedback, reminders in the work place, and improvement of the institutional patient safety climate. Indeed, successful implementation of system change at the healthcare facility level cannot be achieved without staff education about hand transmission and understanding of the advantages of ABHRs to achieve hand hygiene best practices. Furthermore, the commitment of administrators to the continuous procurement of ABHRs and the provision of an appropriate infrastructure for optimal hand hygiene is essential for the long-term sustainability of the results achieved through system change.

The procurement of ABHRs is the critical element of system change. WHO identified precise criteria to take into consideration when selecting ABHR agents at the healthcare facility level for initial procurement, but also for reconsidering adequacy of available products (Table 21.1).[3]

In developing countries, system change can have an even greater impact than in well-resourced settings because of the inadequacy of infrastructure for handwashing. In settings with limited access to water and soap and deficient infrastructure, system change should also involve actions to improve these gaps; thus hand hygiene campaigns can contribute to the improvement of facilities that are useful to improve healthcare delivery and enable best practices in a broader perspective (see Chapter 43). Significant constraints on the introduction of ABHRs can be encountered in developing countries because these products are scarce, and their cost can be even higher than in industrialized countries, rendering them unaffordable. To overcome this problem and facilitate the development of a global approach to hand hygiene improvement in healthcare, WHO proposes the local production

Table 21.1 Criteria for the Selection of Alcohol-Based Handrubs (ABHRs)

Proven efficacy according to ASTM or EN standards for hygienic hand antisepsis
and/or surgical hand preparation

Tested and proven good dermal tolerance

Minimum drying time

Costs of purchase or local production (including raw ingredients, salaries of
dedicated staff, and dispensers)

Aesthetic preferences of HCWs (e.g., fragrance, color, texture, "stickiness," and ease
of use)

Availability, convenience and functioning of dispensers

Ability to prevent microbial contamination

Source: Allegranzi 2013. Reproduced with permission from Elsevier.
ASTM, American Society for Testing and Materials; EN, European Norms.

of two alcohol-based formulations, the antimicrobial efficacy and skin tolerability of which were tested for use for hand antisepsis.[2] Formula improvement is being made for increasing efficacy of the surgical hand preparation. Local production of these formulations was evaluated in 39 sites in 28 countries worldwide with feasibility demonstration in all sites; 54% of sites had already undertaken system change but opted for the local production to replace a previously used ABHR.[5] In 32 sites (82%) the product was well tolerated and accepted by HCWs; the cost was on average USD 1.4 (range: 0.3–4.5) and 0.8 (range: 0.1–1.3) per 100 mL, for the ethanol- and isopropanol-based formulations, respectively.

If ABHRs are already available at the healthcare facility, this does not mean that system change is entirely achieved. In these settings, the focus should be on evaluating if the type of dispensers used and their location ensure appropriateness and ease of access, as well as on monitoring the actual use and acceptance of the agent by HCWs. In specific situations, handwashing is still necessary; therefore, availability of an adequate number of sinks continuously equipped with soap and disposable towels should be ensured. The selection of dispensers according to user-friendliness, facility logistics, and their best ergonomic location, including their good maintenance, are prerequisites to sustain system change. When feasible, the different types of ABHR dispensers (e.g., wall-mounted, bottles placed at the point of care, pocket bottles) should be used in combination to achieve maximum compliance (Figure 21.1). In addition to procurement of ABHR, the integration of dispensing solutions within the patient zone and the selection of dispenser designs that optimize acceptance and usage were identified as being among the key actions to put in place in order to facilitate hand hygiene behavioral change at the point of care.[6]

The implementation of system change can be evaluated through key indicators such as infrastructure in place (ABHR dispenser and sink design and accessibility at the point of care), acceptability and tolerability, and volume of hand hygiene agents used by HCWs. A tool consisting of specific questions and a

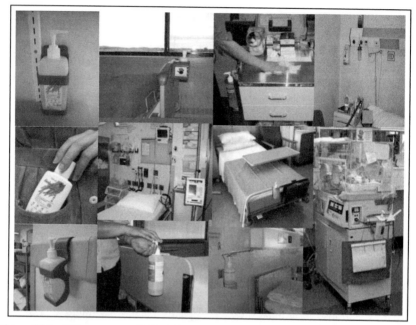

Figure 21.1 Different types of ABHR dispensers. *See plate section for color representation of this figure.*

grid for collecting data on structures and resources in place for hand hygiene at ward level has been developed and made available by WHO.[7] Other investigators have also tested and proposed tools for hand hygiene infrastructure audits. [13,14]

The focus on the preferred recourse to ABHRs within multimodal strategies offers another opportunity: to use ABHR consumption as a surrogate marker for monitoring hand hygiene performance (see Chapter 24). ABHR consumption is usually calculated in litres per 1000 patient-days, and the quantity of product can be translated into estimates of the number of hand hygiene actions by using the average volume used per action as a divider. This information is usually regularly available at the facility level; a WHO tool can help to track ABHR and soap consumption.[8] Another tool has been recently proposed to systematically evaluate the hand hygiene needs in diverse care settings and to estimate the volume of ABHR required for a hand hygiene program.[15]

Several studies have investigated the relation between hand hygiene product consumption and HAI, in particular methicillin-resistant *Staphylococcus aureus* (MRSA) bacteraemia, mostly through time series analysis. In 2010, Sroka and colleagues published a review pooling the results of several studies, which demonstrated that an increase in ABHR consumption significantly correlated with a reduction of MRSA bacteraemia or the incidence of MRSA clinical isolates.[9] More recently, the effect of system change on HAI demonstrated by increased consumption of ABHR in the context of hand hygiene campaigns was reported in several important multicenter studies. In 35 French acute care hospitals ABHR consumption increased from 2 to 21 liters/1000 hospital days in parallel with a significant decrease of MRSA infections.[10] The same temporal association was observed by Stone and colleagues during the roll-out of the "Clean Your Hands" campaign in England and Wales;[11] in the last four quarters of the study, increased procurement of ABHR was independently associated with reduced MRSA bacteremia. Association between significant increase of ABHR consumption over time and reduction of central line-associated bloodstream infection was also reported in a network of ICUs in Colombia.[12]

Feasibility of system change has been shown not only at facility level in many studies[1] but also at the national level. According to information available to WHO, at least 50 campaigns have been launched worldwide at national or subnational level; of these, 46 (92%) have promoted system change on a large scale as the core element of multimodal improvement strategies (see Chapter 36). A global approach to the promotion of ABHR use must also consider cultural and religious concerns raised by some HCWs related to alcohol-containing agents. However, very positive ways of overcoming these barriers are proposed through successful experiences facilitated by WHO in Muslim countries (see Chapter 31).

WHAT WE DO NOT KNOW – THE UNCERTAIN

System change is usually implemented in the context of multimodal hand hygiene improvement strategies that include several components. Its importance to enable behavioral change is indisputable. However, good quality studies assessing the relative impact of system change in the context of multimodal strategies are not available. In addition, recent multimodal approaches have encouraged patient involvement in system change by promoting ABHR usage also among patients, families, and visitors (see Chapter 30). The advantages and potential unintended consequences of this approach should be further investigated.

More research to identify systematic approaches to achieve improvement of ergonomics of system change is needed to optimize the hand hygiene infrastructure both in settings that decide to introduce ABHRs and in facilities where system change is already in place.

More studies are needed to document the cost-effectiveness of ABHR introduction in the context of hand hygiene campaigns in different settings. Available data are still limited but show a great benefit; more solid business case demonstrations in a range of different settings would significantly help convince managers to implement and sustain system change.

Achieving widespread availability of ABHRs worldwide would facilitate substantial behavioral change and enable best hand hygiene practices especially in settings where infection control gaps are many. Limited market coverage, distribution constraints, unaffordable costs, and lack of HCW education hamper system change in developing countries. There is a need for identifying mechanisms to overcome these obstacles and stimulate the private sector to expand market coverage at fair prices. In the context of quality improvement health systems should also be encouraged to prioritize the procurement of ABHRs among essential products.

ABHR local production according to the WHO-recommended formula can be a suitable solution. Although many settings have undertaken local production even at large or national scale by either private companies or governmental factories, this approach has limitations that require advancement and further research.[4] The efficacy of the WHO formulations for use in surgery should be improved; formula modifications have already been identified[16] and should be further clinically tested and evaluated for skin tolerability and HCWs' acceptably. Suitable humectants other than glycerol should be identified because it has been found to influence efficacy, and procurement difficulties have hampered continuity of local production in some countries; formulations including different humectants should then be tested for efficacy and tolerability. Furthermore, sustainable strategies to overcome obstacles in the procurement of ingredients and dispensers should be identified through partnerships, market competition, and other mechanisms. Finally, more data are needed to assess the overall costs of local production, including ingredients, dispensers, and salary and distribution costs, and to compare with local costs of commercially available products.

RESEARCH AGENDA

Further research is needed to enable and improve system change in the context of multimodal hand hygiene improvement strategies. Key research questions are:

- What are the best approaches to facilitate implementation of system change in the context of multimodal strategies?
- What is the relative impact of system change to hand hygiene compliance increase and HAI reduction in the context of multimodal strategies?
- What are the best approaches to improve dispensers' and hand hygiene facilities' location in the healthcare setting?
- Does ABHR usage among patients, families, and visitors contribute to improve HCWs' hand hygiene practices? Are there any unintended consequences of this approach?
- What is the cost-effectiveness of ABHR introduction in the context of hand hygiene campaigns in different settings?
- What are the efficacy, skin tolerability, and HCWs' acceptance of modified WHO formulations?
- What are the best mechanisms and approaches to achieve widespread availability of ABHRs worldwide?

REFERENCES

1. World Health Organization, *WHO Guidelines on Hand Hygiene in Health Care*. Geneva: WHO, 2009.
2. Chamorey E, Marcy P, Dandine M, et al., A prospective multicenter study evaluating skin tolerance to standard hand hygiene techniques. *Am J Infect Control* 2011;**39**:6–13.
3. World Health Organization, *Alcohol-based handrub planning and costing tool*. Geneva: WHO, 2010.
4. Allegranzi B, Sax H, Pittet D. Hand hygiene and healthcare system change within multi-modal promotion: a narrative review. *J Hosp Infect* 2013;**83**:S3–10.
5. Bauer Savage J, Pittet D, Kim EU, et al., Local production of WHO-recommended alcohol-based handrubs: feasibility, advantages, barriers and costs. *Bull World Health Organ* 2013;**91**:963–969.
6. Kendall A, Landers T, Kirk J, et al., Point-of-care hand hygiene: preventing infection behind the curtain. *Am J Infect Control* 2012;**40**:S3–S10.
7. Ward infrastructure survey. Geneva: WHO, 2010.
8. Soap/handrub consumption survey: measuring the consumption of products in association with the implementation of the WHO multimodal hand hygiene improvement strategy. Geneva: WHO, 2009.
9. Sroka S, Gastmeier P, Meyer E, Impact of alcohol hand-rub use on methicillin-resistant Staphylococcus aureus: an analysis of the literature. *J Hosp Infect* 2010;**74**:204–211.
10. Jarlier V, Trystram D, Brun-Buisson C, et al., Curbing methicillin-resistant Staphylococcus aureus in 38 French hospitals through a 15-year institutional control program. *Arch Intern Med* 2010;**170**:552–559.
11. Stone SP, Fuller C, Savage J, et al., Evaluation of the national Clean Your Hands campaign to reduce *Staphylococcus aureus* bacteraemia and *Clostridium difficile* infection in hospitals in England and Wales by improved hand hygiene: four year, prospective, ecological, interrupted time series study. *Br Med J* 2012;**344**:e3005.
12. Barrera L, Zingg W, Mendez F, et al., Effectiveness of a hand hygiene promotion strategy using alcohol-based handrub in 6 intensive care units in Colombia. *Am J Infect Control* 2011;**39**:633–639.
13. Caniza MA, Duenas L, Lopez B, et al., A practical guide to alcohol-based hand hygiene infrastructure in a resource-poor pediatric hospital. *Am J Infect Control* 2009;**37**:851–854.
14. Ahmed K, Audit of hand hygiene at Broadmoor, a high secure psychiatric hospital. *J Hosp Infect* 2010;**75**:128–131.
15. Sicoli S, Hunter L, Shymanski J, et al., Estimating the volume of alcohol-based hand rub required for a hand hygiene program. *Am J Infect Control* 2012;**40**:810–814.
16. Suchomel M, Kundi M, Pittet D, et al., Modified World Health Organization hand rub formulations comply with European efficacy requirements for preoperative surgical hand preparations. *Infect Control Hosp Epidemiol* 2013;**34**:245–250.

Chapter 22

Education of Healthcare Professionals

Elaine Larson,[1] Marie-Noëlle Chraïti,[2] and Wing-Hong Seto[3]

[1] *Columbia University School of Nursing, New York, USA*
[2] *Infection Control Program and WHO Collaborating Centre on Patient Safety, University of Geneva Hospitals, Geneva, Switzerland*
[3] *World Health Organization Collaborating Centre for Infectious Disease, Epidemiology and Control, School of Public Health, The University of Hong Kong, Hong Kong, S.A.R., China*

KEY MESSAGES

- Simplistic, single strategy educational interventions such as an "in-service" program are ineffective.

- Multimodal, institution-wide interventions that include staff education as well as explicit, positive support from leaders show promise for effecting sustained improvement in hand hygiene practices.

- Specific, individual and target-oriented educational strategies to improve hand hygiene adherence are poorly understood and have not been identified.

WHAT WE KNOW – THE EVIDENCE

Of all aspects of hand hygiene, perhaps the most frequently studied over the past five years has been the behavior of healthcare professionals and the impact of education on their hand hygiene practices. In fact, education is a fundamental component of any intervention to improve hand hygiene. This attention is likely a result of increasing recognition that even with the availability of sufficient resources and supplies and excellent products, hand hygiene is dependent on adherence of

Hand Hygiene: A Handbook for Medical Professionals, First Edition.
Edited by Didier Pittet, John M. Boyce and Benedetta Allegranzi.
© 2017 John Wiley & Sons, Inc. Published 2017 by John Wiley & Sons, Inc.

individual clinicians. Additionally, there has been the growing evidence that basic knowledge about infection prevention and control concepts and hand hygiene is still usually poor among healthcare workers (HCWs). This is true for both high-income and developing countries, but particularly relevant for the latter. That being the case, it is important to understand how and why hand hygiene behavior changes among staff and how education might play a part in adherence.

Simplistic, single-unit interventions or traditional in-service education regarding hand hygiene have little, if any, impact on staff behavior and such simple interventions have, for the most part, disappeared in the recent literature. Between 2011 and 2013 at least 10 institution-wide studies using multimodal strategies to improve hand hygiene as recommended in the WHO Guidelines for Hand Hygiene in Health Care[1] have been published, generally with positive results. Strategies reported to be effective include a combination of strong leadership, use of "positive deviants" and role models, staff monitoring, performance feedback, use of workflow diagrams, education, and marketing campaigns.

In addition to the multifaceted approaches used in the majority of successful interventions published, an important recent trend has been a movement away from short-term interventions on single units or in single institutions toward recognition that the larger system in which staff work is likely to have a major impact on practice. Hence, recent interventions to improve hand hygiene more often focus on entire institutions, organizational units, or regions rather than on individual units. In fact, there have been a number of major nationwide campaigns and international efforts[1] to improve hand hygiene – in Canada, the United Kingdom, Australia, Belgium, Germany, and through the International Nosocomial Infection Control Consortium (see Chapter 35). Each of these campaigns, which make education a key component, has been associated with widespread sustained improvements in hand hygiene and, in some cases, reduced rates of certain healthcare-associated infections.[2–5]

Based on what has been learned over the past decade about education and hand hygiene, the following conclusions can be made. First, educational strategies need to be just one component of a larger effort that includes other activities such as audit and feedback, marketing, or other change interventions. Second, education should be planned using theoretical underpinnings regarding what motivates behavior and facilitates sustainable change. Third, in addition to basic educational programs targeted at individuals, interventions may be more effective at the larger systems level because the organizational culture in which one works has a profound effect on hand hygiene expectations.

Recent evidence has also confirmed that an essential component of successful educational programs is a strong and positive leader. Educational interventions with sustained impact generally describe the importance of team leaders and "positive deviants" (individuals who are role models for hand hygiene) as part of organizational improvement strategies. Huis et al. in the Netherlands have taken a particularly rigorous and thoughtful approach in a randomized clinical trial in 67 clinical units in 3 hospitals. They compared a strategy that included the traditional multimodal interventions (education, feedback, reminders) with the same interventions supplemented by involvement of staff teams and leaders using social influence and leadership theory. Based on more than 10,000 hand hygiene opportunities among 2,733 nurses, the strategy which included social influence was about 1.6 times more effective at increasing hand hygiene over a 6-month time period.[6,7] Clearly, explicit and positive leadership is vital to any educational program (see also Chapter 40).

WHAT WE DO NOT KNOW – THE UNCERTAIN

A systematic review published in 2010 found only four studies of interventions to improve hand hygiene among healthcare professionals that met rigorous quality standards.[8] The authors concluded that even though multimodal campaigns seem to have a positive effect, the data are of insufficient quality to reach an unequivocal conclusion. Similarly, Cherry et al.[9] examined almost 9,000 articles regarding educational interventions to improve hand hygiene compliance and found that it was not possible to identify which education strategies were effective because of the variations in the interventions themselves. Further, in general only interventions that report positive results have been published, indicating a strong publication bias. It is unclear exactly what specific educational interventions are likely to be most effective in improving staff hand hygiene practices, and how such interventions are best implemented and disseminated.

Because large campaigns are expensive, it is important to sort out which specific elements are essential for change and whether, in the long term, behavior changes and the organizational culture for such changes are sustained. This is not at all unusual, for promotional fatigue is a phenomenon described in social marketing. While some strategies have been suggested to minimize this phenomenon, it is not clear how often and at what points in time this is likely to occur and what approaches are most successful to avoid it.

Finally, there is little understanding of the basic mechanisms for why an educational intervention works or not. For example, Mortell[10] has suggested a possible theory-practice-ethics gap that might explain hand hygiene behavior. We have only minimal insight into why education, that is, acquisition of knowledge, is often insufficient to change hand hygiene behaviors.

The work of Huis et al.[11] has been based on a solid theoretical foundation and is an example of the types of studies needed to move beyond the simplistic educational and ineffective strategies of the past.

RESEARCH AGENDA

Based on these gaps in our knowledge, a research agenda should include rigorous clinical trials of educational strategies that make it possible to sort out the components that are most effective in the short term as well as the long term, and whether there are differences across settings (e.g., acute care, long-term care, home health) and across healthcare professional categories. Additionally, research is needed to assess the potential impact of hand hygiene education in the basic curriculum of healthcare professionals to determine whether education during training will be more effective or sustainable.

REFERENCES

1. World Health Organization, *WHO Guidelines for Hand Hygiene in Health Care*. Geneva: WHO, 2009. Available at whqlibdoc.who.int/publications/2009/9789241597906_eng.pdf. Accessed March 7, 2017.
2. Grayson ML, Russo PL, Cruickshank M, et al., Outcomes from the first 2 years of the Australian National Hand Hygiene Initiative. *Med J Aust* 2011;**195**:615–619.
3. Reichardt C, Königer D, Bunte-Schönberger K, et al., Three years of national hand hygiene campaign in Germany: what are the key conclusions for clinical practice? *J Hosp Infect* 2013;**83**(Suppl. 1):S11–S16.
4. Stone SP, Fuller C, Savage J, et al., Evaluation of the national Clean Your Hands campaign to reduce Staphylococcus aureus bacteraemia and Clostridium difficile infection in hospitals in England and Wales by improved hand hygiene: four year, prospective, ecological, interrupted time series study. *Br Med J* 2012;**344**:e3005.
5. Rosenthal VD, Pawer M, Leblebicioglu H, et al., Impact of the International Nosocomial Infection Control Consortium (INICC) Multidimensional Hand Hygiene Approach over 13 years in 51 cities of 19 limited-resource countries from Latin America, Asia, the Middle East, and Europe. *Infect Control Hosp Epidemiol*, 2013;**34**:415–423.
6. Huis, A, Schoonhoven L, Grol R, et al., Impact of a team and leaders-directed strategy to improve nurses' adherence to hand hygiene guidelines: a cluster randomised trial. *Int J Nurs Stud* 2013;**50**:464–474.
7. Goto M, Ohl ME, Schweizer ML, et al., Accuracy of administrative code data for the surveillance of healthcare-associated infections: a systematic review and meta-analysis. *Clin Infect Dis* 2014;**58**:688–696.
8. Chudleigh, J, Drey N, Moralejo D, et al., Systematic reviews of hand hygiene in patient care post 2010. *J Hosp Infect*. 2016;**94**:110–111.
9. Cherry MG, Brown JM, Bethell GS, et al., Features of educational interventions that lead to compliance with hand hygiene in healthcare professionals within a hospital care setting. A BEME systematic review: BEME Guide No. 22. *Med Teach* 2012;**34**:e406–e420.
10. Mortell M, Hand hygiene compliance: is there a theory-practice-ethics gap? *Br J Nurs* 2012; **21**:1011–1014.
11. Huis, Holleman G, van Achterberg T, et al., Explaining the effects of two different strategies for promoting hand hygiene in hospital nurses: a process evaluation alongside a cluster randomised controlled trial. *Implement Sci* 2013;**8**:41.

Chapter 23

Glove Use and Hand Hygiene

Marie-Noëlle Chraïti,[1] Benedetta Allegranzi,[2] and Elaine Larson[3]

[1] Infection Control Program and WHO Collaborating Centre on Patient Safety, University of Geneva Hospitals, Geneva, Switzerland

[2] Infection Prevention and Control Global Unit, Department of Service Delivery and Safety, World Health Organization, and Faculty of Medicine, University of Geneva, Geneva, Switzerland

[3] Columbia University School of Nursing, New York, USA

KEY MESSAGES

- Gloves get contaminated as easily as bare hands.
- Gloves do not provide 100% protection.
- Whether gloves are worn or not, hand hygiene guidelines should be followed and hand hygiene should be performed, when indicated.

Hand hygiene is considered the single most effective measure to prevent microbial transmission during healthcare. The strength of this statement is closely linked to appropriate glove use. Since the dissemination of universal precaution recommendations, glove use has been recommended to prevent the transmission of blood-borne pathogens and other infectious agents to healthcare workers (HCWs) and the spread of multi-drug resistant microorganisms from one person to another, particularly during epidemics. Currently, key indications for glove use aimed at preventing microbial transfer are as follows: when exposure to body fluids is anticipated, including contacts with mucous membranes and nonintact skin, and when contact precautions are recommended in addition to standard precautions.[1,2] However, given that glove use is frequently inappropriate and gloves are not changed between patients,[3] a rational approach to glove use and its

Hand Hygiene: A Handbook for Medical Professionals, First Edition.
Edited by Didier Pittet, John M. Boyce and Benedetta Allegranzi.
© 2017 John Wiley & Sons, Inc. Published 2017 by John Wiley & Sons, Inc.

integration with hand hygiene has been proposed in the *World Health Organization (WHO) Guidelines on Hand Hygiene in Health Care*.[2] Based on the evaluation of recommendations from several societies and institutions and according to expert consensus, a question framework to help make the right choice with regards to glove use and removal, and actual indications for donning and removing gloves were identified by WHO.

WHAT WE KNOW – THE EVIDENCE

Gloves are an effective barrier to protect HCWs from microbial transmission when their hands are exposed to body fluids, and to prevent microbial spread within the care environment and to the patient.[4–7] However, gloves do not ensure total protection, regardless of their characteristics (either surgical gloves or examination gloves, sterile or nonsterile), and the material they are made of (latex, vinyl, nitrile, and neoprene mostly).[4,5,7] Microorganisms can pass through gloves; the microbial load depends on the quality of gloves, the mechanical stress applied to the material, the presence of undetected tears and holes, the duration of glove wearing, and the concentration of microbial exposure.[4,6–8]

HCW hands may become contaminated despite glove use as a result of poorly fitting gloves, contamination of hands during glove removal, or by touching contaminated gowns or clothing after glove removal. As reported in several studies, gloves can get contaminated as easily as bare hands when touching patients, their environment, or both.[6,7,9] Thus, when misused, gloves may change from being protective to becoming a means of germ transmission. Thus, gloves should be considered as an adjunct to hand hygiene rather than a substitute. Wearing gloves does not modify indications for hand hygiene and does not replace it.

Unfortunately, however, several studies have reported misuse of gloves, such as failure to change them, and their negative impact on hand hygiene behavior. Scheithauer, for example, reported a twofold lower use of product for hand hygiene when gloves were worn.[10] Glove use has been observed as a predictor for noncompliance with hand hygiene recommendations;[11] Eveillard found a negative correlation between the rate of inappropriate glove use and hand hygiene compliance.[12] HCWs are wearing gloves for two main purposes: to protect themselves and to prevent microbial transmission as part of standard and contact precautions. Misuse of gloves can be associated with HCWs' perception of their own protection, forgetting that wearing gloves is a risk to patients when compliance with indications for hand hygiene and glove on/off is not met.

The issue around the possible benefit of glove use for all contacts with carriers of multi-drug resistant organisms is controversial.[13] The occurrence of an indication for hand hygiene should trigger glove removal in order to perform hand hygiene and to prevent microbial transmission to the patient, to the HCW and into the care environment.

WHAT WE DO NOT KNOW – THE UNCERTAIN

Several studies have demonstrated the benefit of glove use to prevent microbial spread, but minimal research has explored the unintended consequences of glove use. One such consequence is the potential occurrence of healthcare-associated infection (HAI) associated with missed hand hygiene when wearing gloves. This could result in subsequent microbial transfer to the patient, in particular when care involves touching critical sites such as invasive medical devices, non-intact skin and mucous membranes. Furthermore, the proper use of gloves and gloving and ungloving procedures should be better studied and taught (see Figure 23.1). On the other hand, a recent retrospective cohort study among pediatric patients reported a significant positive impact of universal gloving adopted for preventing the seasonal spread of respiratory syncytial virus, on central line-associated bloodstream infections.[14] However, very little information on usual practices of hand hygiene and other infection control measures during the study period is provided.

A recent study explored the impact of glove material on methicillin-resistant *Staphylococcus aureus* (MRSA) transfer by gloved hands and identified glove material and glove hydrophobicity as the two most important factors influencing bacterial transfer.[15] These findings deserve further investigation provided that appropriateness of glove use and of hand hygiene is taken into account. Another aspect that should be investigated is the possibility of disinfecting gloves, for instance by using alcohol-based hand-rubs, and whether this can be done without damaging the quality of gloves. Although a few laboratory-based studies have been conducted with gloves whose external or internal surface has been coated or impregnated with antimicrobial substances, the ability of "antimicrobial gloves" to prevent transmission of pathogens to HCWs or patients has not been established.

Finally, in one study, eliminating the mandatory use of gloves while caring for patients on contact precautions was associated with an increase in hand hygiene compliance, but the impact of such a policy on transmission of healthcare-associated pathogens has not been determined.[16] Further studies of this issue are needed before making changes in existing glove policies.

RESEARCH AGENDA

Further investigations on the following topics would add significant value:

- Glove use with contact precautions is currently recommended. When contact precautions are indicated, is the benefit of appropriately performing hand hygiene according to the WHO "My Five Moments for Hand Hygiene" approach higher than the one attributable to glove use?
- The impact of glove use on hand hygiene practices, and on microbial transmission and healthcare-associated infections.

When the hand hygiene indication occurs before a contact requiring glove use, perform hand hygiene by rubbing with an alcohol-based handrub or by washing with soap and water.

I. HOW TO DON GLOVES:

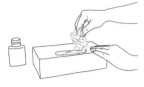

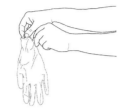

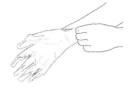

1. Take out a glove from its original box

2. Touch only a restricted surface of the glove corresponding to the wrist (at the top edge of the cuff)

3. Don the first glove

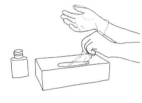

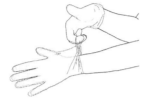

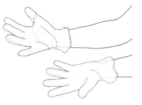

4. Take the second glove with the bare hand and touch only a restricted surface of glove corresponding to the wrist

5. To avoid touching the skin of the forearm with the gloved hand, turn the external surface of the glove to be donned on the folded fingers of the gloved hand, thus permitting to glove the second hand

6. Once gloved, hands should not touch anything else that is not defined by indications and conditions for glove use

II. HOW TO REMOVE GLOVES:

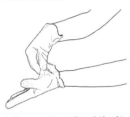

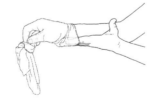

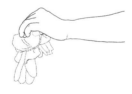

1. Pinch one glove at the wrist level to remove it, without touching the skin of the forearm, and peel away from the hand, thus allowing the glove to turn inside out

2. Hold the removed glove in the gloved hand and slide the fingers of the ungloved hand inside between the glove and the wrist. Remove the second glove by rolling it down the hand and fold into the first glove

3. Discard the removed gloves

4. Then, perform hand hygiene by rubbing with an alcohol-based handrub or by washing with soap and water

Figure 23.1   How to don and remove nonsterile gloves. *Source*: Reproduced with permission from World Health Organization. "WHO Glove Use Information Leaflet", available from www .who.int/gpsc/5may/tools/training-education/en/.

- The potential added value and risks of gloves containing antimicrobial materials.

- Glove disinfection with alcohol-based products rather than changing gloves, particularly in settings with limited resources.

- Behavioral change strategies to improve gloving practices among health-care workers while taking the need for hand hygiene into account.

REFERENCES

1. Centers for Disease Control and Prevention, *CDC Guidelines for Isolation Precaution: Preventing Transmission of Infectious Agents in Healthcare Settings*, 2007. Available at www.cdc.gov/hicpac/ 2007IP/2007isolationPrecautions.html. Accessed March 7, 2017.
2. World Health Organization, *WHO Guidelines for Hand Hygiene in Health Care*. Geneva: WHO, 2009. Part I, Section 23.1; 128.
3. Naderi HR, Compliance with hand hygiene and glove change in a general hospital, Mashhad, Iran, An observational study. *Am J Infect Control* 2012;**40**;e221.
4. Olsen RJ, Lynch P, Coyle MB, et al., Examination gloves as barriers to hand contamination in clinical practice. *JAMA* 1993;**270**:350–353.
5. Tenorio AR, Badri SM, Sahgal NB, et al., Effectiveness of gloves in the prevention of hand carriage of vancomycin-resistant enterococci species by health care workers after patient care. *Clin Infect Dis* 2001;**32**:826–829.
6. Hayden MK, Blom DW, Lyle EA, et al., Risk of hand or glove contamination after contact with patients colonized with vancomycin-resistant enterococcus or the colonized patients' environment. *Infect Control Hosp Epidemiol* 2008;**29**:149–154.
7. Morgan DJ, Liang SY, Smith CL, et al., Frequent multidrug-resistant Acinetobacter baumannii contamination of gloves, gowns, and hands of healthcare workers. *Infect Control Hosp Epidemiol* 2010;**31**:716–721.
8. Harnoss JC, Partecke LI, Heidecke CD, et al., Concentration of bacteria passing through puncture holes in surgical gloves. *Am J Infect Control* 2010;**38**:154–158.
9. Landelle C, Verachten M, Legran P, et al., Contamination of healthcare workers' hands with Clostridium difficile spores after caring for patients with C. difficile infection. *Infect Control Hosp Epidemiol* 2014;**35**:10–15.
10. Scheithauer S, Oberrohrmann A, Haefner H, et al., Compliance with hand hygiene in patients with methicillin-resistant Staphylococcus aureus and extended-spectrum beta-lactamase-producing enterobacteria. *J Hosp Infect* 2010;**76**:320–323.
11. Fuller C, Savage J, Besser S, et al., "The dirty hand in the latex glove": a study of hand hygiene compliance when gloves are worn. *Infect Control Hosp Epidemiol* 2011;**32**:1194–1199.
12. Eveillard M, Joly-Guillou ML, Brunel P. Correlation between glove use practices and compliance with hand hygiene in a multicenter study with elderly patients. *Am J Infect Control* 2012;**40**:387–388.
13. Bearman G, Stevens MP, Control of drug-resistant pathogens in endemic settings: contact precautions, controversies, and proposal for a less restrictive alternative. *Curr Infect Dis Rep* 2012;**14**:620–626.
14. Yin J, Schweizer ML, Herwaldt LA, et al., Benefits of universal gloving on hospital-acquired infections in acute care pediatrics units. *Pediatrics* 2013;**131**:e1515–e1520.

15. Moore G, Dunnill CW, Wilson AP, The effect of glove material upon the transfer of methicillin-resistant Staphylococcus aureus to and from a gloved hand. *Am J Infect Control* 2013;**41**:19–23.
16. Cusini A, Nydegger D, Kaspar T, et al., Improved hand hygiene compliance after eliminating mandatory glove use from contact precautions – is less more? *Am J Infect Control* 2015;**43**:922–927.

Chapter 24

Monitoring Hand Hygiene Performance

Hugo Sax[1] and John M. Boyce[2]

[1] *Division of Infectious Diseases and Infection Control, University Hospital of Zurich, Zürich, Switzerland*

[2] *Hospital Epidemiology and Infection Control, Yale-New Haven Hospital, and Yale University School of Medicine, New Haven, USA*

KEY MESSAGES

- Monitoring hand hygiene performance of healthcare workers represents a key element in patient safety, promotion, and research.

- Different approaches to hand hygiene monitoring exist in parallel today, each featuring advantages and disadvantages, differing also in sophistication and cost, their results not always agreeing.

- Further research is warranted to develop or refine the technique that would produce the best return on investment and the best alignment between measured hand hygiene performance and its effect on infection prevention.

WHAT WE KNOW – THE EVIDENCE

An Ideal Measure of Hand Hygiene Performance

In measuring hand hygiene performance numerically, a binary definition of right and wrong is needed to allow for a meaningful denominator. The My Five Moments for Hand Hygiene, which are rooted in an evidence-based model of hand transmission, provide such definitions (see Chapter 20).[1,2] Importantly,

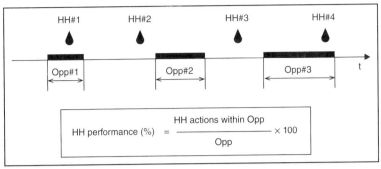

Figure 24.1   Hand hygiene performance calculation legend: The timeline (t) shows graphically three hand hygiene opportunities (Opp#1 to Opp#3) and four hand hygiene actions (HH#1 to HH#4), of which two are within hand hygiene opportunities (HH#1 and HH#4) and two are not (HH#2 and HH#3). The included formula to calculate allows determination of a 66.6% hand hygiene performance for the given example.

this concept builds on the hypothesis that hands can get easily contaminated even when touching a single object/surface. This means that one dimension to be monitored concerns the right moment in time with respect to a sequence of hand-to-surface contacts. As a result, monitoring systems can be divided into those that do rely on such a hand-to-surface sequence denominator and those that do not (Figure 24.1). Another aspect that merits measuring is the thoroughness of each hand hygiene action, as it has been shown that a flawed handrubbing technique or duration results in persistent hand contamination (see Chapter 10).

Hence, an ideal indicator of hand hygiene performance would produce an unbiased and exact numerical measure of how appropriately HCWs practice hand hygiene. Ideally, the method used should not require excessive staffing time and/or resource use for monitoring and still provide sufficient data to maximize the power of the result analysis. Today, such an ideal method does not exist. All current approaches are associated with certain advantages and disadvantages (Table 24.1). They include compliance measures by human observers or automated detection systems, direct counting of hand hygiene actions or indirect estimations.

Direct Observation by Human Observers

Direct observation of hand hygiene behavior during patient care by a validated observer is currently considered the gold standard in compliance monitoring. The human brain of the observer is currently the only available "instrument" to detect all types of hand hygiene opportunities and actions in the sometimes complex and unpredictable sequence of care. Direct observation allows collecting additional information such as glove use, handrubbing technique, application time, and other

Table 24.1 Observation Systems and their Advantages and Disadvantages

Monitoring Approach	Advantages	Disadvantages
Direct observation	• Detect all types of hand hygiene opportunities • Additional observation of hand hygiene duration and quality • Detection of workplace and workflow related issues (ergonomics; work organization) • Individual immediate detailed feedback	• Costly • Prone to various biases (e.g., observer bias, observation bias, selection bias) • Overestimates true performance • Captures only a fraction of the entire hand hygiene activity
Video-based observation	• Can be done offline • Offers HCWs the opportunity to observe themselves • As above, except individualized feedback • May reduce observation bias • May be used for training of observers and HCWs	• Costly • Visual field depending on camera(s) position (usually requires several cameras for a single patient–HCW interaction) • Challenges regarding patient privacy and confidentiality
Self-reporting by HCWs	• Inexpensive; no need for outside observers and extra observation time	• Overestimation of performance through desirability bias and recall/attention bias
Patient observation	• Inexpensive	• Patients' limited knowledge about hand hygiene opportunities • Confusion of traditional rules; may compromise patient–HCW relationship
ABHR consumption	• Inexpensive • Can be made more relevant by using surrogate measures for need of use (e.g., patient-days, etc.)	• True performance cannot be calculated since time of use remains unknown • Stocks on wards may confound results, since usually calculated from delivery data • ABHR used by patients and visitors confound results • Large variations in use observed when ABHR is

Action counting devices in dispensers	• Inexpensive • May be linked to central station for management • Can produce immediate results for motivational feedback to HCWs • Advantages of activity rates of individual dispensers • Can be made more relevant by using surrogate measures for need of use (e.g., patient days, etc.) • Individual or professional category use data possible if combined with identity reader	• True performance cannot be calculated since time/appropriateness of use remains unknown • Significant investment necessary • Does not capture parallel use of mobile ABHR sources; unless those are also equipped with counters
Fully automated monitoring system	• No interobserver bias • Continuous 24/7 monitoring possible • Immediate feedback possible • Real-time reminding possible • May be used in simulators or in real-life scenarios	• Expensive • Fragile technology • Risk of enforcing an ineffective behavior due to technological limitations • Not all established hand hygiene indications are reliably detected, producing asymmetrical improvement • Potential for distrust in HCWs • Potential system-integration challenges with other monitoring and reminding systems (alert fatigue)

ABHR, alcohol-based handrub; HCW, healthcare worker.

quality parameters that affect efficacy such as the wearing of jewelry and finger-nail status. Hand hygiene actions using ABHRs can be distinguished from those requiring handwashing with soap and water.

A major drawback of direct observation concerns the need for trained and validated staff and their many working hours. A typical observation time of 80 hours is required to obtain 500 opportunities in a common acute care setting. An additional major downside of direct observation approaches is that humans are prone to error and bias (Table 24.1). The most important are observation, observer, and selection bias.

Observation bias is generated by the presence of an observer who influences the behavior of the observed HCWs towards a higher compliance or by an increased attention to the topic under study, commonly referred to as the Hawthorne effect. Compliance found to be 45% with overt observations was in reality only 29% when observations were covert.[3] Observation bias can also induce increased recourse to hand hygiene action at times not corresponding to established indications. Observation bias might be eliminated by keeping observations covert. Such observations, however, are not recommended by some experts outside of research projects because they can induce mistrust in the observed HCWs. Furthermore, hiding the true reason for the presence of an observer can hardly be maintained in the case of repeated observations.

If a baseline observation is covert, then the results of overt follow-up observations would be confounded by this change in method. However, it is important to note that covert observers (sometimes called "secret shoppers") are used fairly frequently in some countries; this approach is used in a large number of facilities in the United States.

Observation bias can be attenuated by desensitizing HCWs through the frequent presence of observers or an unobtrusive conduct during observation sessions. On the other hand, a Hawthorne effect can be used deliberately to stimulate hand hygiene compliance in a promotional intention, rather than for obtaining objective quantitative results.

Observer bias refers to the systematic error introduced by interobserver variation in the observation method (Table 24.1). To reduce this bias, observers have to be validated against each other and for their own consistency over time.

Selection bias results from systematically selecting healthcare workers, care settings, observation times, or healthcare sectors with a specific hand hygiene behavior. In practical terms, this bias can be minimized by randomly choosing locations, times during the day/week/year, and HCWs.

If hand hygiene monitoring is used for comparison between healthcare sectors or periods, potential confounding factors should be included in the dataset and corrected for by stratification, adjustment, or keeping them unchanged between the monitoring sets. Typical confounders concern professional category, time of day, and healthcare setting. To exclude chance as an alternative explanation of results, a sample size calculation needs to be performed at the design stage of every hand hygiene observation program to ensure statistical significance.

A special form of direct observation consists of video installations in care environments that send the video feed to observers in a distant location, sometimes even abroad, either in real time or deferred. This technique most certainly reduces the Hawthorne effect.

Patients have been asked to serve as observers, but they may not feel comfortable in a formal role as observers and are not always in a physical or mental condition to execute this task. Finally, self-assessment by HCWs has been demonstrated to markedly overestimate compliance.

The WHO proposes a standardized hand hygiene observation method. All relevant theoretical and practical aspects related to this method are detailed in the *Hand Hygiene Reference Technical Manual* that is included in the Implementation Toolkit of the WHO multimodal hand hygiene promotion strategy (available at www.who.int/gpsc/en/). For analysis and reporting of hand hygiene performance data, refer to Chapter 25.

Detection of Hand Hygiene Actions by Technical Systems

Technical (sometimes electronic) systems are increasingly developed and employed to monitor and ensure hand hygiene performance.[4,5]

Hand hygiene actions are less challenging to detect than hand hygiene opportunities for technical systems. Hand hygiene actions can be deduced from proximity to handrub dispensers or sinks that is captured by electronic sensors based on infrared, ultrasound, or radio frequency technology. Other systems sense high concentration of alcohol in the air during use of alcohol-based handrubs (ABHRs) or read the specific movement patterns during handrubbing with wristband acceleration detectors. The use of dispensers or even pocket-size ABHR bottles can be detected through the movement of levers or caps, or by electronic detection that the product has been dispensed. The accumulating data can be stored in devices worn by HCWs or captured by dispensers or a centrally located hub. Either way, systems may just count hand hygiene actions or provide a time stamp for each; they may additionally identify the person involved.

Even though monitoring the number of hand hygiene actions alone does not allow calculating performance rates, data on hand hygiene actions can be useful to follow usage patterns over time and compare differences in hand hygiene practice between individuals or groups of HCWs or dispenser locations.

To make up for the missing denominator data, some experts use surrogate markers calculated from care activity or severity-of-illness indicators, inpatient days, or outpatient consultations. Such data might directly be used for feedback to individual HCWs or groups. But caution must prevail not to induce a false sense of success in individuals who use hand hygiene at moments that are not considered to actually prevent cross-transmission or infections.

Detection of Hand Hygiene Opportunities by Technical Systems and Combined Systems

Hand hygiene opportunities are much more challenging to detect than hand hygiene action. An opportunity is the time space between two consecutive hand-to-surface exposures that could result in risk-prone cross-transmission of microorganisms and is therefore associated with one or several established hand hygiene actions. Because of the geographical dislocation mostly associated with an opportunity that contains a "before touching a patient" or an "after touching a patient," indication they are somewhat less challenging to detect for technical systems than those concerning the other indications (see also Chapter 20). Usually, an electronic barrier system is used to detect an HCW entering or exiting a patient zone or a patient room. Electronic barriers are established either by infrared, ultrasound, or radio frequency identification (RFID). Some systems can detect HCWs who are designated by active or passive electronic tags. These invisible electronic "curtains" or zones can easily be placed at doors or other gateways, or with more sophisticated systems, around a patient location. The limitation of these systems is that they cannot distinguish if an individual (whether HCW or not) just walks through the "zone" or actually performs a care task that would create a hand hygiene opportunity according to established rules.

Technical solutions designed to detect surrogates of hand hygiene opportunities may additionally be combined with hand hygiene action detection systems. Ideally, such a sophisticated system could produce hand hygiene compliance data. This is usually done by identifying the subject of a hand hygiene action and then determining if this individual walks through an electronic "curtain" within a predefined (short) time period.

When linked over a wired or wireless network, data coming from various system components can be stored, analyzed, and displayed centrally – even in real time.

Before implementation in real care settings, it should be clear that such systems actually improve overall patient safety and do not interfere with good clinical practice in various and sometimes complex care situations. The danger of inducing a HCW behavior that satisfies the system but does not make sense in the face of infectious risk is theoretically possible.[6] On the contrary, hand hygiene promotion may suffer if HCWs believe that such systems do not accurately reflect hand hygiene compliance.

Monitoring of ABHR Consumption: An Inexpensive Surrogate Marker

In the quest for less expensive monitoring approaches, experts have used the consumption of hand hygiene agents such as ABHR, liquid soap, or paper towels to estimate the number of hand hygiene actions.[7,8] To make these monitoring techniques more meaningful, the quantity of handrub was translated into a number of hand hygiene actions by using the average amount per action as a divider. The missing denominator (i.e., the number of hand hygiene opportunities) was either ignored, or substituted by a surrogate measure such as patient-days or workload indicators drawn from a computerized database of nursing activities.

Some studies have shown that the consumption of hand hygiene agents correlated with observed hand hygiene compliance, whereas others have not.[7,8] Thus, the use of this measure as a surrogate for monitoring hand hygiene practices deserves further validation.

Methods based on product consumption cannot determine if hand hygiene actions are performed at the right moment during care or if the technique is correct. The advantages, however, are that they are simple, can be continuous, and provide a global picture that remains unaffected by selection or observer bias and, most likely, observation bias. The amount of ABHR used by healthcare settings has been selected as one of the indicators. Nevertheless, this measure may not exactly reflect product consumption by HCWs, but could include the amount used by visitors or patients, especially if the dispensers are wall-mounted and also located in public areas of the healthcare setting.

WHAT WE DO NOT KNOW – THE UNCERTAIN

Today, a unique, reliable, and robust method to measure hand hygiene performance does not exist. Also, it remains unknown which of the methods described above correlates best with the risk of pathogen transmission. This is especially of concern when comparing the results from measurement of ABHR consumption, a relatively inexpensive monitoring system, with direct hand hygiene observation, a much more costly endeavor; the two systems often do not correlate in their results.

Furthermore, the nature of the relation between measured hand hygiene performance and the different types of HAI, pathogens, and antibiotic resistance remains undetermined. This relation is most likely not linear, meaning that an increase of hand hygiene performance from 30% to 50% does probably not have the same impact on infection rates as an increase from 60% to 90%. It may be that above a given threshold, further improvement is not associated with a more pronounced preventive effect, or that the relation is S-shaped. For this reason it is impossible to produce a universal target goal for hand hygiene performance based on scientific evidence.

Currently, known monitoring systems produce almost exclusively aggregated hand hygiene performance data. Yet, infectious risk in a ward might be different if all HCWs perform at 60% or if some reach 100% performance whereas others remain at 10–20% even if the mean value would be 60% in both cases.

RESEARCH AGENDA

From the missing knowledge cited above the following points constitute a priority research agenda regarding hand hygiene performance monitoring:

- Correlation of different monitoring techniques such as ABHR consumption or direct observations with infectious outcomes to determine the best prediction fit.

- Correlation of different levels of hand hygiene performance with preventive impact to establish a correlation curve; further, performing this in different healthcare settings and endemic infectious situations to produce a meaningful specific threshold, if such exists.

- Production of individual HCW-level hand hygiene performance data to investigate the impact of individual performance in a group of HCWs on the overall infectious outcome; modeling could be an alternative first approach to this question.[9]

- Effectiveness research on the preventive impact would be necessary to evaluate an overall system of monitoring and feedback. To provide HCWs with a risk-based learning opportunity, monitoring systems can be imagined that actually monitor microbiological events (e.g., hand-transmission of multiresistant pathogens) in real time rather than just compliance with behavior rules.

In general, we feel that, given the huge negative impact of HAI and associated burden in health outcomes, lives, and money, research should be much sharper in design and bolder in scope. The necessary resources would have a very high return on investment.

REFERENCES

1. Sax H, Allegranzi B, Uckay I, et al., "My five moments for hand hygiene": a user-centred design approach to understand, train, monitor and report hand hygiene. *J Hosp Infect* 2007;**67**:9–21.
2. Sax H, Allegranzi B, Chraïti M-N, et al., The World Health Organization hand hygiene observation method. *Am J Infect Control* 2009;**37**:827–834.
3. Eckmanns T, Bessert J, Behnke M, et al., Compliance with antiseptic hand rub use in intensive care units: the Hawthorne effect. *Infect Control Hosp Epidemiol* 2006;**27**:931–934.
4. Fisher DA, Seetoh T, Oh May-Lin H, et al., Automated measures of hand hygiene compliance among healthcare workers using ultrasound: validation and a randomized controlled trial. *Infect Control Hosp Epidemiol* 2013;**34**:919–928.
5. Ward MA, Schweizer ML, Polgreen PM, et al., Automated and electronically assisted hand hygiene monitoring systems: a systematic review. *Am J Infect Control* 2014;**42**:472–478.
6. Pineles LL, Morgan DJ, Limper HM, et al., Accuracy of a radiofrequency identification (RFID) badge system to monitor hand hygiene behavior during routine clinical activities. *Am J Infect Control* 2013;**42**:144–147.

7. Boyce JM, Measuring healthcare worker hand hygiene activity: current practices and emerging technologies. *Infect Control Hosp Epidemiol* 2011;**32**:1016–1028.
8. Boyce JM, Hand hygiene compliance monitoring: current perspectives from the USA. *J Hosp Infect* 2008;**70**(Suppl. 1):2–7.
9. Hornbeck T, Naylor D, Segre AM, et al., Using sensor networks to study the effect of peripatetic healthcare workers on the spread of hospital-associated infections. *J Infect Dis* 2012;**206**:1549–1557.

Chapter 25

Performance Feedback

Andrew J. Stewardson[1,2] and Hugo Sax[3]

[1] Infectious Diseases Department, Austin Health and Hand Hygiene Australia, Melbourne, Australia
[2] Infection Control Program and WHO Collaborating Centre on Patient Safety, University of Geneva Hospitals and Faculty of Medicine, Geneva, Switzerland
[3] Division of Infectious Diseases and Infection Control, University Hospital of Zurich, Zürich, Switzerland

KEY MESSAGES

- Performance feedback enhances hand hygiene compliance by demonstrating discordance between perceived and actual hand hygiene behavior.
- Feedback should involve data that healthcare workers will consider pertinent to them.
- Data should be given meaning, whether by peer-comparison, goal-setting, or other methods.

WHAT WE KNOW – THE EVIDENCE

Performance feedback involves providing an individual, or group, with information regarding their own performance with the objective of influencing their practice. In the context of hand hygiene promotion, performance feedback generally means providing healthcare workers (HCWs) with their own hand hygiene compliance data. HCWs generally overestimate their own hand hygiene compliance. Hence, feedback can facilitate improvement by drawing HCWs' attention to the discordance between their perceived and actual performance.

Theoretical Framework

The objective of optimal hand hygiene behavior is to prevent transmission of pathogenic or resistant microorganisms between patients or from nonsterile to

Hand Hygiene: A Handbook for Medical Professionals, First Edition.
Edited by Didier Pittet, John M. Boyce and Benedetta Allegranzi.
© 2017 John Wiley & Sons, Inc. Published 2017 by John Wiley & Sons, Inc.

sterile sites within an individual patient.[1] Thus, from a human factors perspective, hand hygiene faces two overlapping challenges common to many infection prevention activities.[2] First, hand hygiene lacks a direct and observable result. It is highly unlikely that a transmission event or infection will ever be directly attributed to a breach in hand hygiene. Such an outcome will only occur with relative infrequency and will usually only become clinically evident at least days later. Second, hand hygiene is not rewarded with a tangible positive result, but rather with the absence of a negative result. Performance feedback can address both of these barriers to compliance by providing a positive feedback loop between HCWs and their hand hygiene behavior. The mechanism of this strategy can be appreciated with Behavior Change Theory (Figure 25.1).

Control Theory has been proposed as the most pertinent behavior change theory regarding performance feedback.[3] According to Control Theory, behavior is goal driven. In the current context, the goal would be to perform hand hygiene adequately. When a discrepancy between their behavior and their goals is revealed by performance feedback, individuals can be expected to adapt their behavior in order to more closely approximate the goal. Subsequent rounds of feedback and behavior adjustment result in an iterative process that brings the individual progressively closer to his or her goal.

Social psychology provides the complementary theory of "cognitive dissonance."[4] According to this theory, suboptimal hand hygiene compliance data will conflict with a HCW's perceptions of him/herself as providing high-quality care. There are two potential paths by which HCWs can resolve the

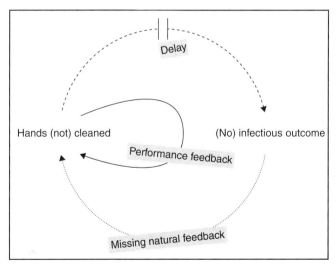

Figure 25.1   In the absence of a direct and observable outcome of hand hygiene, performance feedback provides an important positive feedback loop between healthcare workers and their hand hygiene behavior.

discomfort produced by this cognitive dissonance: by changing their behavior or by "rationalizing away" the poor compliance data. The latter pathway might, for example, include explanations such as being too busy to perform hand hygiene, or that hand hygiene indications are not feasible or are formulated for a healthcare context other than their own.

Both Control Theory and the concept of cognitive dissonance suggest that feedback should be framed in such a manner as to maximize the resulting behavior change, and to minimize the risk of the HCW either "giving up" or "rationalizing away." Typical methods include goal-setting and action-planning. The former involves explicitly fixing an achievable hand hygiene compliance target. The latter involves establishing how this goal can be reached.

Another performance-enhancing dimension of regular feedback is that it conveys an implicit message that hospital leadership considers hand hygiene significantly important such that they provide the resources to collect these data and feed them back. In this way, performance feedback contributes to the development of an institutional safety culture.

A diverse range of different activities can be classified as performance feedback. When formulating a performance feedback intervention, decisions need to be made regarding the feedback recipient, format, source, frequency, duration, and content (Table 25.1).[5] We address these parameters below, with central focus on recipient and content.

Feedback Recipient

Feedback can be provided to the individual HCW. From a practical perspective, this can be best achieved by providing feedback immediately following the observation session.[6] This approach has three key advantages: the feedback is individualized for the HCW, it is provided in real time, and this exchange represents an opportunity to provide targeted hand hygiene education, goal-setting, and action-planning.[7] These advantages are frequently cited as key reasons for the preferability of direct observation over electronic monitoring or use of surrogate markers to monitor hand hygiene. The HCW may have specific questions that can be answered, and workflow issues can be identified and improved. Practical difficulties with this approach of immediate individualized feedback include the fact that HCWs may not have time, and this feedback will by its nature involve a very small number of opportunities for hand hygiene. In addition, only a minority of the total institutional workforce would benefit from this resource-intensive approach.

An alternate means of providing individualized feedback is to record the identity of HCWs observed over a period of time, and then provide aggregate feedback for each HCW. However, with this approach the immediacy of the method described above is lost. Moreover, recording the identity of individual HCWs is usually not feasible for logistical reasons and workplace privacy concerns. Electronic monitoring systems may overcome these barriers in the future, as discussed below.

Table 25.1   Key Parameters and Considerations in Hand Hygiene Performance Feedback

Parameter	Options	Comments
Recipient	Individual Group	Individualized feedback is likely to provide powerful incentive, but it is unlikely to be feasible in an ongoing manner hospital-wide. Group feedback should be provided to a group with a strong sense of collective identity. Aggregate data assists with precision of results
Format	Verbal Written Multisensory	Verbal feedback can be provided during direct observation sessions or at clinical meetings. Written feedback can be provided in the form of letters or emails, posters, or cards, and provides opportunities for infographics. Automated monitoring systems may use auditory, visual, tactile, or combined sensory channels
Source	Infection Control Professional Colleague/Peer Authority Figure	An infection control professional is able to provide expert advice regarding the interpretation of hand hygiene compliance data as well as education about their role in patient safety. Feedback from a colleague may establish new perceptions regarding behavioral norms. Feedback from a clinical supervisor or other authority figure helps establish a culture of hand hygiene excellence
Frequency		Frequency of performance feedback should be tailored depending on target setting and action planning. Frequent feedback of mediocre performance data without action planning might give rise to complacency
Duration	Ongoing Discrete	Most performance feedback systems in hand hygiene have no predetermined end, but a time frame may be based on resource availability or acquisition of a predetermined definition of "mastery." There is evidence of a beneficial on-off effect
Content	Data Goal Setting Peer Comparison Action Plan	The *data* conveyed are most commonly hand hygiene compliance. Other options include a surrogate marker of hand hygiene compliance, hand hygiene technique, or clinical endpoints, such as transmission events or healthcare-associated infections. *Goal setting* requires explicit identification of an achievable and justifiable target. *Peer comparison* or benchmarking can provide motivation to improve. An *action plan* should identify solutions to potential barriers to improved behavior

Performance feedback can also be provided to groups of HCWs. The principal benefit of this approach is to allow feedback of a larger number of observations, and therefore a more precise estimate of hand hygiene compliance. In addition, all HCWs can potentially be reached, whereas this is not feasible with individualized feedback. However, it remains important to define a target group with a strong collective identity. For example, hospital-wide data may be useful for other purposes such as external benchmarking, but is of limited use for performance feedback. An individual HCW is unlikely to alter his/her behavior on the basis of such data, as poor compliance may be easily attributed to "other" sectors of the hospital. How to aggregate the data depends on the organizational structure and data available. For example, ward-level information may be appropriate as the healthcare team within a ward often identifies strongly as a team. An alternate approach is to aggregate data by profession within a defined medical department. This might be helpful, for example, if seeking to improve hand hygiene compliance among physicians.

Feedback Content

The major piece of information to be conveyed is generally hand hygiene compliance. Depending on the context, however, different levels of detail can be provided. For example, compliance might be stratified by indication or profession. Other content might include surrogate indicators of hand hygiene compliance, in particular use of alcohol-based handrub. While hand hygiene compliance is preferable, product consumption data may be useful when direct observation is not feasible. Information regarding hand hygiene technique and correct glove use could also be included, although it usually is not.

Hand hygiene compliance is a process measure. The final endpoint of interest involves patient outcomes. Some researchers have therefore incorporated such endpoints, for example *Staphyloccocus aureus* bloodstream infections, into performance feedback interventions. Due to the nature of this feedback, the recipient will be a HCW group rather than individuals. The argument for this strategy is that it presents information that is more intrinsically meaningful than hand hygiene compliance, and may also stimulate behavior change in multiple domains, such as increased adherence to central or peripheral vascular line protocols as well as improved hand hygiene compliance. The risk, however, is that such clinical endpoints are subject to a range of complex determinants, some of which are beyond HCWs' control. A reasonable approach therefore, may be to provide clinical outcomes as complementary information to hand hygiene compliance rather than instead of it.

As discussed above, provision of data alone without situating it within a problem-solving or goal-setting framework is unlikely to optimize the impact of performance feedback. From this perspective, the actual data can be seen as just the initial, albeit important, component of performance feedback content.

Goal-setting, peer comparison, and action planning may be equally important. For example, compliance results can be used to discuss barriers to compliance, to allow opinion leaders to emphasize the importance of hand hygiene, and to set goals for future performance.[8] Some bodies and institutions have recommended a target hand hygiene compliance of 100%. With Control Theory in mind, one can easily imagine that such a target might be counterproductive by being unrealistically distant from current practice. Added to this is a lack of evidence for such a target, which may allow HCWs to dismiss hand hygiene efforts as lacking a basis in evidence. We propose that a more feasible target is more likely to stimulate behavior change leading to improved hand hygiene compliance.

Feedback Format, Frequency, and Duration

Many different modalities can be used to provide performance feedback. As individualized feedback is generally immediate and verbal, this discussion primarily relates to aggregate feedback. Feedback cards, however, have been used to provide individual feedback. Commonly reported techniques include posters, discussions during team meetings, and group emails or newsletters. A key consideration is to convey the message quickly and clearly. A hand hygiene compliance figure (as percentage or fraction) and graphic demonstrating trends over time can be used. Probably equally important is the context within which the information is provided. As already mentioned, benchmarking against other groups (wards, departments, or the institution as a whole), also referred to as peer-comparison, may add meaning to the data. Electronic or web-based feedback of hand hygiene compliance data provides a flexible and potentially interactive means of conveying performance feedback.

The frequency and duration of performance feedback will, to a large extent, be determined by the other parameters and resource availability. As a general rule, feedback that is provided as soon as possible after data collection will be most effective. Feedback strategies in hand hygiene tend to be ongoing or intermittent in nature, without a specific end-date.

Automated Monitoring Systems

Automated monitoring systems are well suited to providing performance feedback, and it can be expected that they will be increasingly incorporated into hand hygiene monitoring and feedback interventions in high-income countries in the coming years.[9] In their most basic form, such systems can provide information about surrogates for hand hygiene actions. For example, electronic alcohol-based handrub dispensers can be used to audit and feed-back their own use. As with many automated systems, such a method cannot directly provide hand hygiene compliance because the denominator of hand hygiene opportunities is not measured, and cannot discriminate between hand hygiene actions that are or are not indicated. At their most sophisticated level, they would be able to provide real-time, continuous performance feedback that can be individualized or aggregated. Auditory, tactile, or visual feedback signals are used to prompt HCWs to perform hand hygiene when indicated. These issues are discussed in further detail in Chapter 24.

WHAT WE DO NOT KNOW – THE UNCERTAIN

While there exists a rich literature in the field of behavior change psychology related to infection control, many practical and important questions remain unanswered with regard to practical details. Currently, there is insufficient evidence to recommend a specific "optimal" approach to performance feedback for hand hygiene. Therefore, the main parameters (recipient, format, source, frequency, duration, and content) are left to the individual institution to determine and adapt to its own setting. Moreover, once a program is established, we do not know whether the impact can be expected to "wear off," or what measures could be taken to increase and sustain the stimulating effect on performance.

Some researchers have proposed that a decision may be made to end performance feedback once the subject has obtained a predefined state of "mastery" over the behavior.[7,10] This approach would need further investigation prior to implementation, as there is scant evidence that behavior change will be sustained long-term in the absence of ongoing performance feedback.

The cost-effectiveness of performance feedback is also not clear. As it generally depends on direct observation, performance feedback is a resource-intensive intervention,[6] and a trade-off will need to be made between the intensity of feedback provided (as determined by number of observations, frequency of feedback, etc.) and the cost of its conduct. For example, feedback based on few opportunities will be cheaper but more unstable and susceptible to chance variation. While this theoretically represents a threat to effectiveness by deflating the signal-to-noise ratio in feedback data and potentially decoupling HCW effort and compliance results, it is not clear to what extent this is a real problem.

RESEARCH AGENDA

There is a need for further studies to determine how best to apply performance feedback[6] to the field of hand hygiene. Such research should incorporate an underlying behavior change conceptual model, and is likely to involve collaboration between investigators with expertise in infection control, sociology, and psychology. Key questions include identification of important parameters for the effectiveness of performance feedback, as well as the cost-effectiveness of different approaches. The generalizability of research into performance feedback will be limited by numerous contextual features, such as baseline hand hygiene compliance, simultaneous hand hygiene promotion interventions, and organizational structure. Mixed methods studies, including both quantitative and qualitative components, would therefore be likely to provide extremely useful information regarding implementation of performance feedback. Finally, given its great potential for flexible and continuous performance feedback, we expect significant research efforts incorporating automated systems to emerge in the short term.

REFERENCES

1. Sax H, Allegranzi B, Uckay I, et al., "My five moments for hand hygiene": a user-centred design approach to understand, train, monitor and report hand hygiene. *J Hosp Infect* 2007;**67**:9–21.
2. Anderson J, Gosbee LL, Bessesen M, et al., Using human factors engineering to improve the effectiveness of infection prevention and control. *Crit Care Med* 2010;**38** (8 Suppl.):s269–s281.
3. Gardner B, Whittington C, McAteer J, et al., Using theory to synthesise evidence from behaviour change interventions: the example of audit and feedback. *Soc Sci Med* 2010;**70**:1618–1625.
4. Cumbler E, Castillo L, Satorie L, et al., Culture change in infection control: applying psychological principles to improve hand hygiene. *J Nurs Care Qual* 2013;**28**:304–311.
5. Jamtvedt G, Young JM, Kristoffersen DT, et al., Audit and feedback: effects on professional practice and health care outcomes. *Cochrane Database Syst Rev* 2006(**2**):CD000259.
6. Stewardson A, Sax H, Gayet-Ageron A, et al., Enhanced performance feedback and patient participation to improve hand hygiene compliance of healthcare workers in the setting of established multimodal promotion: a single-centre, cluster randomised controlled trial. *Lancet Infect Dis* 2016;**16**:1345–1355.
7. Luke MM, Alavosius M, Adherence with universal precautions after immediate, personalized performance feedback. *J Appl Behav Anal* 2011;**44**:967–971.
8. Fuller C, Michie S, Savage J, et al., The Feedback Intervention Trial (FIT) – improving hand-hygiene compliance in UK healthcare workers: a stepped wedge cluster randomised controlled trial. *PLoS One* 2012;**7**:e41617.
9. Boyce JM, Measuring healthcare worker hand hygiene activity: current practices and emerging technologies. *Infect Control Hosp Epidemiol* 2011;**32**:1016–1028.
10. Alavosius MP, Sulzer-Azaroff B, Acquisition and maintenance of health-care routines as a function of feedback density. *J Appl Behav Anal* 1990;**23**:151–162.

Chapter 26

Marketing Hand Hygiene

Julie Storr[1] and Hugo Sax[2]

[1] *Infection Prevention and Control Global Unit, Department of Service Delivery and Safety, World Health Organization, Geneva, Switzerland*

[2] *Division of Infectious Diseases and Infection Control, University Hospital of Zurich, Zürich, Switzerland*

KEY MESSAGES

- Social marketing (including but not solely focused on the use of reminders) plays an important role in a multimodal hand hygiene improvement strategy, its main benefit being its focus on the needs and wants – that is, worldview – of the customer (healthcare worker).

- If social marketing is to contribute to hand hygiene improvement, there must be a shift away from social advertising to true integration of all principles of social marketing.

- The infection prevention and control community, locally, nationally, and internationally, should harness the power and intelligence of social marketing experts and the social sciences per se, if future gains are to be made in hand hygiene improvement and the necessary influence on healthcare worker behavior secured, resulting in effective, timely hand hygiene for social good.

WHAT WE KNOW – THE EVIDENCE

The use of marketing within healthcare is not a new phenomenon. Social marketing, a subdiscipline of marketing, is concerned with using marketing principles to address social issues. Its incorporation within public health interventions has been documented in developed and developing countries. It aims to bring about voluntary behavior change that is sufficiently scalable to generate wider social or

Hand Hygiene: A Handbook for Medical Professionals, First Edition.
Edited by Didier Pittet, John M. Boyce and Benedetta Allegranzi.

Traditional Approaches	Marketing-Informed Approaches
- Ignores accessibility of information	- Promotes accessibility of information
- Often ambiguous	- Clear unambiguous messages
- Not integrated with natural workflow	- Integration with workflow
- Ignores user perceptions	- Acknowledges user perception
- Difficult to test	- Testable
- Rigid and fixed	- Locally adaptable
- Ignores user-centered design principles	- User-centered design-focused
- Generic	- Population specific

Figure 26.1   Traditional versus marketing-informed approaches.

cultural change.[1] More recently, social marketing has been described as the design, implementation, and control of programs seeking to increase the acceptability of a [positive] social idea or practice in a target group.[2] Social marketing is a behavior science-informed approach to promote social change drawing on psychology, sociology, engineering, and economics.

The main benefit of applying marketing principles to infection prevention and control (IPC) is the mindset that it induces in the leaders and managers who can make a difference. Positioning the implementation of best practices within a marketing framework puts healthcare workers (HCWs) and their needs and wants firmly in the center. Promoting the right thing to do, such as hand hygiene, becomes a matter of exchange with consideration given to HCW return on investment. The key question is this: what do HCWs get for the extra effort needed to comply with best practice rules? Possible answers include professional pride, satisfaction in doing good, working in a stellar institution, tools that facilitate the task, and reduction in learning time. This is radically different from traditional, moralistic, or policy-centric approaches that see IPC procedures as a professional obligation and ignore culture and context. Figure 26.1 summarizes traditional versus marketing-informed approaches.

Advantages of Marketing

Hand hygiene improvement strategies are concerned with changing the attitudes, beliefs, and behaviors of HCWs. The aim is a change from an undesirable behavior, where hand hygiene does not occur at the right moment, to a desirable behavior where hand hygiene occurs at all of the right moments, applying the right technique, contributing to a lower likelihood of microbial cross-transmission and patient harm.

The advantage of using marketing in IPC is its ability to place relevant practices and procedures within a competitive healthcare environment, where HCWs have multiple demands on their attention and time. Understanding IPC (and hand hygiene), within the complex socio-technical system that is healthcare, calls out for the potential advantages that marketing can bring. Table 26.1 outlines some of the key features of marketing.[3]

Table 26.1 Cornerstones of Marketing

1. When applying marketing strategies to infection prevention and control, definitions have to be adapted to the healthcare setting including defining who the customer and consumer are
2. Market research is important in understanding what customers (healthcare workers) want, need, or demand
3. The ultimate goal in marketing hand hygiene is to ensure that healthcare workers perceive hand hygiene as an innovative, intuitive-to-use, and appealing intervention, associated with professionalism, safety, and efficiency
4. All levels of marketing should be targeted
5. A "marketing strategy" can be developed by making use of the marketing mix known as the "4 Ps" (product, price, promotion, and place)
6. Along with the traditional 4 Ps, a fifth, "persistence," is proposed to emphasize the need for specific actions that lead to sustainability in hand hygiene promotion
7. Conceiving hand hygiene through a 5 Ps lens provides a powerful and actionable checklist when engaging in a promotional endeavor
8. Hand hygiene advocacy should profit from the evolution of marketing science towards social marketing, relationship marketing, and viral marketing, leveraging the power of the Internet, and continuing to assimilate new concepts of marketing as they are developed by the industry

Source: Mah 2006. Reproduced with permission from Elsevier.

A number of academic papers exist on marketing hand hygiene improvement, as well as on focusing on using the power of marketing to promote international hand hygiene awareness campaigns, such as World Health Organization's (WHO's) *SAVE LIVES: Clean Your Hands* campaign[4] described in Chapter 38. A systematic review of hand hygiene behavioral interventions found synergies in many modern-day approaches to hand hygiene improvement and social marketing.[5] Another evidence review concluded a positive impact on communicable disease control and cited its successful application in hand hygiene interventions in Europe as proof of success.[6]

Marketing and the Multimodal Strategy

Social marketing could be described as influencing one of the five action areas of WHO's Multimodal Strategy for hand hygiene.[7] The literature since 2009 reveals an increase in papers on implementation of this strategy; however, most focus on reminders in the workplace when attempting to integrate social marketing, with an emphasis on posters at room entrances or remote from the point of care. Lack of emphasis on visual cues at the bedside suggests a misunderstanding among those making decisions and planning programs on hand hygiene improvement. The understanding of marketing in hand hygiene, therefore, must not be reduced to social advertising. There is little sustained effect in displaying posters reminding

HCWs of the benefit of hand hygiene. A more fruitful way is to see marketing as a two-way process in which the right product is designed, using the right messages, according to the needs and requests of the market, that is, HCWs.[8]

Another advance in public health and behavior change is worthy of mentioning. The concept of "nudging" or "nudge theory" has emerged from behavioral economics. It also draws on social psychology, sociology, design, and communication science[9] and is relevant to hand hygiene improvement, particularly with its focus on personal choice and the environmental, cultural, and economic factors that impact on decisions. The authors suggest that many decisions are processed by "mindless choosing" rather than conscious thought, and the tactics employed by nudge theorists aim to influence mindless choosing for social good. How this might translate into hand hygiene has yet to be explored. Nudge theory describes "choice architecture" as the process of designing systems and services in such a way that the "good" choice is the easiest and rewarding one. The overlap here between marketing, behavioral economics, and human factors, discussed in Chapter 27, is evident.

WHAT WE DO NOT KNOW – THE UNCERTAIN

There are six broad knowledge gaps:

1. Absence of published work on the influence of culture on messaging and social marketing across developed and developing countries, as well as between culturally distinct groups of HCWs including the issue of gender.

2. Use of social marketing in hand hygiene implies acceptance of low hand hygiene compliance as a "social problem"; there is limited work in support of this.

3. Better understanding is needed on how successful hand hygiene improvement programs work, in particular their return on investment.

4. An absence of research concerning subcultures and groups within healthcare, that do not believe in the importance or value of hand hygiene as a critical patient safety intervention.

5. Underuse and lack of research on the latest innovations in social media and mobile technology as a way of influencing attitudes, beliefs, and behaviors; it is unclear to what extent these could influence hand hygiene improvement.

6. Further work on the potential for marketing innovations to help healthcare leaders address the adaptive challenges within healthcare systems, including the context and culture.

RESEARCH AGENDA

Influenced by these uncertainties, there remains a need to devote research energy and resources to the following:

- Impact of social marketing, including social and cultural as well as behavioral impact.
- Benefit of segmented, targeted strategies for different groups and cultures within and across healthcare (e.g., professional categories, gender, undergraduate trainees, etc.).
- Impact of message framing, language, and digital communication technologies within social marketing strategies across different cultures and contexts.
- National policy context, including the political commitment to healthcare-associated infection prevention, and its relevance and impact on social marketing interventions.
- Impact of other components of the marketing mix, shifting away from a focus on promotion only.

REFERENCES

1. Kotler P, Zaltman G, Social marketing: an approach to planned social change. *J Mark* 1971;**35**:3–12.
2. Bloom PN, Novelli WD, Problems and challenges in social marketing. *J Mark* 1981; **45**:79–88.
3. Mah MW, Deshpande S, Rothschild ML, Social marketing: a behavior change technology for infection control. *Am J Infect Control* 2006;**34**:452–457.
4. WHO's Save Lives Clean Your Hands campaign. Available at www.who.int/gpsc/5may/en/index.html. Accessed March 7, 2017.
5. Mah MW, Tam YC, Deshpande S, Social marketing analysis of 2 years of hand hygiene promotion. *Infect Control Hosp Epidemiol* 2008;**29**:262–270.
6. MacDonald L, Cairns G, Angus K, et al., *Evidence Review: Social Marketing for the Prevention and Control of Communicable Disease.* Stockholm: ECDC, 2012.
7. World Health Organization, *WHO Guidelines on Hand Hygiene in Health Care.* Geneva: WHO, 2009.
8. Jenner EA1, Jones F, Fletcher BC, et al., Hand hygiene posters: selling the message. *J Hosp Infect* 2005;**59**:77–82.
9. French G, Why nudging is not enough. *J Soc Market* 2011;**1**:154–162.

Chapter 27

Human Factors Design

Lauren Clack and Hugo Sax
Division of Infectious Diseases and Infection Control, University Hospital of Zurich, Zürich, Switzerland

KEY MESSAGES

- Human factors and ergonomics (HFE) is the scientific discipline that seeks to optimize the interactions between humans and their environment. When applied to healthcare, HFE holds the promise to make hand hygiene intuitive, efficient, and sustainable.
- Any systems design project must begin with an evaluation of the current system involving frontline workers, followed by a targeted design process guided by HFE principles and techniques to support physical, cognitive, and social performance.
- Healthcare institutions should seek to establish the organizational structures to support the necessary collaboration between healthcare professionals and HFE experts.

WHAT WE KNOW – THE EVIDENCE

A physician walks out of a patient room under contact precautions with his gloves on. A nurse takes a breath and asks him if he had touched the isolated patient. He crustily replies: "Yes, why?" – Where is the error?

Historically, the medical field has stressed the responsibility of individual clinicians to provide high-quality patient care and avoid adverse events by ensuring error-free practice. This mentality within medical culture expects healthcare workers (HCWs) to be infallible, which is both unrealistic and unsafe. Human factors and ergonomics (HFE) is the scientific discipline that takes a

Hand Hygiene: A Handbook for Medical Professionals, First Edition.
Edited by Didier Pittet, John M. Boyce and Benedetta Allegranzi.
© 2017 John Wiley & Sons, Inc. Published 2017 by John Wiley & Sons, Inc.

systems-approach to understanding the interactions between humans and their environment while accounting for human strengths and limitations.[1] The environment includes the physical environment (workplace layout, tools, lighting, noise), as well as the organizational (policies and regulations related to work organization) and social environment (leadership characteristics, culture), as well as the dynamic interactions between these systems. The goal of this discipline is ultimately to improve two systems outcomes: human well-being and overall system performance.

The value of HFE has long been recognized in many fields such as the nuclear industry, surface transportation, and aerospace systems. More recently, the contributions of HFE have also been increasingly pursued in the healthcare domain and specifically in the realm of patient safety.[2] Two main HFE design approaches have been proposed to this effect, one promoting the design of systems and improved processes to *support HCW performance*,[3] and another advocating the identification and eradication of *system flaws*, also referred to as *latent errors*, in order to mitigate hazards.[4] These approaches are complementary in that through identifying latent errors, systems may be redesigned to better aid human performance, thus they should be considered in parallel.

In the realm of patient safety, hand hygiene performance improvement is an ideal application for a holistic HFE approach. It is well known that current hand hygiene practices remain suboptimal among HCWs in most settings. This low compliance may be related to healthcare environments that lack consideration for HFE design principles. HFE solutions are typically based on the principle of behavioral economy and thus promise a high degree of sustainability.

Supporting Healthcare Workers' Performance

The field of HFE supports human performance through three interrelated domains (Table 27.1).[1] *Physical ergonomics* concerns the design of work environments in order to fit the physical strengths and limitations of humans. *Cognitive ergonomics* is concerned with mental processes, such as memory, perception, reasoning, and emotions, and how these abilities relate to the elements of a system. *Macroergonomics* considers the optimization of the overall socio-technical systems, including social and behavioral aspects. As such, most HFE improvement efforts require the use of inputs from all three domains, while recognizing that in this interactive system, modifications in any single domain will have repercussions on the others.

Eliminating Latent Errors

In the 2000 report, "To Err Is Human," the Institute of Medicine made a strong call to apply HFE intelligence to the healthcare domain to identify and eradicate what were termed "latent errors."[4] These are flaws that are built into the system, in technology and layers of management, that can potentially lead to human errors

Table 27.1 Human Factors Engineering Core Principles

Human Factors and Ergonomics Aim	Human Factors and Ergonomics Principles	Hand Hygiene Application Examples
Supporting physical performance	Keep everything in easy reach Work at proper heights Work in good postures Reduce excessive forces Minimize fatigue Reduce excessive repetition Provide clearance and access Minimize contact stress Provide mobility and change of posture Maintain a comfortable environment	Locate ABHR dispensers at height that is suitable for HCW's anthropometric features (elbow height) Stock ABHR dispensers with adequate amounts of solution, ensure that refill solutions are easily accessible When appropriate, favor the more rapid hand cleansing with ABHR rather than soap and water handwashing Ensure ABHR is skin-friendly Strive for dispensers to provide correct amount of product, ideally according to hand size
Supporting cognitive performance	Standardize common processes and procedures Use stereotypes Link actions with perceptions Present information at the appropriate level of detail Present clear images Use redundancies Use patterns Provide variable stimuli Provide instantaneous feedback Promote emotional design	Standardize placement of dispensers between hospital settings and patient bays Standardize indications for hand hygiene Provide visual cues to remind HCWs of proper moments to handrub; make them coincide with mental models of target population Establish a consistent and highly recognizable visual language to communicate behavior rules Ensure that touchless ABHR dispensers react rapidly Employ user testing to ensure usability of dispensers and any other resources for hand hygiene Design ABHR dispensers to render the user experience of hand hygiene likable on olfactory, haptic, auditory, postural, and visual levels Introduce real-time hand hygiene performance feedback Introduce surveillance feedback on healthcare-associated infection rates Utilize black light technology for hand hygiene training to visualize infectious risk and improve technique

(continued)

Table 27.1 (Continued)

Human Factors and Ergonomics Aim	Human Factors and Ergonomics Principles	Hand Hygiene Application Examples
Supporting social/organizational performance	Identify role models and opinion leaders Set social norms and team-based targets Support salience of social norms in work environment Harness social influence Strengthen leadership Guarantee physical and psychological environment to sustain organizational learning	Identify and support likable and influential persons in the institution who genuinely support the cause of hand hygiene Assure that leaders on all levels know hand hygiene facts and rules in enough detail to be credible Integrate social norm of hand hygiene in as many documents and web contents (on other topics) as possible Consider social perception of hand hygiene actions/omissions (sound, vision, etc.) Ensure that staffing and work organization allow sufficient rest to prevent fatigue and enough time for hand hygiene to be executed (slack time and space for team debriefings and innovation sessions)
Mitigate latent errors	Review errors, adverse events, and near-misses to inform system reform Examine processes of care for potential threats to safety	Apply HFE research and development methods to hand hygiene to reactively and prospectively identify hot spots Consider submitting transmission of multiresistant bacteria or healthcare-associated infections to critical incident reporting systems Consider using barrier mitigation tool such as the Barriers Identification and Mitigation Tool (BIM)*

*Gurses AP, Murphy DJ, Martinez EA, Berenholtz SM, Pronovost PJ. A practical tool to identify and eliminate barriers to compliance with evidence-based guidelines. *Jt Comm J Qual Pat Saf* 2009;**35**:526–532.

ABHR, alcohol-based handrub; HCW, healthcare worker; HFE, human factor and ergonomics.

and only become manifest once holes in the notorious "Swiss cheese" – where layers of cheese represent a system's multiple levels of defense and holes represent opportunities for a process to fail – align.[5]

Human Factors Design Principles and Techniques

HFE benefits from a valuable set of design principles (Table 27.1) that can be applied to support hand hygiene performance and eliminate latent errors. Typical HFE techniques are displayed in Table 27.2. From this knowledge base, multiple opportunities arise in the field of hand hygiene improvement (Figure 27.1).

Original Research in HFE

The following work exemplifies how HFE principles (Table 27.1) and techniques (Table 27.2) can be applied to improve hand hygiene. The strict limitation in mental resources in any given moment and its effect on human performance can be overcome by what is termed *external cognition,* the use of the external environment to reduce required cognitive effort. Nevo et al. used a simulated patient encounter in an actual hospital room to test the impact of visual cues (flashing lights and conspicuous dispenser placement) on hand hygiene performance.[6] Also exploring cues in the external environment, Birnbach et al. found an olfactory cue, fresh fragrance, significantly improved hand hygiene among HCWs.[7] Another study found that although increasing the number of sinks alone did not improve hand hygiene, social norm activation by the presence of peers did have a significant impact on hand hygiene, supporting the argument for a systems approach to improving HCW performance.[8] The HFE approach underlying the "My Five Moments for Hand Hygiene" concept[9] to simplify and standardize processes to reduce cognitive workload, may explain its international success. Clearly, the switch from handwashing to the use of alcohol-based handrubs represents an ergonomic revolution.

WHAT WE DO NOT KNOW – THE UNCERTAIN

Until now, HFE expertise has been underexploited in the realm of patient safety and hand hygiene. While some studies have used evaluative techniques similar to those employed in HFE evaluations, such as questionnaires and surveys, most lack a systems perspective as well as the subsequent design phase and re-evaluation, leaving us to wonder to what extent hand hygiene performance could be ultimately improved. Cost-effectiveness models have demonstrated the benefits of applying HFE in other domains but return on investment for hand hygiene promotion remains to be demonstrated. Strong anecdotal evidence suggests that many low hanging fruit remain for HFE, but harvesting is difficult due to organizational complexity.[10] It remains to be defined where HFE knowhow is best implemented in healthcare organizations.

Table 27.2 Human Factors Engineering Evaluation and Design Techniques

Human Factors Domain	Sub-Domains	Examples of Specific Methods
Evaluation and problem solving	Data collection	Interviews, focus groups, observations, questionnaires; data collection may be qualitative, quantitative, or mixed
	Task analysis	Hierarchical task analysis, critical path analysis, GOMS (goals, operators, methods, and selection rules), verbal protocol analysis (think aloud protocol), cognitive task analysis methods. Task analysis is a basic function in HFE evaluation and problem solving
	Error detection	SHERPA (Systematic Human Error Reduction and Prediction Approach); detection may be prospective, retrospective, or in the form of root-cause analysis
	Situational awareness assessment	Assessment can be in real time, during scenario freeze time, or after the scenario. C-SAS (Cranefield Situational Awareness Scale); SAGAT (Situation Awareness Global Assessment Tool)
	Mental workload assessment	Modified Cooper Harper scale (MCH) technique, Subjective Workload Assessment Technique (SWAT), NASA-TLX (Task Load Index), physiological measures. Assessment may be predictive or evaluative
Design process	Gather design input	Literature review, harvesting existing designs
	Front-end analysis	Interviews, focus groups, questionnaires, observations, personas, eye tracking, time/motion study, think aloud protocols, story telling
	Conceptual, participatory design	Co-creation, workshops
	Iterative design and usability testing	Prototyping, design scenario analysis, walk through, think-aloud protocols, Wizard of Oz experiment

GOMS, Goals, Operators, Methods, and Selection Rules;
SHERPA, Systematic Human Error Reduction and Prediction Approach;
C-SAS, Cranfield Situational Awareness Scale;
SAGAT, Situation Awareness Global Assessment Tool.

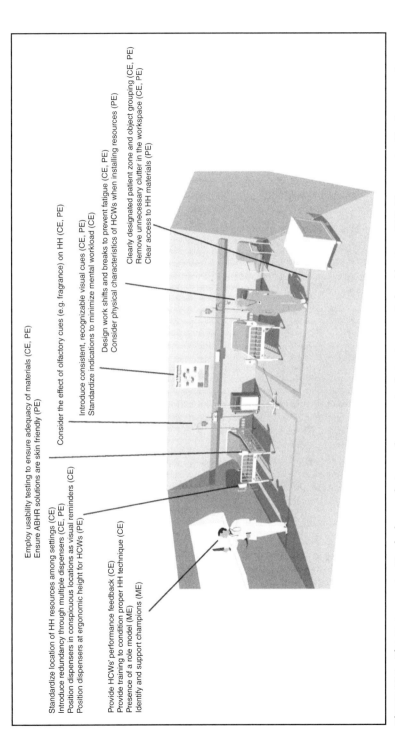

Employ usability testing to ensure adequacy of materials (CE, PE)
Ensure ABHR solutions are skin friendly (PE)

Consider the effect of olfactory cues (e.g. fragrance) on HH (CE, PE)

Standardize location of HH resources among settings (CE)
Introduce redundancy through multiple dispensers (CE, PE)
Position dispensers in conspicuous locations as visual reminders (CE)
Position dispensers at ergonomic height for HCWs (PE)

Introduce consistent, recognizable visual cues (CE, PE)
Standardize indications to minimize mental workload (CE)

Design work shifts and breaks to prevent fatigue (CE, PE)
Consider physical characteristics of HCWs when installing resources (PE)

Clearly designated patient zone and object grouping (CE, PE)
Remove unnecessary clutter in the workspace (CE, PE)
Clear access to HH materials (PE)

Provide HCWs' performance feedback (CE)
Provide training to condition proper HH technique (CE)
Presence of a role model (ME)
Identify and support champions (ME)

Figure 27.1 The many opportunities for human factors and ergonomics design to promote hand hygiene (HH). The opportunities for supporting healthcare worker (HCW) hand hygiene performance through human factors engineering can be applied at three levels: PE, physical ergonomics; CE, cognitive ergonomics; and ME, macroergonomics. ABHR, alcohol-based handrub. *See plate section for color representation of this figure.*

RESEARCH AGENDA

Although interest in HFE has increased steadily in the past years, most health-care institutions still lack the organizational structures to support the necessary collaboration between healthcare professionals and HFE experts. HFE needs to be considered earlier in the design process of any project, by involving HFE experts in collaboration with front-end clinicians, and making full use of the specific HFE toolset. The approach should be truly systemic and effectively support physical, cognitive, and social/organizational human performance. In this vein, it is reasonable to believe that we will see an exponential growth in HFE research and engineering to promote hand hygiene, patient safety, and HCW job satisfaction in the coming years.

In all its brevity and commonplaceness, the scenario at the beginning of this chapter holds many HFE aspects as this chapter suggests. The failure to perform hand hygiene after touching the patient might be due to a lack of a convenient place to dispose of gloves in the patient room, a wrong mental model, missing signage, ineffective training, weak social norm activation, or ignoring fatigue, any of which are accessible for HFE evaluation and design.

REFERENCES

1. International Association of Ergonomics, (2000) Definition of Ergonomics IAE, 2000. Available at www.iea.cc/whats/index.html. Accessed March 7, 2017.
2. Hignett S, Carayon P, Buckle P, et al., State of science: human factors and ergonomics in healthcare. *Ergonomics* 2013;**56**:1491–1503.
3. Karsh BT, Holden RJ, Alper SJ, et al., A human factors engineering paradigm for patient safety: designing to support the performance of the healthcare professional. *Qual Saf Health Care* 2006:**15**(Suppl. 1):i59–i65.
4. Kohn LJ, Corrigan JM, Donaldson M, *To Err Is Human: Building a Safer Health System*. Washington DC: National Academies Press, 2000:312.
5. Reason J, *Human Error*. Cambridge: Cambridge University Press, 1990.
6. Nevo I, Fitzpatrick M, Thomas R-E, et al., The efficacy of visual cues to improve hand hygiene compliance. *Simul Healthc* 2010;**5**:325–331.
7. Birnbach DJ, King D, Vlaev I, et al., Impact of environmental olfactory cues on hand hygiene behavior in a simulated hospital environment: a randomized study. *J Hosp Infect* 2013;**85**:79–81.
8. Lankford MG, Zembower TR, Trick WE, et al., Influence of role models and hospital design on hand hygiene of health care workers. *Emerg Infect Dis* 2003;**9**:217–223.
9. Sax H, Allegranzi B, Uckay I, et al., "My five moments for hand hygiene": a user-centred design approach to understand, train, monitor and report hand hygiene. *J Hosp Infect* 2007;**67**:9–21.
10. Clack L, Kuster SP, Giger H, et al., Low-hanging fruit for human factors design in infection prevention – still too high to reach? *Am J Infect Control* 2014;**42**:679–681.

Chapter 28

Institutional Safety Climate

Enrique Castro-Sánchez,[1] Alison Holmes,[1] and Didier Pittet[2]

[1] *National Institute for Health Research, Health Protection Research Unit in Healthcare Associated Infection and Antimicrobial Resistance, Imperial College London, London, UK*
[2] *Infection Control Program and WHO Collaborating Centre on Patient Safety, University of Geneva Hospitals and Faculty of Medicine, Geneva, Switzerland*

KEY MESSAGES

- Hand hygiene improvement must be embedded within wider institutional safety climate initiatives.
- Perceptions of institutional safety are shaped by multiple factors, including managerial decision making, norms, policies, and procedures as well as expectations to comply with those.
- It is recommended to promote an adequate safety climate in a concerted and focused organizational effort, that is carried out concurrently with each step of hand hygiene improvement proposals.

Organizations striving to offer quality care must encourage a comprehensive safety culture that includes hand hygiene improvement initiatives. To achieve sustained success in this area, leaders must carefully balance their demands for excellence while providing support and resources; implementation plans must be inclusive and focused; staff and patients must be encouraged to communicate and collaborate together; and any failures must be seen as opportunities to learn and achieve success. Embracing these steps is central to the advance of perceptions of patient safety that in turn will inspire hand hygiene excellence.

Hand Hygiene: A Handbook for Medical Professionals, First Edition.
Edited by Didier Pittet, John M. Boyce and Benedetta Allegranzi.
© 2017 John Wiley & Sons, Inc. Published 2017 by John Wiley & Sons, Inc.

WHAT WE KNOW – THE EVIDENCE

Hand hygiene initiatives that focus solely on technical elements or emphasize individual healthcare worker responsibility are unlikely to generate effective and sustainable hand hygiene improvements. For these to take place, the World Health Organization (WHO) multimodal hand hygiene promotion strategy has recognized that cultural, social, and organizational factors appear to be equally necessary to achieve successful progress in compliance with recommendations (see Chapter 33). Hand hygiene interventions must be embedded within the institutional patient safety agenda that lies at the core of organizational activity.

What is the Institutional Safety Climate?

The institutional safety climate refers to the environment and perceptions of patient safety issues at the healthcare setting and facility, in which hand hygiene improvement is considered a high priority.[1] Although safety climate and safety culture have often been used interchangeably, it may be useful to consider the subtle differences between the two terms. While organizational culture encompasses the set of norms, values, and basic assumptions prevalent within the entire organization, the notion of institutional safety climate is more specific and refers to the employees' perceptions of safety aspects of the organization's culture.[2] Such perceptions about the attention to patient safety will be shaped by multiple factors, including managerial decision making and style, institutional safety norms, policies, and procedures, as well as the expectations to comply with those. Identifying the significance of safety expectations can explain how the mere presence of policies and guidelines would not be sufficient to ensure appropriate safety behaviors, as illustrated often when reviewing patient safety failures. Due to these multiple factors, different perceptions about institutional safety can be highly variable between different professional groups, hierarchical levels, or organizational roles, and are likely to fluctuate over time. The inconsistency between groups and temporal variability demands that continued and renewed institutional safety activities be in place, as shared cultures are unlikely to emerge without explicit and consistent efforts to nurture them. It is vital to acknowledge how a successful institutional safety climate encompasses any recommended hand hygiene procedures, but is not limited to them, and conceptualizes organizational and clinical activity that strives to maintain and continuously improve comprehensive patient safety. The WHO Hand Hygiene Self-Assessment Framework (2010, see Appendix) illustrates this idea of total engagement with quality hand hygiene practices permeating a whole organization (see Chapter 34).[3–5]

The successful implementation of institutional safety climate requires a shift in the structural focus — from point-of-care issues (e.g., availability of products, staff education) to wider, strategic drivers of excellent practice. However, the diversity of factors that influence safety perceptions impairs the development and implementation of effective interventions. Furthermore, current available evidence to support interventions remains limited, and recent reviews have highlighted how healthcare organizations may have also underestimated the assets and commitment required to introduce and maintain safety initiatives successfully.[6]

Such lack of engagement may be due to the long-term vision required to cultivate a culture and perceptions of safety, in contrast to other low-hanging tasks yielding immediate benefits following simpler organizational improvements (e.g., ensuring the supply of alcohol-based handrub, introducing regular training, etc.). Fostering an organization's safety climate may appear as the final step among the components proposed in the WHO strategy, with the suggestion that any attention given to this step should occur only after all other elements have been achieved. Although it may be true that developing the institutional safety climate would be a key priority for healthcare organizations at advanced stages of hand hygiene improvement, it would be misguided to ignore the institutional safety climate as essential at all stages in order to maintain the motivation and momentum for any success already achieved.

A variety of measurement tools have been developed with the aim to identify the underlying safety culture of a given organization. Although using these tools can be beneficial to gain a strategic overview of the organizational safety readiness,[7] some caution has to be exercised when appraising the results obtained. It is unlikely that a single survey, even if extensively conducted, would be able to characterize the richness and features of existing patient safety subcultures that may exist on individual wards, hospitals, or healthcare centers. Further, as existing tools reflect or describe particular cultural traits, it is necessary to evaluate the validity of any scores derived from the tools when applied to settings other than the original ones. Finally, it would be desirable to supplement any findings from the survey with qualitative data that can facilitate an understanding of contextual factors and support the implementation of any quality-improvement initiatives.[8] Some of the most widely used institutional safety tools include:

1. Patient Safety Climate in Healthcare Organizations:[9] this tool was developed by Stanford University and the US Agency for Healthcare Research and Quality Research in 2007. It considers safety-related issues from a holistic perspective (at the individual, unit, and overall organization level). However, its use outside the United States has been limited.

2. Safety Attitudes Questionnaire (SAQ),[10] one of the most rigorously validated tools (at least in the United States) which emphasizes safety climate and team attitudes towards safety. The repeated application of this tool may be ideal to identify changes in the institutional patient safety climate over time, perhaps to examine the impact of improvement programs.

3. The Hospital Survey on Patient Safety Culture[11] has been predominantly used in US hospitals, allowing for an integration of individual, unit, and organizational level factors to describe the organizational safety culture. Similar to the SAQ, it is able to signal variations over time to identify the success of interventions.

What are Some of the Elements Required to Encourage a Successful Institutional Safety Climate?

Some elements required to support an environment that increases awareness at all levels about patient safety matters (including hand hygiene) as a high priority include the active participation of leaders, the awareness of individuals to change and improve their practice, and the contribution of patients and patient organizations.

a. Active Participation of Leaders
Traditionally, hand hygiene improvement strategies have concentrated on adjusting the behaviors of healthcare professionals (i.e., a focus on the individual level) or the introduction of new technologies or facilities (i.e., a focus on the organizational level). Still, those approaches would not be able to resolve barriers such as negative role models, a poor safety culture, and lack of managerial involvement. It would be very unlikely, if possible at all, for any healthcare setting to adopt a given quality improvement or patient safety initiative without the agreement and support from institutional leaders.

Clearly, successful hand hygiene initiatives benefit from explicit and visible endorsement and participation from organizational leaders. For instance, the interest of clinical managers in hand hygiene activities, including the dissemination of feedback and evaluations, has been identified as a critical and one of the most powerful incentives for all stakeholders involved (see also Chapter 40). In other settings, the institutional leadership is demonstrated at a higher level, with politicians including ministers of health, attending the launch of hand hygiene improvement initiatives.[12] These endorsements by key figures shape not only the opinions and beliefs about the value of hand hygiene improvements held by an organization, but also those of the wider health community including perceptions from competing or rival institutions.

As healthcare is delivered through collaborations of multiple professionals from different backgrounds, the attitudes displayed by organizational leaders diffuse to middle managers, ward and team leaders, and ultimately frontline staff. Conversely, feedback about the success or failure of a hand hygiene improvement initiative can also be directed in the opposite direction. For example, hand hygiene achievements could be included in institutional dashboards and performance reports, with leadership engagement demonstrated by monitoring hand hygiene compliance rates and the communication of rates to managers and staff. Additionally, leaders can steer the incentives or penalties used to encourage any preferred attitudes or practices. For example, supportive rather than punitive tactics are generally considered more effective in sustaining institutional safety climate programs.[13] But while the recognition of achievements is preferred to punishing noncompliant individuals or underperforming units, some projects have explored the use of "violation letters" composed jointly by administrators and infection control clinicians and endorsed by hospital board members.[14]

Ultimately, leaders are essential not only to articulate a vision and climate of safety, maintaining enthusiasm, and inspiring ethical, purposeful, and safe clinical practice, but also to ensure that cohesion of clinical and administrative teams is not damaged when staff leave or are replaced, reducing the risks derived from the loss of the education and experience accumulated by those individuals and preserving what could be thought of as "institutional hand hygiene resilience."

b. Awareness of Individual Healthcare Workers of the Need to Improve Their Practice

The successful implementation of system change at the healthcare facility level cannot be achieved without staff education about hand transmission of pathogens and hygiene standards, the commitment of managers and commissioners to the sustained procurement of ABHRs, and the provision of an appropriate infrastructure for optimal hand hygiene. However, the inclusion of these elements will not guarantee the success of an initiative, and for such an accomplishment the sustained participation of staff is indispensable. Unfortunately, this has been proven to be a much more problematic task.

What solutions have then been proposed to maintain the engagement towards hand hygiene improvement initiatives? Some of the successful methodologies have incorporated different insights from behavioral sciences with additional activities to reinforce the social element of teamwork.[15] For example, positive deviance has produced significant increases in compliance and improvements on HAIs.[16] In the positive deviance framework, positive deviants include frontline staff recognized as role models due to their consistent and effective hand hygiene practice. These role models resolve problems such as noncompliance with guidelines in collaboration with others. In turn, organizational leaders and managers focus on supporting frontline workers in implementing the new, proposed solutions into their routines.

In addition to these role models, other social factors influencing the participation of staff on institutional safety initiatives include peer pressure and hand hygiene preceptors and buddies, among others (Table 28.1).

Finally, social marketing and communication principles (see also Chapter 26) have been used to maintain the interest of healthcare workers towards hand hygiene initiatives, linking proficient hand hygiene practice to accountability, safety, and professionalism.[17]

Table 28.1   Some Factors Encouraging Staff Commitment to Institutional Safety

- Adequate lead-in time and duration of intervention
- Multiprofessional involvement in design, implementation, and evaluation
- Shift in responsibility towards safety initiatives from specific individuals or roles to all staff
- Use of rewards rather than punitive incentives

Source: Gurse 2009. Reproduced with permission from The Joint Commission.

Table 28.2   Some Barriers to Patient and User Involvement in Safety Initiatives

---

- **Sociocultural**: preventing patients from asking healthcare workers about their hand hygiene compliance due to perceived roles about what is expected from patients as well as healthcare workers
- **Boundaries**: patients may feel anxious to look like they are policing staff and worrying about receiving worse care if they ask about hand hygiene compliance. On the other hand, they may assume also that it is not their responsibility to ask about hand hygiene compliance
- **Self-efficacy**: including willingness to be empowered as key participants; knowledge and skills about hand hygiene appropriateness. In order to obtain such knowledge, patients' health literacy about hand hygiene may play a key role

---

c. Contribution and Participation of Patients and Service Users
The inclusion of patient and service user contributions in hand hygiene improvement initiatives has gained traction in recent years (see also Chapter 30). It is now considered a paramount aspect in the field of institutional safety, reflecting the contribution of patients as peers in the shared decision-making process, with very successful initiatives encouraging participation of patients in institutional safety programs.[18] For example, an explicit invitation to ask staff about hand hygiene was associated with an increased willingness by parents of hospitalized children to remind staff to perform hand hygiene.[19] Such encouragement may have wider benefits outside the domain of safety, decreasing social barriers related to healthcare workers' professional status and seniority.

Although guidelines suggest that engagement of patients in hand hygiene practices appears to be a suitable strategy, there exist unresolved questions. Patient participation may only take place if an organization is already well prepared and with an appreciation that not every patient may be willing or able to join the efforts. Organizational, cultural, and structural barriers preventing the participation of patients have been identified (Table 28.2), suggesting that unless those factors are addressed, organizations will fail to motivate patients to engage with improvement initiatives. Patient characteristics, clinical situation, and willingness have to be appraised before assuming their involvement, and adequate safeguards have to exist to guarantee care of similar quality for those who are not able or decline to be involved in a hand hygiene initiative. It seems clear that for patient engagement strategies to be successful, healthcare workers and organizations cannot just give permission for patients and relatives to participate.

WHAT WE DO NOT KNOW – THE UNCERTAIN

Despite the progress made, further challenges in the achievement and sustainability of institutional patient safety initiatives remain unaddressed. For example, in terms of leader participation, it is still unclear how to engage leaders, including political figures, in safety improvement initiatives, and how best to equip clinicians with the skills to transmit the importance of life- and cost-saving hand hygiene initiatives to leaders and decision makers (see also Chapter 40).

The dynamics of team and organizational networks must be further explored to examine the impact of key influencers who are not official leaders, in order to gain their support and galvanize improvement proposals. Similarly, it is crucial to understand how clinicians and healthcare workers balance public expressions of commitment and endorsement to hand hygiene initiatives from leaders with other competing demands, and how the resources allocated may frame such expressions of commitment. But if the identification of a given institutional safety climate requires the measurement of employees' perceptions using diverse tools, could this in itself then induce a certain safety climate Hawthorne effect? In addition, how might perceptions change following critical incidents?

Finally, and reflecting upon the underestimation of resources required to introduce engagement with safety initiatives, it may be apt to describe the experiences of those units and organizations who tried but failed to produce adequate or sustainable effects, highlighting the critical steps.

RESEARCH AGENDA

As mentioned, addressing the determinants of patients' participation is essential to encourage their involvement. In addition to those, more progress is needed to optimize the ways in which to provide information to service users, patients, and relatives about the importance of suitable institutional safety initiatives, including hand hygiene. The incipient patient participation in hand hygiene promotion strategies appears to be limited to interactions at the point of care, but studies should further evaluate the benefit of including user feedback during the design and implementation stages of the initiatives. Interestingly, there are few studies focusing on the role and impact of visitors and informal caregivers in hand hygiene improvement initiatives; is it then necessary to develop initiatives that serve to remind patients of their potential role in hand hygiene? There is a need to examine the ethical framework used to foster patient participation in hand hygiene initiatives. It seems pertinent to reflect upon any dilemmas that this approach may present to vulnerable individuals, and in areas with limited material or human resources (see also Chapter 43) where there may be potential for subtle exploitation. Finally, describing the perceptions of service users and patients about a given safety climate can add richness to organizational initiatives, but there could be challenges to collect and integrate these perceptions onto the existing tools.

REFERENCES

1. World Health Organization, *WHO Guidelines on Hand Hygiene in Health Care.* Geneva: WHO, 2009. Available at whqlibdoc.who.int/publications/2009/9789241597906_eng.pdf. Accessed March 7, 2017.

2. Gershon RR, Stone PW, Bakken S, et al., Measurement of organizational culture and climate in health care. *J Nurs Adm* 2004;**34**:33–40.

3. World Health Organization, *Hand Hygiene Self-Assessment Framework*. Geneva: WHO, 2010. Available at www.who.int/gpsc/country_work/hhsa_framework_October_2010.pdf. Accessed March 7, 2017.

4. Stewardson AJ, Allegranzi B, Perneger TV, et al., Testing the WHO Hand Hygiene Self-Assessment Framework for usability and reliability. *J Hosp Infect* 2013;**83**:30–35.

5. Allegranzi B, Conway L, Larson E, et al., Status of the implementation of the World Health Organization multimodal hand hygiene strategy in United States of America health care facilities. *Am J Infect Control* 2014;**42**:224–230.

6. Morello RT, Lowthian JA, Barker AL, et al., Strategies for improving patient safety culture in hospitals: a systematic review. *BMJ Qual Saf* 2013;**22**:11–18.

7. McCarthy D, Blumenthal D, Stories from the sharp end: Case studies in safety improvement. *Milbank Q* 2006;**84**:165–200.

8. Singer SJ, Falwell A, Lin S, et al., Relationship of safety climate and safety performance in hospitals. *Health Serv Res* 2009;**44**:399–421.

9. Singer S, Meterko M, Baker L, et al., Workforce perceptions of hospital safety culture: development and validation of the patient safety climate in healthcare organizations survey. *Health Serv Res* 2007;**42**:1999–2021.

10. Sexton JB, Helmreich RL, Neilands TB, et al., The Safety Attitudes Questionnaire: psychometric properties, benchmarking data, and emerging research. *BMC Health Serv Res* 2006;**6**:44.

11. Blegen MA, Gearhart S, O'Brien R, et al., AHRQ's hospital survey on patient safety culture: psychometric analyses. *J Patient Saf* 2009;**5**:139–144.

12. Allegranzi B, Gayet-Ageron A, Damani N, et al., Global implementation of WHO's multimodal strategy for improvement of hand hygiene: a quasi-experimental study. *Lancet Infect Dis* 2013;**13**:843–851.

13. Hysong SJ, Teal CR, Khan MJ, et al., Improving quality of care through improved audit and feedback. *Implement Sci* 2012;**7**:45.

14. Chou T, Kerridge J, Kulkarni M, et al., Changing the culture of hand hygiene compliance using a bundle that includes a violation letter. *Am J Infect Control* 2010;**38**:575–578.

15. Pittet D, Simon A, Hugonnet S, et al., Hand hygiene among physicians: performance, beliefs, and perceptions. *Ann Intern Med* 2004;**141**:1–8.

16. Marra AR, Guastelli LR, Araújo CMP, et al., Positive deviance: a program for sustained improvement in hand hygiene compliance. *Am J Infect Control* 2011;**39**:1–5.

17. Forrester LA, Bryce EA, Mediaa AK, Clean Hands for Life: results of a large, multicentre, multifaceted, social marketing hand-hygiene campaign. *J Hosp Infect* 2010;**74**:225–231.

18. Landers T, Abusalem S, Coty MB, et al., Patient-centered hand hygiene: the next step in infection prevention. *Am J Infect Control* 2012;**40**(4 Suppl. 1);S11–S17.

19. Buser GL, Fisher BT, Shea JA, et al., Patient willingness to remind health care workers to perform hand hygiene. *Am J Infect Control* 2013;**41**:492–496.

Chapter 29

Personal Accountability for Hand Hygiene

Robert M. Wachter[1] and Peter Pronovost[2]

[1] *Department of Medicine, University of California, and University of California San Francisco Medical Center, San Francisco, USA*

[2] *Armstrong Institute for Patient Safety and Quality, Johns Hopkins, and Patient Safety and Quality, The Johns Hopkins University School of Medicine, Baltimore, USA*

KEY MESSAGES

- Infection prevention and control has become a central theme of the patient safety movement, and has benefited from the attention, resources, and systems focus that this has created.

- As one of the most important evidence-based practices in infection prevention (and in patient safety), hand hygiene has received a tremendous amount of attention. In many countries, there are now significant policy initiatives that are designed to put emphasis on performance.

- While "better systems" are a crucial component of any program to improve hand hygiene compliance, it is important to support and enforce both individual and organizational accountability for performance. In fact, hand hygiene may be an ideal test case for the healthcare system to work through the complex issues related to accountability.

The patient safety movement has elevated the field of infection prevention. Prior to the year 2000, many hospitals had infection control officers who tried to promote good infection-prevention practices, monitored antibiotic resistance patterns, and kept an eye out for emerging infectious risks. But in most countries, the motivations for physicians and other healthcare professionals to comply with the recommendations of infection preventionists – ranging from hand hygiene to isolation

Hand Hygiene: A Handbook for Medical Professionals, First Edition.
Edited by Didier Pittet, John M. Boyce and Benedetta Allegranzi.
© 2017 John Wiley & Sons, Inc. Published 2017 by John Wiley & Sons, Inc.

precautions – were relatively weak, in part because many clinicians did not make the connection between following such recommendations and harming their own patients. Front-line clinicians did not see infection prevention, or the patient harm created when it was not practiced, as their problem. Added to this lack of tangible connection between preventive practices and harm was the virtual absence of pressure from the broader system to promote compliance.

WHAT WE KNOW – THE EVIDENCE

The emergence of an international effort to improve patient safety approximately 15 years, ago – introduced in the United States by the Institute of Medicine's *To Err is Human*, and in the UK by *An Organisation with a Memory* – changed the perceptions of individual clinicians, patients, administrators, and policy makers.[1,2] Finally, the idea of healthcare-associated harms moved onto the radar screen of the healthcare system, and infectious risks became one of the major harms targeted by the nascent safety movement. The reasons for this were many, but included the fact that such harms are more easily measured than many others (such as diagnostic or medication errors); that there are several practices, including hand hygiene but others as well, with a strong evidence base; and that the infrastructure supporting infection prevention (from standard definitions of infections to trained professionals to data collection to connection to local or national prevention-oriented agencies) was already present in many hospitals.[3]

In fact – and perhaps surprisingly – infection prevention became a central focus of the patient safety movement. In the United States, this trend accelerated after the publication of the Keystone study, which demonstrated that a program blending the use of checklists with efforts to change culture and feedback information on infection rates to clinicians led to a striking decrease in central-line-associated bloodstream infections.[4]

Although hand hygiene had already been identified as a crucial practice by the infection prevention community, it benefited from the additional attention it received by its inclusion under the broad umbrella of patient safety. And the field's emphasis on "systems thinking" – that most errors are committed by competent, caring people; thus the best way to prevent them is to create systems to catch the errors before they cause harm – also led to major improvements, many of which are documented throughout this book. These include the decision to emphasize alcohol-based handrubs rather than soap and water, the placement of dispensers in convenient places around the facility, educational campaigns surrounding hand hygiene, and even audit and feedback programs. Today, such system thinking is leading to the development and deployment of new technologies, such as those that alert caregivers if they approach a patient without first actuating the alcohol-based handrub dispenser.[5]

While the linkage of the patient safety movement with infection prevention has undoubtedly been salutary, we have raised a cautionary note in recent years: that the movement's emphasis on a "no blame," systems-oriented culture is leading to lax enforcement of certain practices that should be inviolable, in part because this approach has largely viewed clinicians as separate from, not as part of, the system.[6,7] Here too, prime among these practices is hand hygiene.

One of the definitions of a profession is that it is self-policing.[8] The need for this comes from society's appreciation that the professionals possess specialized knowledge that non-experts lack, thus putting the profession in the best position to create and enforce its own rules. It also comes from the assumed beneficence of a profession, particularly a healing profession like medicine, in which the practitioners are expected to place the welfare of their patients above their own. The public and policy makers expect medical professionals to enforce reasonable, evidence-based safety standards, but will reluctantly step in when they feel that the profession is not taking this charge seriously or is too tolerant of bad apples.[9]

Yet the public's expectation that the medical profession (and other clinicians such as nurses) will be self-policing with regard to evidence-based safety practices may come into conflict with a paradigm that has emphasized "no blame" as the appropriate response to errors. But this tension is less significant than it might at first appear. As David Marx has pointed out in his popularization of the concept of "Just Culture," a no-blame response is only appropriate for errors that involve slips and innocent mistakes.[10] It is *not* appropriate for willful violation of reasonable safety standards, such as hand hygiene.

As the public has come to understand the risks of healthcare ("100,000 deaths per year from medical errors" is a common mantra in the United States, though the actual number is likely far higher), its tolerance for a no-blame approach has waned, particularly in the face of relatively low hand hygiene rates in many hospitals and high rates of severe healthcare-associated infections (HAIs), many of which could be prevented by better hand hygiene practices. As we wrote in 2009 in the *New England Journal of Medicine*,

Part of the reason we must [begin to enforce certain safety standards] is that if we do not, other stakeholders, such as regulators and state legislatures, are likely to judge the reflexive invocation of the "no blame" approach as an example of guild behavior — of the medical profession circling its wagons to avoid confronting harsh realities, rather than as a thoughtful strategy for attacking the root causes of most errors. With that as their conclusion, they will be predisposed to further intrude on the practice of medicine, using the blunt and often politicized sticks of the legal, regulatory, and payment systems.

Having our own profession unblinkingly deem some behaviors as unacceptable, with clear consequences, will serve as a vivid example of our professionalism and thus represent our best protection against such outside intrusions. But the main reason to find the right balance between "no blame" and individual accountability is that doing so will save lives.[6]

There are multiple accountabilities when it comes to hand hygiene. While it is easy and natural to focus on personal accountability – that of the individual clinician who has to make the choice whether to engage in hand hygiene – Bell and colleagues have highlighted the importance of collective accountability: accountability at the level of the individual clinician, the healthcare team, and the institution.[11] When clinicians fail to perform hand hygiene, it is important to consider system factors before immediately moving to enforce individual accountability measures. Have clinicians been adequately educated? Are hand hygiene product dispensers filled and functioning, and are they located in easy-to-use places? Do nurses have the time to perform hand hygiene as many times as needed? Safe organizations approach complex issues like hand hygiene compliance with a balanced and open approach: low rates should not immediately be assumed to be personal failings, nor should they immediately be assumed to be systems problems. Just as patient care depends on making the right diagnosis before recommending a therapeutic plan, so too does a strong hand hygiene program. In addition, the organization should create a culture in which peers can monitor and critique each other; peer norms can be a powerful force to increase compliance with hand hygiene.

WHAT WE DO NOT KNOW AND RESEARCH AGENDA

We now understand that high hand hygiene compliance rates are a key driver of patient safety. There are also few safety practices that are so inexpensive, so effective, and have such little risk of harm or unanticipated consequences. As such, they serve as a useful marker for an organization's and an individual's overall commitment to patient safety. According to this reasoning, if we can't get hand hygiene right, how are we ever going to achieve high rates of compliance with important safety practices that are much harder to accomplish? And, just as hand hygiene is a marker of patient safety, it can also be a model for accountability. Healthcare systems should develop, implement, and evaluate accountability systems for hand hygiene. Once they have sorted out the many clinical, educational, economic, and political issues that will invariably arise, they should then spread the model to other patient safety practices with strong supporting evidence.

REFERENCES

1. Committee on Quality of Health Care in America, Institute of Medicine, *To Err is Human: Building a Safer Health System*. Washington, DC: National Academy Press, 2000.
2. Department of Health, *An Organisation with a Memory*, 2000. Available at webarchive .nationalarchives.gov.uk/20130107105354/http:/www.dh.gov.uk/prod_consum_dh/ groups/dh_digitalassets/@dh/@en/documents/digitalasset/dh_4065086.pdf. Accessed March 7, 2017.
3. Gerberding JL, Hospital-onset infections: a patient safety issue. *Ann Intern Med* 2002; **137**:665–670.
4. Pronovost P, Needham D, Berenholtz S, et al., An intervention to decrease catheter-related bloodstream infections in the ICU. *N Engl J Med* 2006;**355**:2725–2732. [Erratum, *N Engl J Med* 2007;**356**:2660.]
5. Boyce JM, Update on hand hygiene. *Am J Infect Control* 2013;**41**(5 Suppl.):S94–S96.

6. Wachter RM, Pronovost PJ, Balancing "no blame" with accountability in patient safety. *N Engl J Med* 2009;**361**:1401–1406.

7. Wachter RM, Personal accountability in healthcare: searching for the right balance. *BMJ Qual Saf* 2013;**22**:176–180.

8. ABIM Foundation, Medical professionalism in the new millennium: a physician charter. *Ann Intern Med* 2002;**136**:243–246.

9. Shojania KG, Dixon-Woods M. "Bad apples": time to redefine as a type of systems problem? *BMJ Qual Saf* 2013;**22**:528–531.

10. Marx D, *Patient Safety and the "Just Culture": A Primer for Health Care Executives*. New York: Columbia University Press, 2001.

11. Bell SK, Delbanco T, Anderson-Shaw L, et al., Accountability for medical error: moving beyond blame to advocacy. *Chest* 2011;**140**:519–526.

Chapter 30

Patient Participation and Empowerment

Yves Longtin,[1] Susan E. Sheridan,[2] and Maryanne McGuckin[3]

[1] Infection Control and Prevention Unit, Jewish General Hospital, and McGill University, Montreal, Canada
[2] World Alliance for Patient Safety, World Health Organization, Geneva, Switzerland
[3] Patient-Centered Outcomes Research Institute, Washington, USA

KEY MESSAGES

- Inviting patients to participate in hand hygiene promotion is advocated by numerous organizations worldwide as a way to improve staff hand hygiene compliance.

- Numerous studies have shown that this avenue is associated with an increase in hand hygiene compliance.

- Some aspects need to be further explored to better identify the optimal methods of involving patients.

Patient participation is a concept that reinforces the patient's right to safety, right to chose and right to be heard.[1,2] In recent decades, patients' involvement in their care – traditionally passive –has become more active.[1] Patients are increasingly solicited to participate in new areas such as self-treatment of chronic diseases,[1] the design and dissemination of research,[3] and the prevention of medical adverse events.[4]

Hand Hygiene: A Handbook for Medical Professionals, First Edition.
Edited by Didier Pittet, John M. Boyce and Benedetta Allegranzi.
© 2017 John Wiley & Sons, Inc. Published 2017 by John Wiley & Sons, Inc.

Patient participation in the promotion of safe hand hygiene practices is among the most promising avenues. Healthcare workers' (HCWs') hand hygiene compliance remains alarmingly low despite intensive promotion, and patient involvement has been suggested as a way to improve their practices.[5] This strategy fits into the broader objective of creating an institutional safety climate (see Chapter 28), which is one component of a successful hand hygiene campaign according to the World Health Organization (WHO).[5]

McGuckin and colleagues were among the first to explore this field.[2] In most programs, patients are invited to remind their caregivers to perform hand hygiene before caring for them or to thank them for performing hand hygiene. Many different organizations including the WHO Patients for Patient Safety and the US Joint Commission call for greater patient involvement. This chapter reviews the principles underlying patient participation in hand hygiene promotion and identifies barriers and facilitators. Tips for implementation, areas of uncertainty, and an agenda for research are also proposed.

WHAT WE KNOW – THE EVIDENCE

Definitions and Terminology

Some uncertainty remains regarding the proper terminology to use.[1,2] Various terms such as "patient participation," "patient empowerment," "patient involvement," "patient collaboration," and "patient engagement" are used interchangeably. Some of these have been borrowed from sociology and psychology, and the fine distinction between these terms is beyond the scope of this chapter. We will use preferentially "participation" and "empowerment" in this chapter. Overall, the choice of terminology to use should take into account community and cultural specificities.[5]

Despite an abundant literature, no single definition of patient participation and empowerment in hand hygiene is universally accepted.[1,2,5] Based on previous publications, one could tentatively define it as "a set of behaviors by patients, family members and health professionals and a set of organizational policies that foster the inclusion of patients and family members in improving hand hygiene practices."[6]

Patient Willingness to Participate and Actual Participation Rate

Numerous studies have shown that a high proportion of patients (60–90%) believe they should be involved in hand hygiene promotion,[2] although other studies have observed lower proportions. Willingness is highest when theoretical concepts are presented (e.g., "do you think that patients should be involved?") and

lower when the question is more practical (e.g., "will you remind a HCW to perform hand hygiene the next time you notice omission?").[7] Many of these studies
were single-center surveys with a limited number (100–300) of respondents.
Also, desirability bias (i.e., patients providing an answer that reflects societal
norms rather than their own personal belief) and sampling bias (i.e., interviewing
the most able patients and excluding those who cannot or decline to answer)
may overestimate the level of willingness.

The proportion of respondents who actually participate and ask about hand
hygiene is also relevant. The proportion of patients who report having participated
is invariably lower than the proportion of patients who declare being willing to
ask.[1,7] Many factors could explain why some patients fail to progress from the
motivational stage to the volitional stage. Intention does not always translate into
the corresponding action in health-related matters. Skills, coping mechanisms, and
situational circumstances, among other factors, influence a patient's capacity to
translate willingness into real actions.

Efficacy of Patient Participation in Hand Hygiene

It is challenging to evaluate some aspects of the impact of patient participation
programs on patient safety. Even though the ultimate objective is to prevent
healthcare-associated infections, patients' impact on actual infection rates
has not been demonstrated yet because of methodological difficulties. Hence,
researchers have used surrogate indicators to evaluate the impact of these
programs, the most popular being caregiver hand hygiene compliance rate. Many
publications – mostly before-and-after quasi-experimental studies – have shown
improvements in hand hygiene compliance associated with patient participation
programs.[2] Studies with more elaborate designs such as cluster-randomized
controlled trials are still very rare. Also, the impact of patient participation
on hand hygiene compliance is difficult to measure using the recognized gold
standard – direct observation by trained observers – because the mere presence
of the observer acts as a reminder and has a sizeable Hawthorne effect. The use
of automated monitoring systems and hand-cleansing product consumption can
also be used to evaluate compliance rates.[2]

Another outcome commonly used to assess the effectiveness of patient participation is the proportion of patients who do remind their caregivers. However,
this indicator also has some limitations. For example, a hypothetical patient whose
nurse would comply perfectly with hand hygiene indications would not have to
intervene. A study evaluating the success of a participation program through the
rate of patient intervention would erroneously conclude that it does not work
because the patients did not remind their caregivers.

Also, some caregivers may change their behavior and start cleansing their
hands in front of patients to avoid being reminded.[8] Such change in behavior
would prevent patients from asking about hand hygiene and limit patients' opportunities to ask. Finally, a single patient intervention can have a long-lasting effect

on the caregiver, who may remain more attentive to hand hygiene long after a patient has intervened. This long-lasting impact of patient empowerment cannot be accounted for in studies that use actual patient intervention as an outcome.

Barriers

Despite all the potential benefits of patient participation, there are some obstacles at the patient, caregiver, and institution levels that must be overcome in order for patients to truly become partners in their care.

Patient-Related Obstacles

LOW PATIENT MOTIVATION. The importance of promoting hand hygiene is not readily obvious to some patients, who may believe that staff compliance is good. From the patient's perspective, poor quality of care is more often linked with other quality indicators such as waits and delays than with lapses in hand hygiene.[6] Hence, many patients may be poorly motivated to help prevent it. Also, many patients may not see promoting hand hygiene as one of their roles.[1,4] Reluctance to participate may be linked to fear of embarrassment and reprisals or fear of being tagged a "difficult patient."

Some patient characteristics influence willingness. Outgoing, extroverted patients are more willing to participate than introverted ones.[1] Patients who are younger or those who have been afflicted with a healthcare-associated infection are generally more willing to ask.[7] There may also be a gender gap, with a greater propensity in women to ask about hand hygiene.[9]

Furthermore, patient willingness is influenced by the type of caregiver, with a lower degree of readiness to ask physicians than nurses.[1,9] Finally, patients' willingness is influenced by their perception of caregiver's attitude towards being asked.[9] Patients are unwilling to ask if they feel they are not authorized to do so.[1,2]

LOW PATIENT ABILITY. Along with low motivation, lack of sufficient knowledge regarding hand hygiene may be the most important barrier to their involvement.[9] Although hand hygiene indications may seem simple to caregivers, this concept may appear overly complex to patients. Patients have struggled understanding other basic medical concepts such as surveillance of postoperative wound infections. The patients' health status also impacts their degree of involvement. Understandably, acute sickness and pain can divert their attention away from caregivers' hand hygiene practices. Sedation, confusion, and hearing, speech, or visual impairments can limit their capacity to participate.[4] The opportunity to intervene is also often lacking. The optimal moment to perform hand hygiene – and hence for patients to participate – is immediately before a caregiver touches a patient.[5] This situation may occur at a moment that may not lend itself to a question from the patient. Patients may have difficulty to intervene without interrupting the caregivers' discourse or actions. Patients' capacity to discuss a potentially sensitive topic must not be underplayed. Asking about hand hygiene is perceived by many patients as challenging.[9]

Caregiver-Related Obstacles

Obstacles to patient participation also exist at the caregiver level. A significant proportion of caregivers – up to a third in one study – may be unwilling to empower patients.[8] Many maintain a paternalistic vision and do not see patient participation as part of the patient's role. They may also harbor misconceptions and perceive these programs as a way to "police" them and as a threat to their competency. They may react negatively and defensively to being asked.[8] The fear of litigation and a perception of lack of time to both encourage patients to ask about hand hygiene and to provide an answer are also common deterrents to patient participation in their care.[1]

Lack of caregiver training in patient engagement is a significant hurdle. Many campaigns overlook the importance of training caregivers in addition to patients. Less than 20% of tools created for patient engagement campaigns are targeted to health professionals.[6]

Systemic and Organizational Barriers

Some structural and organizational aspects of healthcare institutions are also important determinants. The culture of an institution, its size, its academic or for-profit status, the presence of unions, and the strength of its leadership can impact the success of a patient participation campaign.[6] The degree of ease with which one can initiate change, the culture of safety, and the level of internal alignment (i.e., the consistency in goals across all levels of the organization) are also very important.

Previous experience in the field of patient participation will impact an institution's motivation to undertake a campaign on patient participation in hand hygiene.[6] On the other hand, the lack of continuity of care can be a challenge to the establishment of a suitable patient-caregiver relationship.[4] Placing alcohol-based handrub solution dispensers away from the patient's sight (e.g., in corridors rather than at the point of care) is another structural barrier to patient participation.

STRATEGIES TO OVERCOME BARRIERS. Fortunately, even though many barriers exist, numerous solutions have been identified to facilitate patient participation.[2] Patients' reluctance to intervene can be overcome by explicitly authorizing them to participate.[1,9] The use of badges by individual caregivers is an effective nonverbal strategy to invite patients. The use of visual reminders such as leaflets and posters can be useful.[2] Patients' low health literacy can be corrected by providing sufficient information regarding "why" and "how" they can participate.

Patient engagement can also be increased by improving the quality of the patient-caregiver relationship.[4] Caregivers can learn to adopt a more active listening style. Use of reinforcing nonverbal behaviors such as sitting to discuss with the patient and making eye contact can help improve the relationship. Caregivers' empathy and their attention to clarifying patients' concerns and beliefs also foster patient-centered care.

A clear institutional commitment to the involvement of patients is required to reinforce the merits, importance, and relevance of such programs and convince patients and caregivers that their input is desirable. Additional strategies that can facilitate patient participation can be found in the Table 30.1.

Other Forms of Patient Participation
Other forms of participation have been described in addition to patients reminding caregivers to perform hand hygiene. Patients can act at the organizational level and steer patient-safety groups to increase awareness regarding hand hygiene. They can sit on councils and advisory boards to advise on the creation of safety policies. They can also partner in the design of research related to patient participation in hand hygiene to ensure that it is relevant, meaningful, and useful.[3] Through patient organizations such as Patients for Patient Safety and Consumers Advancing Patient Safety, they can lobby for funding or improved facilities, provide patient case studies, educate patients, and conduct patient surveys and focus groups. Patients can also observe hand hygiene practices for consistency with guidelines, in particular in areas ill suited to direct observation by trained observers such a outpatient clinics.

Patient Relatives' Participation
Patient relatives are powerful allies who can also be involved in hand hygiene promotion. They can play a role in advocating for patient safety and remind caregivers to cleanse their hands. Family members, especially parents of children,[10] may be more vocal about patient safety than the patients themselves. In contrast to patients, who are less likely to participate in the context of a poor patient-caregiver relationship, relatives who are less satisfied by the level of care may be keener to prevent or correct errors.[4,10,11]

Steps in Creating a Patient Participation Campaign
A successful patient participation program requires a multimodal strategy.[5] The goal is to convince, enlist, and educate all the various stakeholders (including patients and their families, caregivers, and the institution's decision makers) of its merit and validity. Placing a few posters inviting patients to ask about hand hygiene without rallying all stakeholders will fail to yield satisfactory results. A list of steps and tips to implement a successful campaign can be found in the Table 30.1.

WHAT WE DO NOT KNOW – THE UNCERTAIN

Some aspects of patient participation in hand hygiene promotion remain unstudied. Its impact on patient satisfaction has not been fully elucidated. There is a need

Table 30.1   Checklist for Developing a Patient Participation Program

Background

- Patient participation and empowerment programs add to but do not replace a full-scale hand hygiene promotion program. Ensure that a multimodal hand hygiene promotion campaign (such as the one recommended by WHO) is in place in your institution. This includes system change, support from the institution, education, observation and feedback, and promotion
- Patient participation programs may require the implementation of a series of complementary interventions to be truly successful. Institutions may need to use a combination of tools and strategies to truly empower patients and obtain the buy-in of caregivers and decision makers
- This table describes the main steps to implement a patient participation campaign and provides tips and advice that may be followed to increase patient and caregiver uptake

Step 1. Review the literature

1.1 Review guidelines, scientific articles and review articles on the topic to identify facilitators and barriers that may be relevant to your institution.[1] In its international guidelines on hand hygiene, the World Health Organization provides a detailed strategy for involving patients in hand hygiene promotion

1.2 Institutions can find numerous resources created by national and international organizations that provide guidance on how to set up a campaign.[2–4] These solutions can provide the basis for the development of a local campaign

1.3 The use of promotional video can give patients the skills and knowledge to be empowered[5]

Step 2. Define the objectives of the campaign and convene on a simple message

2.1 Set up the campaign by defining its objectives ("what"), the means ("how"), and the interlocutors ("whom")

2.2 Anticipate and address the potential barriers and constraints to implementation and sustainability, and emphasize the facilitators. Emphasizing the altruistic aspect of the campaign (i.e., this is the "right thing" to do) may help rally a proportion of the caregivers

2.3 Frame the message so that the ultimate goal and purpose of the intervention (improving patient care) is never lost from sight

2.4 A unique message that targets both audiences may be used, but specific messages that target patients and caregivers individually may be needed to address their specific concerns and interrogations regarding the campaign

2.5 Use plain language that is simple enough for patients to understand. Some terms that may seem simple to caregivers (such as medical errors and infections) may not be understood by the target audience

2.6 Ensure that the campaign focuses on patients' needs and perspectives rather than the needs of the institution. Patients are unlikely to participate if they don't see how they can benefit from it

Table 30.1   (*Continued*)

2.7 Define the audience. Focusing on patients who are less acutely sick (e.g., patients with chronic, stable conditions such as hemodialysis populations) and patients who are frequent hospital visitors may be judicious

2.8 Plan the patient participation campaign while taking into consideration the available resources, including funding, time for training of both staff and patients, and physical spaces

2.9 Identify and elicit the collaboration of patient organizations. The international Alliance of Patient Organizations[6] and the WHO Patients for Patient Safety[7] can provide assistance in identifying organizations with whom to work

Step 3. Create tools to disseminate the campaign's key messages

3.1 Tools must be created that are complementary and address the various audiences. Different, complementary tools and materials may need to be prepared to reach all these audiences. The materials must address both "what'" is the intent of the campaign (i.e., the content) and 'how" to communicate better

3.2 Design and create tools that enlist both patients and caregivers. This may include posters, leaflets, testimonial videos, brochures, posters, screensavers, etc. Caregivers can wear badges to visibly demonstrate their commitment and legitimize patient intervention

3.3 Ensure that the tools help patients understand the underlying rationale for the campaign to increase motivation, but also provide information about how to do it and provide them with strategies to help them engage in a conversation with their caregivers

3.4 The material must be visually appealing and easy to read and understand. Select a font size that is sufficiently large and easy to read, use headings to break up the text, leave white spaces, and use visuals to capture and maintain interest

3.5 Consider translating the tools into other languages depending on your patient population

3.6 Create tools to help caregivers welcome patient input and participation. These tools should help caregivers understand the goals of the campaign, and provide them with strategies on how to communicate with patients on hand hygiene and patient participation

3.7 Obtain patient input throughout the tool development to select strategies that are most likely to influence willingness to participate. The tools should be tested on patients to determine whether they find them clear and easy to understand. Many studies published so far do not report involving or consulting patients in the development of the intervention

3.8 Ensure the presence of alcohol-based handrub at the point of care (i.e., well within patient sight) to facilitate patient intervention

Step 4. Obtain support from every level of your organization

4.1 Identify champions within your institution and involve them in setting up a campaign

4.2 Emphasize the importance of patient participation by mentioning external respected bodies that actively promote patient involvement such as the WHO, the Institute of Medicine, and the US Centers for Disease Control and Prevention

(*continued*)

Table 30.1   *(Continued)*

4.3 Highlight the fact that patient participation campaigns will help the institution comply with legislation, national policies, and accrediting organizations such as the US Joint Commission, which set up goals for hospitals to involve patients and their families in their own care as a patient safety strategy

4.4 Mention that patient participation programs are an opportunity to increase the institution's visibility and reputation in the community

4.5 Mentioning the occurrence of a sentinel event (i.e., an adverse event linked to hand hygiene omission that could have potentially been prevented through patient participation) can be a strong motivator for change

4.6 Once the support from the decision makers is obtained, disseminate this information to all employees to reinforce the importance of the program, for example through the local newsletter or through a communication from the director that is addressed to all workers

Step 5. Collect data and provide feedback

5.1 Collecting data will allow the institution to assess progress, identify areas for improvement, and help secure sustainability. The types of data that can be collected include patient and healthcare worker satisfaction surveys and hand hygiene compliance audits

Step 6. Make plans to ensure sustainability of the program

6.1 Patient participation may be short-lived if the available resources and support are not sustained in the long term. Identify strategies to secure long-term commitment from the institution to the project (leadership support, financial and labor resources, etc.)

[1] www.ahrq.gov/research/findings/final-reports/ptfamilyscan/ptfamilyscan.pdf.
[2] www.who.int/gpsc/5may/5may2013_patient-participation/en/index.html.
[3] www.ahrq.gov/questions/.
[4] www.jointcommission.org/speakup.aspx.
[5] www.cdc.gov/handhygiene/Patient_materials.html.
[6] www.patientsorganizations.org.
[7] www.who.int/topics/patient_safety/en/.

to find how campaigns must be articulated to overcome all the above-mentioned barriers. As most studies were conducted in settings with low baseline hand hygiene compliance rates, its efficacy in institutions with reasonably high compliance is unknown. Publication bias (i.e., the preferential reporting of studies with positive outcomes) cannot be ruled out.

Caregivers' perceptions of these campaigns have received little interest. It is possible that workers who do not comply with hand hygiene will also refuse to empower patients. How these "opponents" can undermine the success of an entire program is unknown. As patients cannot easily predict whether a given caregiver is "for" or "against" patient participation, they may err on the side of caution by refraining to ask any caregiver about hand hygiene. Finally, few studies have focused on the alternative forms of participation such as patient observers and participation at the organization level.

RESEARCH AGENDA

There is a need to identify new strategies to involve the more vulnerable patients who may be less capable of participating and at an increased risk of developing an infection.[11] More research is required to identify factors that motivate decision makers to involve patients. There is a need to measure the relative contribution of direct patient intervention and the impact of "silent" empowerment (i.e., the increase in staff hand hygiene compliance due to increased patient awareness without them having to intervene verbally). The ethical ramifications of patient participation must be further studied, and additional cost-effectiveness analysis should be performed.[4] Furthermore, as virtually all studies were conducted in high-income countries, research is needed in low- and middle-income countries.[1,4] Further studies using appropriate study designs[12] are needed to better understand the optimal strategies to use to involve patients and foster a safety climate.

REFERENCES

1. Longtin, Y, Sax H, Leape LL, et al., Patient participation: current knowledge and applicability to patient safety. *Mayo Clin Proc* 2010;**85**:53–62.
2. McGuckin M, Govednik J, Patient empowerment and hand hygiene, 1997–2012. *J Hosp Infect* 2013;**84**:191–199.
3. Patient-Centered Outcomes Research Institute. Available at www.pcori.org/about-us/landing/. Accessed March 7, 2017.
4. Doherty C, Stavropoulou C, Patients' willingness and ability to participate actively in the reduction of clinical errors: a systematic literature review. *Soc Sci Med* 2012;**75**:257–263.
5. World Health Organization, *WHO Guidelines on Hand Hygiene in Health Care*. Geneva: WHO, 2009.
6. Maurer M, Dardess P, Carman, KL, et al., *Guide to patient and family engagement: environmental scan report*. (Prepared by American Institutes for Research under contract HHSA 290-200-600019). AHRQ Publication No. 12-0042-EF. Rockville, MD: Agency for Healthcare Research and Quality, May 2012.
7. Reid, N, Moghaddas J, Loftus M, et al., Can we expect patients to question health care workers' hand hygiene compliance? *Infect Control Hosp Epidemiol* 2012;**33**:531–532.
8. Longtin Y, Farquet N, Gayet-Ageron A, et al., Caregivers' perceptions of patients as reminders to improve hand hygiene. *Arch Intern Med* 2012;**172**:1516–1517.
9. Davis, RE, Koutantji M, Vincent CA, How willing are patients to question healthcare staff on issues related to the quality and safety of their healthcare? An exploratory study. *Qual Saf Health Care* 2008;**17**:90–96.
10. Bellissimo-Rodrigues F, Pires D, Zingg W, et al., Role of parents in the promotion of hand hygiene in the paediatric setting: a systematic literature review. *J Hosp Infect* 2016;**93**:159–163.
11. McGuckin M, Shubin A, McBride P, et al., The effect of random voice hand hygiene messages delivered by medical, nursing, and infection control staff on hand hygiene compliance in intensive care. *Am J Infect Control* 2006;**34**:673–675.
12. Stewardson A, Sax H, Gayet-Ageron A, Enhanced performance feedback and patient participation to improve hand hygiene compliance of healthcare workers in the setting of established multimodal promotion: a single-centre, cluster randomised controlled trial. *Lancet Infect Dis* 2016;**16**:1345–1355.

Chapter 31

Religion and Hand Hygiene

Jaffar A. Al-Tawfiq[1] and Ziad A. Memish[2]

[1] Saudi Aramco Medical Services Organization, Dhahran, Saudi Arabia
[2] Former Deputy Health Minister, College of Medicine, Alfaisal University, Riyadh, Saudi Arabia

KEY MESSAGES

- Religious influence on hand hygiene should be considered when develop-ing hand hygiene promotion strategies.
- The interaction of religion and cultural norms should be specifically exam-ined for better understanding of healthcare workers' perception of hand hygiene.
- Future research should include the differences of hand hygiene practice as a result of religion as reflected by the practice of different followers of the same faith.

WHAT WE KNOW – THE EVIDENCE

The practice of handwashing with soap and water or handrubbing using an alcohol-based handrub (ABHR) is influenced by many social, cultural, and religious beliefs.[1] The complex interaction between religion and hand hygiene practices among healthcare workers (HCWs) is not well studied.[2] In the Hindu faith, hands are rubbed with ash or mud followed by rinsing with water, not soap as it is believed to contain animal fat.[3] However, handwashing is practiced in Hinduism before any worship or ceremony, and other activities.[3] The practice of hand hygiene is specifically mentioned in Judaism, Islam, and Sikhism, where it is performed for ritual and symbolic reasons.[3] In Buddhism, there are no specific

Hand Hygiene: A Handbook for Medical Professionals, First Edition.
Edited by Didier Pittet, John M. Boyce and Benedetta Allegranzi.
© 2017 John Wiley & Sons, Inc. Published 2017 by John Wiley & Sons, Inc.

indications for hand hygiene except for washing hands after each meal.[3] In Judaism, hands are washed after waking in the morning.[3] Christianity does not include specific indications for handwashing except before the ritual sprinkling of holy water before consecration of the bread and wine, and handwashing after touching the holy oil.[1,3] The concept of hand hygiene in Sikhism is well known in certain acts such as before wound dressing. Islam puts considerable importance on personal hygiene in general and on hand hygiene in particular.[4] Clear instructions on when hands should be cleaned are given by Islam.[5] In Muslim teaching, the different hands are used for different purposes, with distinction between attending to personal matters such as micturition or defecation and those for eating.[6] There are specific teachings for cleaning hands before daily prayers, before and after any meal, after using the toilet, and after handling soiled items.[1,5,7,8] A summary of the indications for hand hygiene in different religions is shown in Table 31.1. Understanding the role of religion in hand hygiene is an important teaching point to educate HCWs.[9]

Alcohol-Based Handrubs and Religion

The use of ABHRs is considered an important strategy to promote hand hygiene among HCWs. The use of alcohol is prohibited and/or considered an offense in some religions (Table 31.2).[1,2]

The use of ABHRs by some HCWs is affected by religious beliefs.[10–12] In a publication on this topic, it was noted that ABHRs were used by HCWs in more than 200 public hospitals in Saudi Arabia.[13] The concern of the use of ABHRs may also stem from the potential absorption of alcohol through the skin. The use of ABHRs resulted in an isopropyl alcohol level of 0.5–1.8 mg/L.[14] In contrast, another study did not detect any isopropanol absorption after intense alcohol-based handrubbing 30 times per hour (see Chapter 16 for complete discussion).[15]

WHAT WE DO NOT KNOW – THE UNCERTAIN

The exact influence and impact of religion on hand hygiene practice in healthcare settings is not well known. We do not know the exact influence of religion on the practice of hand hygiene among HCWs who are adhering well to religious instructions. It is important to know if strict adherence to hand hygiene is enhanced among followers of any particular religion. Such findings would help to streamline the educational processes. It is not clear what cultural versus religious factors are actually contributing to hand hygiene compliance rates.

RESEARCH AGENDA

The exact influence of different religions on hand hygiene in healthcare settings should be further examined by identifying factors that promote and factors that

Table 31.1 Specific Indications for Hand Hygiene According to the Most Widely Represented Religions Worldwide

Religion	Specific Indications for Hand Hygiene	Reason/Purpose
Buddhism	After each meal	Hygienic/cleansing
	To wash the hands of the deceased	Symbolic
	At the New Year, young persons pour water over elders' hands	Symbolic
Christianity	Before the consecration of bread and wine	Ritual
	After handling holy oil (Catholics)	Hygienic/cleansing; ritual
Hinduism	During worship (*puja*) (water)	Ritual
	End of prayer (water)	Ritual
	After any unclean act (toilet)	Hygienic/cleansing
Islam	Repeating ablutions at least 3 times with running water before prayers (5 times/day)	Ritual
		Hygienic/cleansing
		Hygienic/cleansing
	Before and after any meal	Hygienic/cleansing
	After going to the toilet	Hygienic/cleansing
	After touching a dog, shoes, or a cadaver	Ritual
	After handling anything spoiled	
Judaism	Immediately after awakening in the morning	Ritual
	Before and after each meal	Hygienic/cleansing
	Before praying	Ritual
	Before the beginning of Shabbat	Ritual
	After going to the toilet	Hygienic/cleansing
Orthodox Christian	After putting on liturgical vestments before the ceremony	Ritual
	Before the consecration of bread and wine	Ritual
Sikhism	Early in the morning	Hygienic/cleansing
	Before every religious activity	Ritual
	Before cooking and entering the community food hall	Hygienic/cleansing
	After each meal	Hygienic/cleansing
	After taking off or putting on shoes	Hygienic/cleansing

Source: World Health Organization (2009). Reproduced with permission from the World Health Organization.

may hinder hand hygiene. Due to the uncertainty of the acceptance of ABHRs among all faiths, it is important to conduct surveys among different faiths and in different regions to elucidate beliefs and potential obstacles for the use of products in healthcare settings. The development of hand hygiene guidelines should involve scholars from different religions.

Table 31.2   Alcohol Prohibition in Some Religions

Religion	Alcohol Prohibition	Reason for Alcohol Prohibition	Alcohol Prohibition Potentially Affecting the Use of Alcohol-Based Handrub
Buddhism	Yes	Kills living organisms (bacteria)	Yes, but surmountable
Christianity	No	—	—
Hinduism	Yes	Causes mental impairment	No
Islam	Yes	Causes disconnection from a state of spiritual awareness or consciousness	Yes, but surmountable
Judaism	No	—	—
Orthodox Christian	No	—	—
Sikhism	Yes	Unacceptable behavior disrespectful to the faith; considered an intoxicant	Yes, possibly

Source: World Health Organization (2009). Reproduced with permission from the World Health Organization.

REFERENCES

1. World Health Organization, *WHO Guidelines on Hand Hygiene in Health Care*. Geneva: WHO, 2009.
2. Allegranzi B, Memish ZA, Donaldson L, et al., World Health Organization Global Patient Safety Challenge Task Force on Religious and Cultural Aspects of Hand Hygiene; World Alliance for Patient Safety, Religion and culture: potential undercurrents influencing hand hygiene promotion in health care. *Am J Infect Control* 2009;**37**:28–34.
3. Mishra B, Sarkar D, Srivastava S, et al., Hand hygiene – Religious, cultural and behavioral aspects. *Univ J Educ Gen Stud* 2013;**2**:184–188.
4. Lawrence P, Rozmus C, Culturally sensitive care of the Muslim patient. *J Transcult Nurs* 2001;**12**:228–233.
5. Katme AM, Muslim teaching gives rules for when hands must be washed. *Br Med J* 1999;**319**:520.
6. Watts G, You need hands. *Lancet* 2006;**367**:1383–1384.
7. Muftic D, Maintaining cleanliness and protecting health as proclaimed by Koran texts and hadiths of Mohammed SAVS. *Med Arh* 1997;**51**:41–143.
8. Brooks N, Overview of religions. *Clin Cornerstone* 2004;**6**:7–16.
9. Valenzeno L, Alibali MW, Klatsky R, Teachers' gestures facilitate students' learning: a lesson in symmetry. *Contemp Educ Psychol* 2003;**28**:187–204.
10. Jumaa PA, Hand hygiene: simple and complex. *Int J Infect Dis* 2005;**9**:3–14.

11. Pittet D, Boyce JM, Revolutionising hand hygiene in health-care settings: guidelines revisited. *Lancet Infect Dis* 2003;**3**:269–270.

12. Boyce JM, Pittet D, Guideline for Hand Hygiene in Health-Care Settings. Recommendations of the Healthcare Infection Control Practices Advisory Committee and the HIC-PAC/SHEA/APIC/IDSA Hand Hygiene Task Force. Society for Healthcare Epidemiology of America/Association for Professionals in Infection Control/Infectious Diseases Society of America. MMWR Recomm Rep 2002;**51**(RR-16):1–45.

13. Ahmed QA, Memish ZA, Allegranzi B, et al., WHO Global Patient Safety Challenge, Muslim health-care workers and alcohol-based handrubs. *Lancet* 2006;**367**:1025–1027.

14. Turner P, Saeed B, Kelsey MC, Dermal absorption of isopropyl alcohol from a commercial hand rub: implications for its use in hand decontamination. *J Hosp Infect* 2004;**56**:287–290.

15. Brown TL, Gamon S, Tester P, et al., Can alcohol-based hand-rub solutions cause you to lose your driver's license? Comparative cutaneous absorption of various alcohols. *Antimicrob Agents Chemother* 2007;**51**:1107–1108.

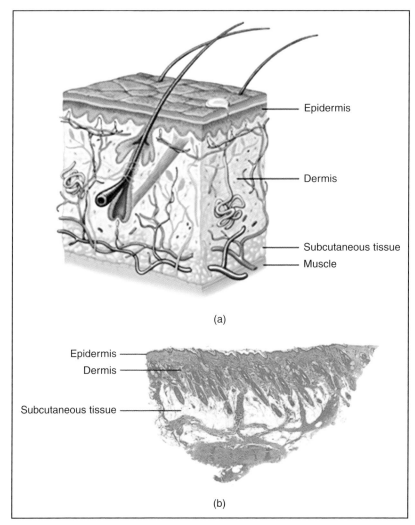

Epidermis

Dermis

Subcutaneous tissue
Muscle

(a)

Epidermis
Dermis

Subcutaneous tissue

(b)

Figure 3.1 The anatomical layers of the skin. *Source*: Shier 2004. Reproduced with permission from McGraw-Hill.

Hand Hygiene: A Handbook for Medical Professionals, First Edition.
Edited by Didier Pittet, John M. Boyce and Benedetta Allegranzi.
© 2017 John Wiley & Sons, Inc. Published 2017 by John Wiley & Sons, Inc.

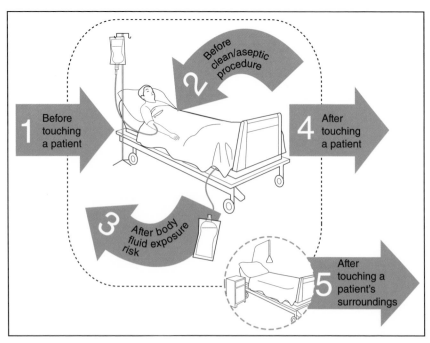

Figure 20.1 Unified visuals for My Five Moments for Hand Hygiene. *Source*: Reproduced with permission from the World Health Organization

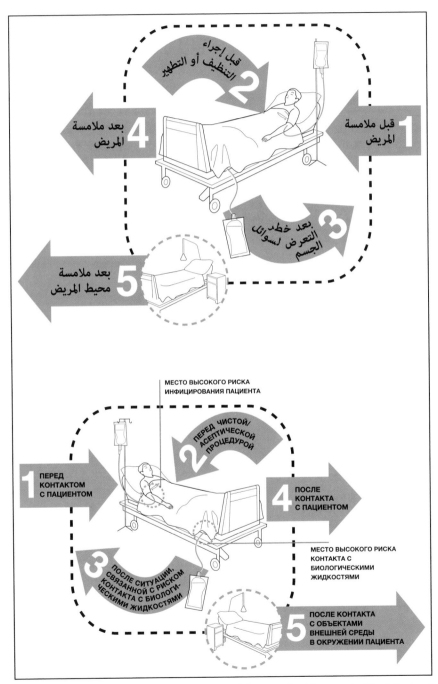

Figure 20.2 Translations and local adaptations of the "My Five Moments for Hand Hygiene" visual. *Source*: Reproduced with permission from the World Health Organization

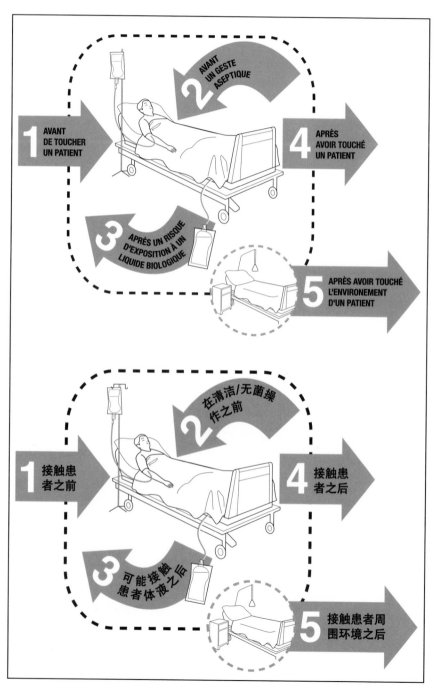

Figure 20.2 (*Continued*)

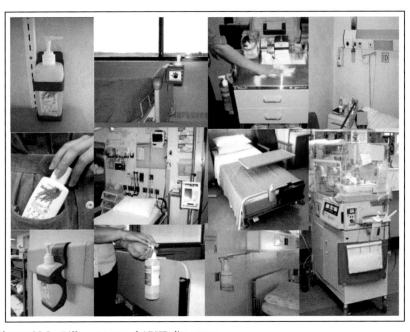

Figure 21.1 Different types of ABHR dispensers.

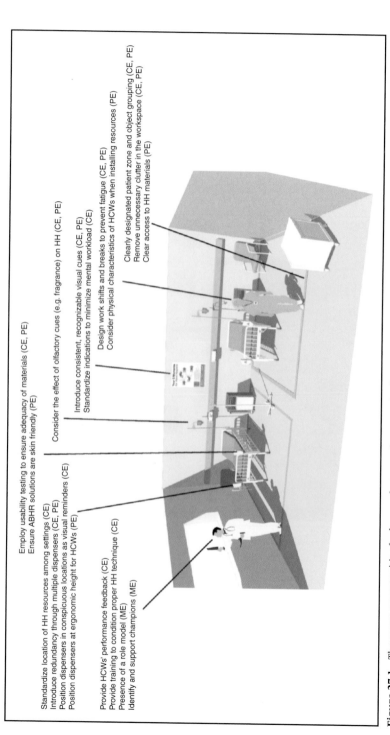

Employ usability testing to ensure adequacy of materials (CE, PE)
Ensure ABHR solutions are skin friendly (PE)

Consider the effect of olfactory cues (e.g. fragrance) on HH (CE, PE)

Introduce consistent, recognizable visual cues (CE, PE)
Standardize indications to minimize mental workload (CE)

Design work shifts and breaks to prevent fatigue (CE, PE)
Consider physical characteristics of HCWs when installing resources (PE)

Clearly designated patient zone and object grouping (CE, PE)
Remove unnecessary clutter in the workspace (CE, PE)
Clear access to HH materials (PE)

Standardize location of HH resources among settings (CE)
Introduce redundancy through multiple dispensers (CE, PE)
Position dispensers in conspicuous locations as visual reminders (CE)
Position dispensers at ergonomic height for HCWs (PE)

Provide HCWs' performance feedback (CE)
Provide training to condition proper HH technique (CE)
Presence of a role model (ME)
Identify and support champions (ME)

Figure 27.1 The many opportunities for human factors and ergonomics design to promote hand hygiene (HH). The opportunities for supporting healthcare worker (HCW) hand hygiene performance through human factors engineering can be applied at three levels: PE, physical ergonomics; CE, cognitive ergonomics; and ME, macroergonomics. ABHR, alcohol-based handrub.

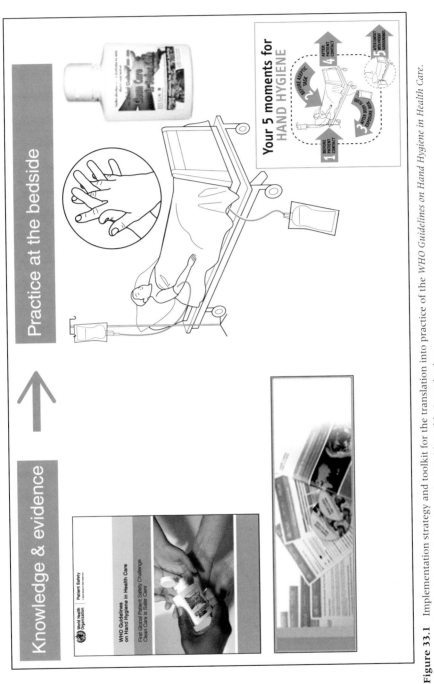

Figure 33.1 Implementation strategy and toolkit for the translation into practice of the *WHO Guidelines on Hand Hygiene in Health Care*.
Source: Reproduced with permission from the World Health Organization.

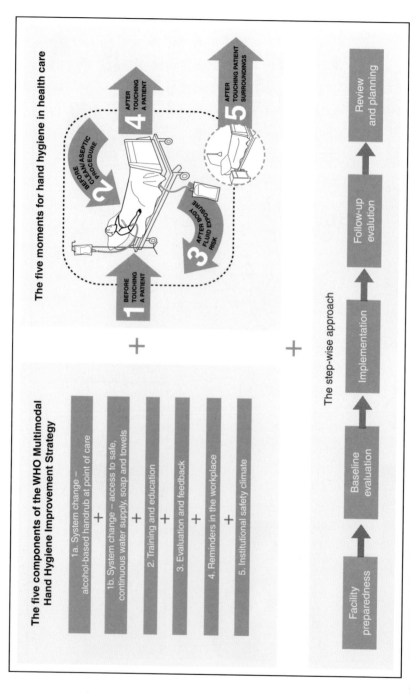

Figure 33.2 WHO Multimodal Hand Hygiene Improvement Strategy Implementation Model. *Source:* Reproduced with permission from the World Health Organization.

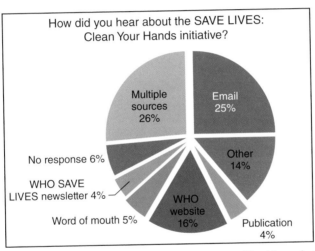

Figure 38.1 Categories associated with how campaign registered healthcare facilities hear about *SAVE LIVES: Clean Your Hands* – 2010.

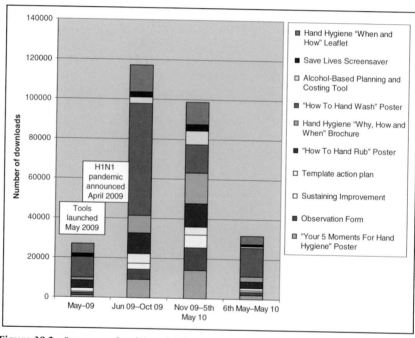

Figure 38.2 Summary of tool download activity for 2009 and 2010 and key events that may have influenced these.

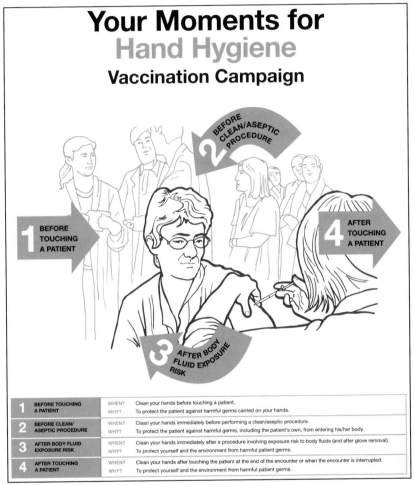

Figure 42D.1   Hand hygiene indications in the context of a vaccination campaign. Hand Hygiene in Outpatient and Home-Based Care and Long-Term Care Facilities: A Guide to the Application of the WHO Multimodal Hand Hygiene Improvement Strategy and the "My Five Moments for Hand Hygiene" Approach. WHO, 2012. *Source*: Reproduced with permission from the World Health Organization.

Additional figures illustrating other care situations in outpatient settings are available in the guidance document cited above.

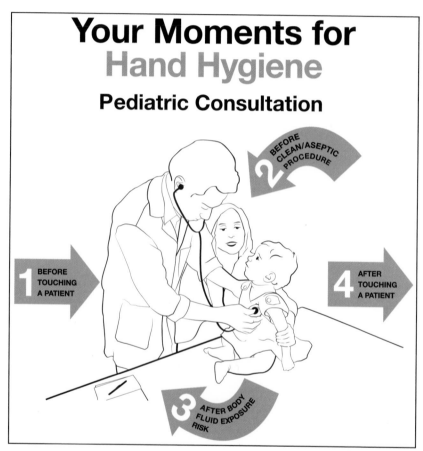

Figure 42D.2   Hand hygiene indications during a pediatric consultation. Hand Hygiene in Outpatient and Home-Based Care and Long-Term Care Facilities: A Guide to the Application of the WHO Multimodal Hand Hygiene Improvement Strategy and the "My Five Moments for Hand Hygiene" Approach. WHO, 2012. *Source*: Reproduced with permission from the World Health Organization.

Additional figures illustrating other care situations in outpatient settings are available in the guidance document cited above.

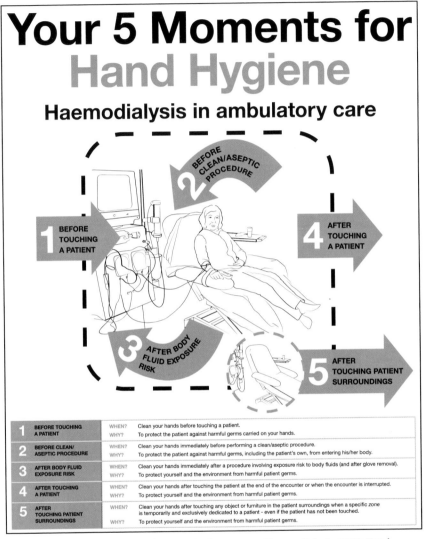

Figure 42E.1 Hand hygiene indications in the context of haemodialysis. WHO Hand Hygiene in Outpatient and Home-Based Care and Long-Term Care Facilities: a Guide to the Application of the WHO Multimodal Hand Hygiene Improvement Strategy and the My Five Moments for Hand Hygiene Approach 2012. *Source*: Reproduced with permission from the World Health Organization.

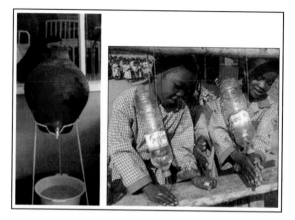

Figure 43.2 Examples of using various types of handwashing facilities in LMI countries where there is a lack of access to a piped water supply. *Source*: Reproduced with permission from the Centers for Disease Control and Prevention, www.cdc.gov.

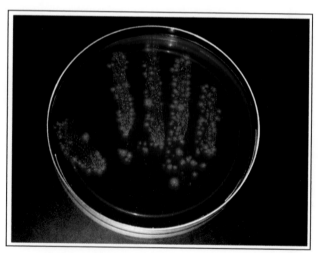

Figure 44B.1 Hand imprint culture of *Clostridium difficile* on sterile gloves after contact with a *C. difficile*-associated diarrhea-affected patient's groin. *Source*: Reprinted from Bobulsky G et al. with permission from C.J. Donskey.[2]

Chapter 32

Hand Hygiene Promotion from the US Perspective: Putting WHO and CDC Guidelines into Practice

Katherine Ellingson

Oregon Health Authority, Public Health Division, Healthcare-Associated Infections Program, Portland, USA

KEY MESSAGES

- For accreditation by the Joint Commission, facilities in the United States are required to implement hand hygiene recommendations from the Centers for Disease Control and Prevention or World Health Organization guidelines, which are largely convergent. Clarifications and updates to these guidelines can be found in a 2014 compendium published by the Society of Healthcare Epidemiology of America, but more research is needed to determine optimal hand hygiene technique, product use, and measurement strategies.

- Multimodal implementation approaches to hand hygiene improvement are imperative, and healthcare facilities in the United States participate indirectly or directly in a number of different implementation campaigns, including, but not limited to, the WHO *SAVE LIVES: Clean Your Hands* campaign.

- Healthcare facilities in the United States have experimented with a variety of hand hygiene measurement modalities; and currently guidelines recommend using multiple methodologies to gain a complete picture of hand hygiene practices. A national standard for measurement would be helpful,

Hand Hygiene: A Handbook for Medical Professionals, First Edition.
Edited by Didier Pittet, John M. Boyce and Benedetta Allegranzi.
© 2017 John Wiley & Sons, Inc. Published 2017 by John Wiley & Sons, Inc.

but determining what that standard should be requires further evaluation of existing methods, including the emerging automated measurement technologies.

WHAT WE KNOW – THE EVIDENCE

In United States (US) healthcare facilities, hand hygiene is widely accepted as a central component of infection prevention and control. Evidence-based recommendations for when and how to perform hand hygiene reside in the US Centers for Disease Control and Prevention (CDC) and World Health Organization (WHO) guidelines, published in 2002 and 2006 (draft)/2009, respectively.[1,2] These guidelines differ in the amount of details provided in background and implementation sections, but evidence-based recommendations are nearly identical. Recommendations from CDC and WHO guidelines, along with updates from more recently published scientific studies, are summarized in a 2014 compendium by the Society for Healthcare Epidemiology of America (SHEA).[3] Despite the existence of multiple nationally and internationally recognized guidelines to support hand hygiene in healthcare settings – and substantial gains in adherence since the introduction of alcohol-based handrubs (ABHRs) in the early 2000s – hand hygiene adherence among healthcare personnel in the United States and other similarly resourced countries remains disappointingly low.[4]

Recent implementation of multimodal hand hygiene improvement strategies, however, has shown promise (see Chapter 33).[5] In place of a single national hand hygiene campaign, US healthcare facilities have implemented various types of programs to enhance accessibility of hand hygiene products, educate healthcare personnel, remind staff and visitors to clean hands, and measure and feed-back performance. From one perspective, the lack of a national standard for implementing hand hygiene improvement strategies in the US is problematic; it limits benchmarking and interfacility comparisons, prevents a national assessment of hand hygiene aptitude, and complicates participation in global hand hygiene campaigns. Yet diversity in implementation has also allowed for experimentation and creative thinking in the US approach to hand hygiene in healthcare settings. Given that hand hygiene among healthcare personnel has been a persistent challenge for more than 150 years, innovative approaches in the US can yield valuable lessons for the global healthcare community. Regarding the implementation of the hand hygiene multimodal improvement strategy recommended by WHO, a survey conducted in 2011 in a sample of US healthcare facilities showed an advanced or intermediate level of progress by using a standardized assessment tool[6] (see Chapter 34). However, the authors highlighted that further improvement should be achieved, in particular by embedding hand hygiene in a stronger institutional safety climate and optimizing the staffing levels dedicated to infection prevention. This chapter provides an overview of existing CDC and WHO guidelines including recent updates, summarizes various approaches to hand hygiene improvement in US healthcare facilities, and discusses future directions in hand hygiene and implementation science research.

CDC AND WHO GUIDELINES

In general, healthcare facilities in the United States base their hand hygiene policies on CDC and WHO guidelines. Both guidelines include an evidence grade for each specific recommendation: IA, IB, IC, or II. Category IA recommendations are strongly supported by well-designed experimental, clinical, or epidemiological studies; Category IB recommendations are supported by certain experimental, clinical, or epidemiological studies with a strong theoretical rationale; Category IC recommendations are required by regulation; and Category II recommendations are supported by suggestive clinical or epidemiological studies or a theoretical rationale. The Joint Commission on Accreditation of Healthcare Organizations, i.e Joint Commission (JC) since 2007, which has accredited over 3,300 (of approximately 5,700) hospitals in the US – has issued a National Patient Safety Goal that "facilities comply with current WHO or CDC hand hygiene guidelines." Specifically, JC requires that healthcare facilities implement all Category I recommendations, and that Category II recommendations be considered, though not required. JC directs healthcare facilities to choose either the WHO or CDC guideline and implement recommendations at their facility. Recommendations are highly consistent between guidelines (see Table 32.1), although the evidence grades differ slightly for some recommendations; this is primarily a result of different publication dates allowing more or fewer scientific studies to be considered. While the indications for routine hand hygiene are consistent between CDC and WHO guidelines, the only recommended practice differences include: 1) prohibition of artificial nails in high-risk settings (CDC) versus prohibition of artificial nails in all settings (WHO); and 2) prewashing hands with an antimicrobial soap before use of an alcohol-based presurgical rub (CDC) versus no need for prewashing hands before use of an ABHR for surgical hand preparation unless hands are visibly soiled (WHO).[1,2]

In addition to the above-mentioned CDC and WHO guidelines, specific recommendations for hand hygiene also appear in other CDC guidelines, including the 2007 Guidelines for Isolation Precautions, the 2011 Guideline for the Prevention and Control of Norovirus Gastroenteritis Outbreaks in Healthcare Settings, as well as other guidelines for the prevention of specific device- and procedure-associated healthcare-associated infections (HAIs). Table 32.1 summarizes recommendations for when to perform hand hygiene (i.e., indications) contained in various CDC guidelines as well as in WHO guidelines. Importantly, the WHO's highly promoted Five Moments for Hand Hygiene (see Chapter 20), which was introduced with the publication of the Guide to Implementation alongside the WHO guidelines,[7] is consistent with the indications recommended in both guidelines. The Five Moments framework is a tool for educating healthcare personnel about hand hygiene indications in a way that is arguably more

Table 32.1   Summary of Recommended Indications for Routine (i.e., Excluding Surgical Hand Preparation) Hand Hygiene from the Centers for Disease Control and Prevention (CDC) and World Health Organization (WHO) Guidelines

	CDC Guidelines[*]	WHO (2006 – Draft Form; 2009 – Final)[**]
Wash hands with either nonantimicrobial or antimicrobial soap and water in the following clinical care situations:		
When hands are visibly soiled	Y (IA), HH-2002	Y (IB)
After known or suspected exposure to *Clostridium difficile*	Y (II), ISO-07	Y (IB, during outbreaks)
After known or suspected exposure to patients with infectious diarrhea during norovirus outbreaks	Y (II), NV-2011	ND
If exposure to *Bacillus anthracis* is suspected or proven	Y (II), HH-2002	Y (IB, spore-forming organisms)
Rub hands with ABHR in the following situations:[***]		
Before direct patient contact	Y (1B), HH-2002	Y (IB)
Before handling medication	ND	Y (IB)
Before donning sterile gloves to insert an invasive device	Y (IB), HH-2002	Y (IB, before handling)
Before and after handling respiratory devices, urinary catheters, and intravascular catheters (palpating, replacing, accessing, repairing, or dressing)	Y (IA), PNEU-2003 Y (IB), CAUTI-2009 Y (IB), BSI-2011	Y (IB, before handling)
After direct patient contact	Y (IB), HH-2002	Y (IB)
After removing gloves	Y (IB), HH-2002	Y (IB)
After contact with blood, body fluids, mucous membranes, nonintact skin, and wound dressings if hands not visibly soiled	Y (IA), HH-2002 Y (1A), PNEU-2003	Y (IA)
After contact with inanimate objects in the patients' immediate environment	Y (II), HH-2002	Y (IB)
If moving from a contaminated body site to a clean body site	Y (II)	Y (IB)

[*]Includes published guidelines from CDC on hand hygiene (HH-2002), isolation precautions (ISO-2007), management of norovirus outbreaks in healthcare (NV-2011), prevention of catheter-associated urinary tract infections (CAUTI-2009), prevention of pneumonia in healthcare settings (PNEU-2003), and prevention of intravascular catheter-related infections (BSI-2011).

[**]Y, Yes, N, No, ND, Not Discussed. Designations as IA, IB, and II refer to CDC and WHO use of the following evidence grades: IA = strongly recommended for implementation and strongly supported by well-designed experimental, clinical, or epidemiological studies; IB = strongly recommended for implementation and supported by certain experimental, clinical, or epidemiological studies and a strong theoretical rationale; and II = suggested for implementation and supported by clinical or epidemiological studies or a theoretical rationale.

[***]If ABHR is not available, clean hands with soap and water (WHO), or with antimicrobial soap and water (CDC).

dynamic and easier to remember than a list of recommended indications (see Chapter 20). Although there are more than five indications for hand hygiene in the CDC and WHO guidelines, the Five Moments framework highlights these indications in a visual format that reminds healthcare personnel of the most critical hand hygiene opportunities during the course of patient care.

WHAT WE DO NOT KNOW AND RESEARCH AGENDA

The CDC and WHO guidelines are considered comprehensive documents, but there remain several areas of controversy and recommendations that could be informed by a focused research agenda and enhanced rigor. There are many Category I recommendations in both guidelines, but few are based on randomized trials or epidemiologically rigorous observational studies, in part because of ethical considerations in randomizing control groups, and in part because investment in hand hygiene research has lagged behind other healthcare topics. Publication of the 2014 SHEA compendium provided an opportunity to clarify the state of the science and bring areas of controversy to light. The topics listed below are prominent examples of hand hygiene–related topics that would benefit from more attention and investment from the research community.[3]

Hand Hygiene Product Selection

The majority of published studies comparing the efficacy of ABHR to antimicrobial or nonantimicrobial soap and water reported that ABHRs are superior to soap and water in killing a wide range of bacteria and viruses. An area of frequent confusion and controversy is the use of ABHR in situations where *Clostridium difficile* or norovirus are present (see also Chapters 44B and 44D). In vitro and in vivo studies have shown that ABHR does not kill *C. difficile* spores, and handwashing with soap and water, though superior to ABHR, is also suboptimal. While these studies seemingly support preferential use of soap and water over ABHR for *C. difficile*, discouraging ABHR use may have unintended adverse consequences; other studies have shown that the presence of ABHR increases hand hygiene adherence, which has an impact on the spread of other epidemiologically important organisms. Because there is no literature showing that either ABHR or soap and water leads to actual clinical decreases in the incidence of *C. difficile* infection (and glove use does decrease incidence), SHEA suggests shifting the focus from hand hygiene method to strict adherence to contact precautions. Similarly for norovirus, where studies show contradictory results regarding the superiority of soap and water versus ABHR, the messaging in the SHEA compendium is: "Given the low-quality and contradictory evidence combined with the sporadic nature of norovirus outbreaks, focus should be on stressing adherence to glove use and hand hygiene rather than on specific products or methods." Further clarification on appropriate hand hygiene product selection, including the relevance of various experimental studies to clinical settings will be important for standardizing messaging and promoting safest practices.

Both CDC and WHO guidelines review the efficacy of various hand hygiene products in background sections, but recommendations only contain language about ABHR and "nonantimicrobial or antimicrobial soaps"; the recommendations do not address different types of antimicrobials contained in soaps or other waterless hand hygiene products. The SHEA compendium, however, recommends against use of triclosan-containing soaps, which have been heavily marketed in US healthcare settings. Justification for this recommendation includes nonsuperiority compared to ABHR and soap, reports of contamination, promotion of resistance, and potential public health impact of triclosan bioaccumulation. In general, hand hygiene products are evaluated as safe and effective for use based on tolerability of the product on healthcare worker hands. A broader universe of health outcomes should be considered in assessing antimicrobial products. Additionally, future research on hand hygiene products should incorporate study designs that consider realistic clinical situations when artificial contamination with microorganisms and controlled hand hygiene regimens are used.

Technique

The CDC guideline emphasizes following product-specific recommendations for appropriate hand hygiene technique and to wash hands for at least 15 seconds. The WHO emphasizes technique over time requirement, although the approximate time requirements for WHO-recommended handrubbing technique is 20–30 seconds and for handwashing is 40–60 seconds. Recent studies suggest that 15 seconds might be insufficient for meeting standards for high-quality antisepsis and that physical coverage of hands with hand hygiene product is often substandard (see also Chapter 10). Questions remain about whether rigid adherence to a step-by-step protocol for hand hygiene technique (like the WHO "How to Handrub" technique, see Chapter 10) is any more effective than instructing HCWs to cover their hands with product (the "reasonable application" approach). More research is needed to clarify optimal hand hygiene technique protocols. If the reasonable application approach is found to be most effective, then there must also be standards for how much product is to be used; the current studies using this approach had protocols with 3 mL of product, but other studies have shown that most dispensers provide far less than 3 mL (ranging from 0.6 to 1.3 mL per actuation). WHO guidelines recommend the application of a palmful amount of ABHR, which makes sense and is consistent with different HCWs' hand sizes worldwide. While smaller volumes have been shown to meet recommended log reductions,[8] these volumes have not been widely incorporated into research protocols. Standardized research protocols that mirror clinical realities will greatly enhance the body of evidence for hand hygiene technique.

Hand Adornments: Rings and Nails

Neither the WHO nor CDC nor SHEA takes a stance on wearing rings in non-surgical healthcare settings. In WHO Guidelines, rings are not accepted, but the wedding ring is tolerated. Although one study in 2007 found that the presence of rings did not negatively impact the effectiveness of ABHRs, this area deserves more attention as it is a frequent question without any evidence assessment in nationally or internationally recognized guidelines. To date, no evidence-based guidance on shellac (gel) nails or nail art exists. Policies regarding nail enhancements hinge on whether they are considered artificial nails or not. A conservative approach treats these adornments as artificial nails, in which case they should not be allowed in high-risk areas (CDC) or in any healthcare area (WHO). Further research to clarify the transmission potential of these popular nail adornments would help provide a stronger evidence base for future recommendations.

Glove Use

One common area of controversy in US healthcare settings is whether hand hygiene should be required immediately prior to donning nonsterile gloves. Both CDC and WHO guidelines strongly emphasize performing hand hygiene prior to direct patient contact, but neither guideline specifies exactly when that hand hygiene episode should take place relative to donning gloves. Reports of healthcare personnel getting cited by regulatory agencies for not performing hand hygiene immediately prior to donning nonsterile gloves have raised questions about how to approach this issue. Technically, personnel should only be cited if they do not perform hand hygiene before patient contact. Two studies suggest that hand hygiene may be unnecessary immediately before donning nonsterile gloves. The WHO guidelines include specific language about hand hygiene and glove use: "glove use is not a substitute for hand hygiene." In other terms, opportunities for hand hygiene occur regardless of glove use; if a specific patient care situation requires glove use, the hand hygiene action aimed at patient protection will happen immediately before donning gloves. Other studies reporting contamination of unused gloves raise concerns of glove box contamination by unclean hands. Clearer messaging on this issue is needed, and engineering solutions should be explored to reduce potential contamination of boxed unused gloves (see also Chapter 23).

Implementation of Hand Hygiene Improvement Programs

According to a recent meta-analysis, implementation of a multimodal program – including enhanced access to ABHR, education, reminders, feedback on adherence, and administrative support – is the best way to improve hand hygiene adherence.[5] Healthcare facilities in the US have implemented or adapted elements of a number of different multimodal programs, including the WHO *SAVE LIVES: Clean Your Hands* campaign (www.who.int/gpsc/5may/en/), the Institute for Healthcare Improvement's Guide to Improving Hand Hygiene (www.ihi.org/ resources/Pages/Tools/HowtoGuideImprovingHandHygiene.aspx), and The Joint Commission Center for Transforming Healthcare's targeted solutions tool (www .centerfortransforminghealthcare.org/tst_hh.aspx). While over 2,000 healthcare facilities in the US have joined the WHO campaign, which draws heavily on the WHO Guide to Implementation,[7] there has been non-universal adoption of the WHO campaign in the United States as there has been in other countries. Lack of a national campaign is a common critique of hand hygiene in the US, yet there have been many local efforts to form coalitions among healthcare facilities to improve hand hygiene. Several states have implemented campaigns; South Carolina launched a statewide hand hygiene campaign that formally integrates into the WHO materials (www.scha.org/grime-scene-investigators- south-carolina); New Hampshire also has a statewide campaign ("High Five" www.healthynh.com/index.php/hand-hygiene-high-5-for-a-healthy-nh.html) that promotes locally developed or adapted materials; and Maryland has a statewide initiative to "strengthen and complement work already being done to improve hand hygiene" by providing standard tools for data entry and opportunities to learn from peer facilities. Within each state, different health systems may adopt their own campaigns and promotion efforts. The result is a non-coordinated campaign from the national perspective, but it is unclear that abandoning local efforts in favor of a national standard is the right direction either.

One barrier to establishing a single national standard for hand hygiene is that optimal methods for hand hygiene monitoring have not been established, although the US has pioneered several new and innovative approaches[9] (see also Chapter 24). According to the Joint Commission, there are five main approaches to monitoring hand hygiene adherence including direct observation, technology-assisted direct observation, product volume or event count measurement, advanced technologies for automated monitoring, and self-reporting.[10] Aside from self-report, which is not recommended, the SHEA compendium recommends using a combined measurement approach appropriate to the facility's resources and commitment to using data productively; using different approaches (e.g., direct observation as well as indirect event count monitoring) can help provide information on specific practices as well as overall trends. Advanced technologies for automated monitoring are still under development or in various stages of evaluation. Automated monitoring systems offer promise in that they reduce the resource burden on human observers and can in theory provide consistent data over time for benchmarking. These systems, which often use sensor-based technology to characterize hand hygiene opportunities and hand hygiene events, have been piloted mainly in academic research institutions. Recent reviews of these technologies found that limited data were currently available to support the adoption of a specific automated monitoring system.[11,12] In particular, most of the systems currently available measure hand hygiene performance at patient room entry and exit, and thus they fail to identify standard indications at the point of patient care when microbial transmission most likely occurs (e.g., the WHO Five Moments; see Chapter 20).[11] We refer the reader to Chapter 24 for a complete review on this topic. There are many ongoing efforts to refine and evaluate these new technologies, which if adopted nationally as part of quality improvement systems, could provide some consistent benchmarking. In the meantime, local hand hygiene measurement and promotion initiatives, as well as participation in larger national and global campaigns, should be encouraged as a critical element of patient safety.

REFERENCES

1. Boyce JM, Pittet D, Guideline for hand hygiene in health-care settings: recommendations of the Healthcare Infection Control Practices Advisory Committee and the HIPAC/SHEA/APIC/ IDSA Hand Hygiene Task Force. *Am J Infect Control* 2002;**30**:S1-S46.
2. Pittet D, Allegranzi B, Boyce J, The World Health Organization Guidelines on Hand Hygiene in Health Care and their consensus recommendations. *Infect Control Hosp Epidemiol* 2009;**30**:611–622.
3. Ellingson K, Haas J, Aiello A, et al., Strategies to prevent healthcare-associated infections through hand hygiene. *Infect Control Hosp Epidemiol* 2014;**35**:937–960.
4. Erasmus V, Daha TJ, Brug H, et al., Systematic review of studies on compliance with hand hygiene guidelines in hospital care. *Infect Control Hosp Epidemiol* 2010;**31**:283–294.
5. Schweizer ML, Reisinger HS, Ohl M, et al., Searching for an optimal hand hygiene bundle: a meta analysis. *Clin Infect Dis* 2014;**58**:248–259.
6. Allegranzi B, Conway L, Larson E, et al., Status of the implementation of the World Health Organization multimodal hand hygiene strategy in United States of America health care facilities. *Am J Infect Control* 2014;**42**:224–230.
7. World Health Organization, *WHO A Guide to the Implementation of the WHO Multimodal Hand Hygiene Improvement Strategy.* Geneva: WHO, 2009.
8. Macinga DR, Edmonds SL, Campbell E, et al., Efficacy of novel alcohol-based hand rub products at typical in-use volumes. *Infect Control Hosp Epidemiol* 2013;**34**:299–301.
9. Boyce JM, Measuring healthcare worker hand hygiene activity: current practices and emerging technologies. *Infect Control Hosp Epidemiol* 2011;**32**:1016–1028.
10. The Joint Commission, *Measuring Hand Hygiene Adherence: Overcoming the Challenges,* 2009. Available at www.jointcommission.org/assets/1/18/hh_monograph.pdf. Accessed March 7 2017.
11. Ward MA, Schweizer ML, Polgreen PM, Gupta K, Reisinger HS, Perencevich EN, Automated and electronically assisted hand hygiene monitoring systems: a systematic review. *Am J Infect Control.* 2014;**42**:472–478.
12. World Health Organization, *Systematic literature review of automated/electronic systems for hand hygiene monitoring.* Geneva: WHO, 2013. Available at www.who.int/gpsc/5may/monitoring_feedback/en/. Accessed March 7, 2017.

Chapter 33

WHO Multimodal Promotion Strategy

Benedetta Allegranzi[1] and Didier Pittet[2]

[1] Infection Prevention and Control Global Unit, Department of Service Delivery and Safety, World Health Organization, and Faculty of Medicine, University of Geneva, Geneva, Switzerland

[2] Infection Control Program and WHO Collaborating Centre on Patient Safety, University of Geneva Hospitals and Faculty of Medicine, Geneva, Switzerland

KEY MESSAGES

- The *WHO Multimodal Hand Hygiene Improvement Strategy* aims at translating the World Health Organization (WHO) hand hygiene recommendations into practice at the point of care.

- The strategy involves the implementation of five key components at the facility level and is accompanied by a range of tools per each component.

- Implementation of the WHO strategy has been shown to be feasible and sustainable across a range of settings in different countries and leads to significant improvement of key hand hygiene indicators.

With the launch of the First Global Patient Safety Challenge *"Clean Care is Safer Care"* in 2005, the World Health Organization (WHO) committed to promote hand hygiene improvement in healthcare to support the reduction of healthcare-associated infection (HAI) worldwide. This effort led to the development of the first evidence-based global hand hygiene guidelines in 2006, issued as a final document in 2009.[1] Among the peculiarities and added values of these guidelines was the fact that WHO and international experts contributing to this project put together experience and expertise to develop, pilot test, and finalize a multimodal strategy and a comprehensive set of tools to translate the WHO hand hygiene recommendations into practice at the bedside in different healthcare settings worldwide (Figure 33.1). These were issued at the same time as the final guidelines; this approach has significantly contributed to the success of the WHO hand hygiene promotion strategy and its uptake in many countries and thousands of facilities worldwide.

Hand Hygiene: A Handbook for Medical Professionals, First Edition.
Edited by Didier Pittet, John M. Boyce and Benedetta Allegranzi.
© 2017 John Wiley & Sons, Inc. Published 2017 by John Wiley & Sons, Inc.

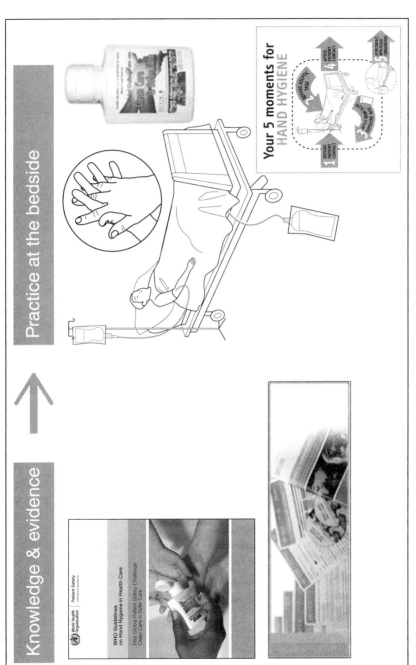

Figure 33.1 Implementation strategy and toolkit for the translation into practice of the *WHO Guidelines on Hand Hygiene in Health Care. Source:* Reproduced with permission from the World Health Organization. *See plate section for color representation of this figure.*

WHAT WE KNOW – THE EVIDENCE

The development of the *WHO Multimodal Hand Hygiene Improvement Strategy*[2] was based on the literature on implementation science, behavioral change, spread methodology, diffusion of innovation, and impact evaluation. The core of the strategy was conceived at the University of Geneva Hospitals and Faculty of Medicine and proved to be effective to significantly reduce HAI hospital-wide and to be cost-effective.[3,4] In its draft version, the WHO strategy accompanied by a package of draft implementation tools was tested between 2006 and 2008 in a range of facilities in several countries with different cultural and economic levels, backgrounds, health systems, and degrees of implementation of infection control (see below). Following the demonstration of its effect to significantly increase healthcare workers' (HCWs') hand hygiene compliance and knowledge, and its feasibility and sustainability, the strategy was finalized according to the lessons learned and issued in 2009 as a standardized approach for worldwide implementation and adaptation.[2]

The multimodal strategy consists of five components to be implemented in parallel (Table 33.1 and Figure 33.2). Tools to facilitate implementation of each component (Table 33.1) are available in several languages to any healthcare facility or country willing to roll out a hand hygiene promotion campaign. The strategy aims at facilitating infrastructure and HCWs' behavioral change at the point of care in the context of a favorable institutional safety climate.

System change represents a number of actions aimed at ensuring that the necessary equipment and supplies for hand hygiene are available and in working condition (see Chapter 21).[5] Based upon scientific evidence of antimicrobial efficacy, rapidity of action, skin tolerability, and ease of use when needed, as well as users' preferences, alcohol-based handrubs (ABHRs) are the best products to be used for hand hygiene in healthcare.[1] Therefore, a primary element of system change is that a facility must make ABHR of adequate quality continuously available at the point of care. The lack of running water, soap, and single-use towels are other conditions that need to be overcome to enable adequate hand hygiene practices. Thus, while evaluating actions for system change, the facility should also consider the installation of an adequate number of sinks at the point of care, the continuous provision of water, soap, and disposable towels, and possibly the use of automated sinks. Specific recommendations within the WHO hand hygiene guidelines urge both healthcare administrators and governments to enable system change.[1] Several WHO tools (Table 33.1) are available to direct and support them in making prompt and appropriate system changes.

Education of front-line staff on the importance of hand hygiene and when and how it should be performed is a pillar of a hand hygiene improvement strategy (see Chapter 22).[6] Education should also target other HCWs including administrators and cleaning personnel in order to convince them of the importance to support hand hygiene promotion. Future trainers should also be briefed on the key messages to be spread and should be supported to become familiar with the tools

Table 33.1 Components of the WHO Hand Hygiene Multimodal Improvement Strategy and Associated Implementation Tools

Strategy Component	Definition	Associated Implementation Tools
1. System Change	Ensuring that the necessary infrastructure is in place to allow HCWs to practice hand hygiene. This includes two essential elements: 1. Access to a safe, continuous water supply as well as to soap and towels 2. Readily-accessible alcohol-based handrub at the point of care	• Ward Infrastructure Survey • Alcohol-based Handrub Planning and Costing Tool • Guide to Local Production: WHO-recommended Handrub Formulations • Soap Handrub Consumption Survey • Protocol for Evaluation of Tolerability and Acceptability of Alcohol-Based Handrub in Use or Planned to be Introduced: Method 1 • Protocol for Evaluation and Comparison of Tolerability and Acceptability of Different Alcohol-based Handrubs: Method 2
2. Training/ Education	Providing regular training on the importance of hand hygiene, based on the My Five Moments for Hand Hygiene approach and on the correct procedures for handrubbing and handwashing to all HCWs	• Slides for the hand hygiene coordinator • Slides for education sessions for trainers, observers, and healthcare workers • Hand hygiene training films • Slides accompanying the training films • Hand Hygiene Technical Reference Manual • Hand Hygiene Why, How and When brochure • Glove Use Information leaflet • Your Five Moments for Hand Hygiene poster • Frequently asked questions • Key scientific publications • Sustaining improvement – additional activities for consideration by healthcare facilities

(continued)

Table 33.1 (*Continued*)

Strategy Component	Definition	Associated Implementation Tools
3. Evaluation and Feedback	Monitoring hand hygiene practices and infrastructure, along with related perceptions and knowledge among HCWs, while providing performance and results feedback to the staff	• Hand Hygiene Technical Reference Manual • Observation tools: Observation Form and Compliance Calculation Form • Ward Infrastructure Survey • Soap/Handrub Consumption Survey • Perception Survey for Health-Care Workers • Perception Survey for Senior Managers • Hand Hygiene Knowledge Questionnaire for Health-Care Workers • Protocol for Evaluation of Tolerability and Acceptability of Alcohol-based Handrub in Use or Planned to be Introduced: Method 1 • Protocol for Evaluation and Comparison of Tolerability and Acceptability of Different Alcohol-based Handrubs: Method 2 • Data Entry Analysis Tool • Instructions for Data Entry and Analysis • Data Summary Report Framework • Hand Hygiene Self-Assessment Framework

4. Reminders in the Workplace	Prompting and reminding HCWs about the importance of hand hygiene and about the appropriate indications and procedures for performing it	• Your Five Moments for Hand Hygiene poster • How to Handrub poster • How to Handwash poster • Hand Hygiene: When and How leaflet • *SAVE LIVES: Clean Your Hands* screensaver • 5 May 2014 – WHO 5 Moments for Hand Hygiene screensaver • Hand Hygiene and Antimicrobial Resistance posters • My Five Moments for Hand Hygiene – Focus on Caring for a Patient with a Urinary Catheter poster • My Five Moments for Hand Hygiene – Focus on Caring for a patient with a Central Venous Catheter poster • My Five Moments for Hand Hygiene – Focus on Caring for a Patient with a Peripheral Venous Catheter poster • My Five Moments for Hand Hygiene – Focus on Caring for a Patient with an Endotracheal Tube poster • My Five Moments for Hand Hygiene – Focus on caring for a patient with a post-operative wound • Hand Hygiene and the Surgical Patient Journey Infographic • Reminders produced by WHO every year on May 5 (www.who.int/gpsc/5may/en

(continued)

Table 33.1 (*Continued*)

Strategy Component	Definition	Associated Implementation Tools
5. Institutional Safety Climate	Creating an environment and the perceptions that facilitate awareness-raising about patient safety issues while guaranteeing consideration of hand hygiene improvement as a high priority at all levels Including: • Active participation at both the institutional and individual levels • Awareness of individual and institutional capacity to change and improve (self-efficacy) • Partnership with patients and patient organizations	• Template Letter to Advocate Hand Hygiene to Managers • Template Letter to Communicate Hand Hygiene Initiatives to Managers • Guidance on Engaging Patients and Patient Organizations in Hand Hygiene Initiatives • Sustaining Improvement – Additional Activities for Consideration by Health-Care Facilities • *SAVE LIVES: Clean Your Hands* Promotional DVD • Tips for patients to participate in hand hygiene improvement • Tips for implementing a successful patient participation program • Hand Hygiene Self-Assessment Framework

Source: Reproduced with permission from the World Health Organization.

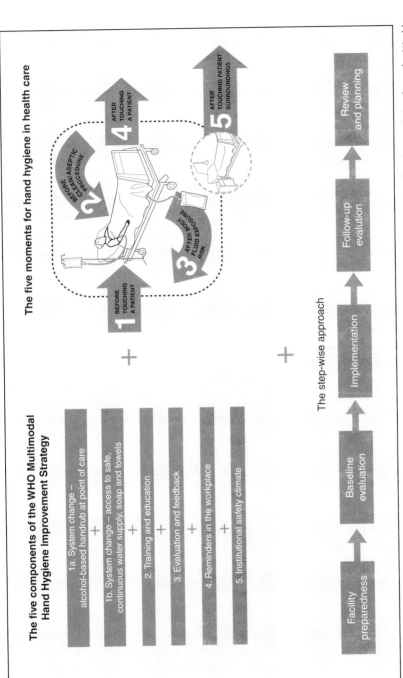

Figure 33.2 WHO Multimodal Hand Hygiene Improvement Strategy Implementation Model. *Source:* Reproduced with permission from the World Health Organization. *See plate section for color representation of this figure.*

available for training; if feasible, formal training of the trainers is recommended (so-called train-the-trainers programs). The main technical principles conceived and fostered by WHO are centered on the concepts of patient zone and the My Five Moments for Hand Hygiene (see Chapter 20).[7] The latter have been proven to be very instrumental in raising HCWs' attention and making them understand, remember, and effectively focus on the essential moments when and why to perform hand hygiene at the point of care. Practical training on the correct technique and duration to achieve maximum hand decontamination is also of utmost importance because serious gaps in knowledge and practices are widespread in these regards. To support training, WHO developed standard PowerPoint presentations, leaflets, and brochures available in several languages and Hand Hygiene Training films/videos (Table 33.1); an additional educational video on hand hygiene was published in the *New England Journal of Medicine*[8] and is available at www .who.int/gpsc/5may/hand_hygiene_video/en/ in more than 10 languages. Facilities should consider implementing a system of checking on the competence of all HCWs who have received hand hygiene training. Utilizing the WHO hand hygiene knowledge survey could fulfill the purpose of checks on competences. Evaluation of staff ability to correctly perform hand hygiene could also take the form of a practical hand hygiene demonstration in relation to correct hand hygiene techniques at the appropriate moments.

Evaluation and feedback of key hand hygiene infrastructure, process, knowledge, and performance indicators is the third component of the WHO strategy. It is an integral part of the strategy and should not be seen as a component separated from implementation or only to be used for scientific purposes. Key indicators should be assessed before starting a hand hygiene campaign and then periodically (at least annually, but ideally more frequently) during and after the implementation period. Providing regular feedback to the concerned HCWs and senior managers using local data on the key hand hygiene indicators and possibly also on outcome indicators (e.g., HAIs) is a very powerful approach to raise awareness about defective practices and achieve improvement. In addition to specific monitoring tools measuring the above-mentioned indicators (see Table 33.1), WHO developed a comprehensive instrument (the WHO Hand Hygiene Self-assessment Framework) for the evaluation of the status of hand hygiene activities in healthcare facilities according to the WHO multimodal strategy (see Chapter 34).[9] More details about hand hygiene monitoring can be also found in Chapters 24 and 25.

Reminders in the workplace are key tools to prompt and remind HCWs about the need for performing hand hygiene and the appropriate indications and procedures. They are also means of informing patients and visitors of the hand hygiene best practices that they should expect during care delivery. Posters are the most common type of reminders and these should be placed as close as possible to the point of care (see Table 33.1). The image of the WHO My Five Moments for Hand Hygiene (see Chapter 20)[7] not only provides technical information, but it has become a visual branding of hand hygiene promotion that many people can recognize around the world. Good maintenance and a regular refreshment of posters' content are very important aspects to achieve maximum impact with these tools.

The establishment or strengthening of institutional safety climate is the fifth and overarching component in which the WHO strategy should be embedded (see Chapter 28). HAI and antimicrobial resistance transmission need to be seen as an institutional patient safety problem and even more broadly as a social problem. Therefore, the healthcare community, consisting of individual HCWs, managers, and the institution as a whole, should take responsibility at all levels and should show clear commitment, reliability, and accountability for hand hygiene improvement as a patient safety solution. Patients should also be involved in the creation of this climate, according to cultural sensitivities and social dynamics (see Chapters 30 and 31).[10]

Scientific evidence and global experience shows that each component of the WHO strategy is crucial, and in general no component can be considered optional if the objective is to achieve effective and sustainable impact. However, the implementation strategy itself is designed to be adaptable without jeopardizing its fidelity and intended outcome; therefore, depending on the local situation and available resources, some components might be given more emphasis than others or might be practically implemented in different ways. Examples are provided in the WHO Guide to Implementation.[2]

WHO suggests implementing the multimodal strategy by using a stepwise approach, especially in facilities where a hand hygiene program has not yet been implemented (Table 33.2).[1,2] This allows appropriate locally tailored planning based upon evaluations to gradually implement a comprehensive hand hygiene program. Figure 33.2 illustrates the conceptual combination of WHO multimodal hand hygiene improvement strategy, the My Five Moments for Hand Hygiene approach, which is key to the strategy implementation, and the stepwise approach.

Finally, to provide more guidance on implementation of the strategy based upon comprehensive evaluation of the local situation using the WHO Hand Hygiene Self-Assessment Framework,[9] WHO developed specific action plans depending on the identified level of progress (www.who.int/gpsc/5may/EN_PSP_GPSC1_5May_2012/en/).

The WHO Multimodal Hand Hygiene Improvement Strategy[2] was tested across a range of settings in different countries using a quasi-experimental study conducted between 2006 and 2008 in six pilot sites in five countries. The implementation proved to be feasible and sustainable across a range of settings in different countries and led to significant improvements of hand hygiene infrastructure and HCWs' compliance, perception, and knowledge.[11,12]

Finally, the systematic review and network meta-analysis by Luangasanatip and colleagues demonstrates the key role of the WHO multimodal approach in successful hand hygiene promotion in recent years.[13]

Table 33.2 Step-Wise Approach for the Implementation of the WHO Hand Hygiene Multimodal Improvement Strategy

Strategy Component	Definition
Step 1: Facility preparedness – readiness for action	Ensuring the preparedness of the institution. This includes obtaining the necessary resources (both human and financial), putting infrastructure in place, identifying key leadership to head the program including a coordinator and his/her deputy Proper planning must be done to map out a clear strategy for the entire program
Step 2: Baseline evaluation – establishing knowledge of the current situation	Conducting baseline evaluation of hand hygiene practice, perception, knowledge, and the infrastructures available
Step 3: Implementation – introducing the improvement activities	Implementing the improvement program Ensuring the availability of an alcohol-based handrub at the point of care is vitally important, as is conducting staff education and training and displaying reminders in the workplace Well-publicized events involving endorsement and/or signatures of commitment from leaders and individual healthcare workers will generate great participation
Step 4: Follow-up evaluation – evaluating the implementation impact	Conducting follow-up evaluation to assess the effectiveness of the program
Step 5: Ongoing planning and review cycle – developing a plan for the next 5 years (minimum)	Developing an ongoing action plan and review cycle, while ensuring long-term sustainability

WHAT WE DO NOT KNOW – THE UNCERTAIN

The WHO strategy has been implemented in thousands of facilities around the world, as reported through the WHO *SAVE LIVES: Clean Your Hands* campaign (www.who.int/gpsc/5may/registration_update/en/). It is essential to gather more reports and publications about the variations in implementation of the strategy and its impact in different settings.

Among the publications related to the strategy's effectiveness, most are quasi-experimental studies comparing time periods before and after the strategy implementation with regards to several indicators, especially hand hygiene compliance. Studies assessing HAIs and transmission of antimicrobial-resistant pathogens as outcome indicators are less frequent. Indeed, it would be very interesting to gather more research on this, ideally through (cluster) randomized, controlled studies (see Chapter 6). The recent report by Luangasanatip and colleagues is informative in this respect.[13]

Furthermore, although each strategy component is considered essential, it would be useful to know their relative impact and which one might have a stronger effect on hand hygiene compliance and other indicators in a specific setting. This proves to be difficult, given the multimodal nature of the strategy, to be typically delivered as a set of interventions in parallel. For instance, within the WHO pilot sites, the strategy was clearly shown to be effective to increase HCWs' knowledge on hand hygiene and HAIs. HCWs' training was certainly a key determinant, if not the most important, to achieve these results. However, feedback (strategy component 3) of local hand hygiene compliance results accompanied by data interpretation on specific hand hygiene indications might also have had a role in determining knowledge improvement. Furthermore, bedside mentoring by influential leaders playing role modeling (strategy component 5) could also contribute to increased knowledge in addition to traditional education. Whether additional components (e.g., goal setting, reward incentives, accountability) should be considered as additional elements [13] or as part of the five core elements of the WHO strategy deserves further research.

Cluster-randomized, stepped wedge approaches gradually introducing different strategy components at different times and controlling for confounders could allow more accurate evaluation (see also Chapter 6).

However, although this research would probably bring additional evidence, by definition these study designs would hamper the multimodal approach.[13] In addition, randomization occurring at ward level within a single facility would bring the risk of cross-contamination between control and intervention wards (i.e., movement of staff between wards, workplace reminders, leadership, etc.).[14] Furthermore, without a transparent and facility-wide approach of the campaign, the development of an institutional safety climate, an essential component of the WHO strategy would be impeded.

Another area which has not been appropriately evaluated is the cost-effectiveness of the strategy implementation,[13] although some simple cost estimates have been conducted during pilot testing and proved to be very feasible. For instance, the cost of local production of the WHO formulation in a tertiary care hospital in Mali was only about US$0.30 per 100 mL, representing 0.006% of the total annual hospital budget. More sophisticated cost-effectiveness studies evaluating the whole strategy and calculating the benefit of preventing healthcare-associated infections (HAIs) would be very useful to support local sustainment of a campaign and further spread of the approach in other facilities[13] (see also Chapter 39).

Finally, appropriate qualitative evaluations to determine barriers and facilitators of the WHO strategy implementation would be interesting and very helpful to guide further dissemination and adoption. In addition, studies to understand the

predictive implementation factors leading to sustainability would be very beneficial; in particular, it would be essential to identify successful approaches to keep
HCWs and decision makers motivated to continue to put efforts into the strategy
implementation and refreshment over time.

RESEARCH AGENDA

Further research is needed to:

- Identify and describe successful and creative local adaptations of the WHO
  strategy.
- Establish the relative importance of the specific components of the WHO
  multimodal hand hygiene improvement strategy, as well as eventual additional components, to induce HCWs' behavioral change and determine sustained outcome improvement.
- Establish the effect of specific strategy components on selected different
  types of indicators.
- Estimate the cost-effectiveness of the whole WHO strategy implementation
  in different settings.
- Develop qualitative approaches to determine barriers and facilitators of the
  WHO strategy implementation.
- Identify best approaches to ensure and maintain sustainability of the strategy implementation and its positive results.

REFERENCES

1. World Health Organization, *WHO Guidelines on Hand Hygiene in Health Care.* Geneva: WHO,
   2009.
2. World Health Organization, *WHO Guide to Implementation of the WHO Multimodal Hand
   Hygiene Improvement Strategy.* Geneva: WHO, 2009. Available at www.who.int/gpsc/5may/
   tools/en/. Accessed March 7, 2017.
3. Pittet D, Hugonnet S, Harbarth S, et al., Effectiveness of a hospital-wide programme to
   improve compliance with hand hygiene. *Lancet* 2000;**356**:1307–1312.
4. Pittet D, Sax H, Hugonnet S, et al., Cost implications of successful hand hygiene promotion.
   Infect Control Hosp Epidemiol 2004;**25**:264–266.
5. Allegranzi B, Sax H, Pittet D, Hand hygiene and healthcare system change within
   multi-modal promotion: a narrative review. *J Hosp Infect* 2013;**83**(Suppl. 1):S3–S10.
6. Mathai E, Allegranzi B, Seto WH, et al., Educating healthcare workers to optimal hand
   hygiene practices: addressing the need. *Infection* 2010;**38**:349–356.
7. Sax H, Allegranzi B, Uckay I, et al., 'My five moments for hand hygiene': A user-centred
   design approach to understand, train, monitor and report hand hygiene. *J Hosp Infect*
   2007;**67**:9–21.

8. Longtin Y, Sax H, Allegranzi B, et al., Videos in clinical medicine. Hand hygiene. *N Engl J Med* 2011;**364**:e24.

9. World Health Organization, *WHO Hand Hygiene Self-Assessment Framework.* Geneva: WHO, 2010. Available at www.who.int/gpsc/5may/hhsa_framework/en/. Accessed March 7, 2017.

10. McGuckin M, Govednik J, Patient empowerment and hand hygiene, 1997–2012. *J Hosp Infect* 2013;**84**:191–199.

11. Allegranzi B, Sax H, Bengaly L, et al., Successful implementation of the World Health Organization hand hygiene improvement strategy in a referral hospital in Mali, Africa. *Infect Control Hosp Epidemiol* 2010;**31**:133–141.

12. Allegranzi B, Gayet-Ageron A, Damani N, et al., Global implementation of WHO's multimodal strategy for improvement of hand hygiene: a quasi-experimental study. *Lancet Infect Dis* 2013;**13**:843–851.

13. Luangasanatip N, Hongsuwan M, Limmathurotsakul D, et al., Comparative efficacy of interventions to promote hand hygiene in hospital: systematic review and network meta-analysis. *BMJ* 2015;**315**:h37281.

14. Stewardson A, Sax H, Gayet-Ageron A, et al., Enhanced performance feedback and patient participation to improve hand hygiene compliance of health-care workers in the setting of established multimodal promotion: a single-centre, cluster randomised controlled trial. *Lancet Infect Dis* 2016;**16**:1345–1355.

Chapter 34

Monitoring Your Institution (Hand Hygiene Self-Assessment Framework)

Benedetta Allegranzi,[1] Andrew J. Stewardson,[2,3] and Didier Pittet[3]

[1] *Infection Prevention and Control Global Unit, Department of Service Delivery and Safety, World Health Organization, and Faculty of Medicine, University of Geneva, Geneva, Switzerland*

[2] *Infectious Diseases Department, Austin Health and Hand Hygiene Australia, Melbourne, Australia*

[3] *Infection Control Program and WHO Collaborating Centre on Patient Safety, University of Geneva Hospitals and Faculty of Medicine, Geneva, Switzerland*

KEY MESSAGES

- The Hand Hygiene Self-Assessment Framework (HHSAF) is a validated, systematic tool designed to obtain a situation analysis of hand hygiene promotion and practices within an individual healthcare facility (HCF), based upon the key elements of the WHO Multimodal Hand Hygiene Improvement Strategy.

- The HHSAF acts as a diagnostic tool, identifying key issues requiring attention and improvement. The results can be used to facilitate development of an action plan for the HCF's hand hygiene promotion program or campaign.

- Repeated use of the HHSAF allows documentation of progress over time. Several countries and HCFs use the HHSAF as part of their regular hand hygiene campaign evaluation and for monitoring hand hygiene promotion as a key national patient safety and quality of care indicator.

Hand Hygiene: A Handbook for Medical Professionals, First Edition.
Edited by Didier Pittet, John M. Boyce and Benedetta Allegranzi.
© 2017 John Wiley & Sons, Inc. Published 2017 by John Wiley & Sons, Inc.

Hand hygiene activities and practices have become a key indicator of patient safety and quality of care in health systems worldwide, at both national and healthcare facility (HCF) level. Hand hygiene monitoring and performance feedback are essential elements of most successful strategies to achieve behavioral change amongst healthcare workers (HCWs; see Chapter 24). Different indicators of hand hygiene practices have been identified and used over the last decades, the most popular being the direct and indirect monitoring of HCWs' compliance and alcohol-based handrub (ABHR) consumption (see Chapter 24). Given this important focus on hand hygiene in infection prevention and control programs, World Health Organization (WHO) has developed an instrument for the evaluation of the status of hand hygiene activities in HCFs worldwide.

WHAT WE DO KNOW – THE EVIDENCE

The Hand Hygiene Self-Assessment Framework (HHSAF)[1] was developed by WHO with input by international experts as a systematic self-assessment tool to provide a situation analysis of hand hygiene resources, promotion, and practices within healthcare facilities. The tool was developed in three phases: initial drafting, usability testing, and reliability testing.[2] For usability testing, 26 facilities in 19 countries completed the draft HHSAF and a feedback survey. For inter-rater reliability testing, two users in each facility independently completed the HHSAF. The results supported the usability and reliability of this tool in the assessment of hand hygiene promotion activities at HCF level.[3] Based on this pilot study, the tool underwent revision; it was finalized and launched in 2010.

The HHSAF is structured in five sections, which reflect the five components of the WHO Multimodal Hand Hygiene Improvement Strategy[4] (see Chapter 33). These are system change, training and education, evaluation and performance feedback, reminders in the workplace, and institutional safety climate. Indicators appropriate for each component were identified based on available evidence and expert consensus. Twenty-seven indicators were included (see Appended tool at the end of the book before Index). The innovative approach of this tool rests in the scoring system associated with the responses for each indicator and based on the five components. The sum of maximum values for all indicators in each section is 100 points, resulting in a maximum overall score of 500 points. Based on its overall score, a HCF is assigned to one of four levels of progress (see Table 34.1). HCFs scored as *Advanced* can undergo further assessment according to 20 additional criteria, and a HCF is defined as reaching the *Leadership* level if it satisfies at least 12 of these latter criteria.

The HHSAF is an excellent tool for baseline evaluation of hand hygiene activities within a HCF when planning a hand hygiene campaign.[4] By completing the HHSAF and carefully analyzing the detailed information included in each section, the team in charge of organizing the campaign can identify the priorities for action. Given the organization and scoring in sections that correspond to components of the multimodal strategy, the tool facilitates the maintenance of

Table 34.1 Levels of Hand Hygiene Implementation Progress Defined by the WHO Hand Hygiene Self-Assessment Framework (HHSAF)

Level of Progress	HHSAF Score	Definition
Inadequate	≤125	Hand hygiene practices and promotion are deficient. Significant improvement is required
Basic	126–250	Some measures are in place, but not at a satisfactory standard. Further improvement is required
Intermediate	251–375	An appropriate hand hygiene promotion strategy is in place, and hand hygiene practices have improved. It is now crucial to develop long-term plans to ensure that improvement is sustained and progresses
Advanced	>375	Hand hygiene promotion and optimal hand hygiene practices have been sustained and/or improved, helping to embed a culture of safety in the healthcare setting
Leadership*		The healthcare facility is considered as a reference center for and contributes to the promotion of hand hygiene through research, innovation and information sharing

*The healthcare facility reached the Advanced level and in addition meets at least 12 out of 20 leadership criteria and at least one leadership criterion per each category.

an appropriate balance among the strategy components. Information provided by use of the HHSAF should be fed into the general template action plan proposed by WHO in the Guide to Implementation[4] for developing a hand hygiene campaign or any local adaptation or campaign planning framework. WHO has also developed three specific action plans to assist translation of HHSAF results into action. The three templates are designed for HCFs achieving an inadequate/basic, intermediate, or advanced/leadership results. In addition, each indicator in the HHSAF includes reference to the WHO hand hygiene tools that can be used to support implementation and improvement related to that specific indicator.

By using the HHSAF intermittently over time, the HCF can keep track of the changes following the campaign implementation and progressively set new targets for improvement. The HHSAF results and score can be integrated within the campaign communication strategy and used as a social mobilization tool to leverage HCWs' and institutional engagement to achieve the desired targets.

As part of the activities to support the *SAVE LIVES: Clean Your Hands* campaign for May 5, 2012, WHO launched a global survey based on the HHSAF.[5,6] The aims were to have an overview of hand hygiene activities in different countries and facilities and to understand what parts of the WHO hand hygiene improvement strategy were more widely implemented and which ones were less easily achieved. Overall, 2,119 healthcare settings from 69 countries (mainly located in upper-middle or high-income countries) submitted complete results to WHO using a web-based survey. Most facilities were general, nonteaching, public hospitals, delivering acute or mixed (acute and long-term) care. The overall mean score reflected *intermediate* level of hand hygiene implementation progress (292.5 ± 100.6). Most facilities were at *intermediate* or *advanced* levels (65%), with a high proportion qualifying for the leadership level. Among the HHSAF sections, the lowest scores concerned evaluation and performance feedback on hand hygiene activities and the institutional patient safety climate. The highest mean score was found in Western Pacific countries and the lowest in African countries. The average level of progress was *intermediate* in all regions, except in Africa where it was *basic*. Several countries conducted the survey nationwide, and WHO shared the country data and/or results with national authorities. These were therefore able to use the survey results to evaluate and further develop their ongoing hand hygiene campaign. A specific subanalysis of the data was performed for HCFs participating from the United States, most of which had an advanced or intermediate level of progress.[7] In this sample, the total HHSAF score was found to be significantly higher in facilities with staffing levels of infection control professionals exceeding 0.75/100 beds than for those with lower ratios ($P = 0.01$) and for those participating in regional hand hygiene campaigns ($P = 0.002$).

Several countries continue to use the HHSAF as part of their regular hand hygiene campaign evaluation and for monitoring hand hygiene as a key national patient safety and quality of care indicator. It is also used as the main tool for short-listing and selecting hospitals to be awarded with the Hand Hygiene Excellence Award (www.hhea.info) issued by the Aesculap Academy every year in Europe, Latin America, and Southeast Asia, and from 2017 in Africa, the Middle East, and North America.

WHAT WE DO NOT KNOW – THE UNCERTAIN

The WHO HHSAF includes the inherent limitations of a self-reported evaluation tool, and it was not primarily conceived and validated to make external comparison or benchmarking.

The appropriateness of use of the HHSAF for comparing facilities of different sizes and complexity is unknown, and no evidence is available so far on best methods for benchmarking. In addition, it is unclear how to account for socio-economic status when interpreting results from different HCFs and countries, and how to integrate resource availability with the HHSAF results when planning for improvement actions.

RESEARCH AGENDA

Further research is needed to:

- Identify appropriate benchmarking variables for comparing facilities of different sizes and complexity.
- Identify best methodological approaches for comparing HHSAF results from HCFs in countries with different socio-economic background and resource availability.

- Develop semi-automated and electronic tools to facilitate regular and easy completion of the HHSAF at HCF level.

REFERENCES

1. World Health Organization, *WHO Hand Hygiene Self-Assessment Framework*. Geneva: WHO, 2010. Available at www.who.int/gpsc/5may/hhsa_framework/en/. Accessed March 7, 2017.
2. Allegranzi B, Stewardson A, Grayson L, et al., Background and features of the WHO Hand Hygiene Self-Assessment Framework. First International Conference on Prevention and Infection Control (ICPIC) 2011. Geneva, Switzerland, June 29 to July 2, 2011.
3. Stewardson AJ, Allegranzi B, Perneger TV, et al., Testing the WHO Hand Hygiene Self-Assessment Framework for usability and reliability. *J Hosp Infect* 2013;**83**:30–35.
4. World Health Organization, *WHO Guide to Implementation of the WHO Multimodal Hand Hygiene Improvement Strategy*. Geneva: WHO, 2009.
5. World Health Organization, *WHO Hand Hygiene Self-Assessment Framework Global Survey. Summary Report*. Geneva: WHO, 2012. Available at www.who.int/gpsc/5may/hhsa_framework/en/. Accessed March 7, 2017.
6. Allegranzi B, Gayet-Ageron A, Sax H, et al., Tracking the progress of hand hygiene indicators in healthcare facilities worldwide. 52nd Interscience Conference on Antimicrobial Agents and Chemotherapy (ICAAC 2012). San Francisco, September 9–12, 2012.
7. Allegranzi B, Conway L, Larson E, et al., Status of the implementation of the World Health Organization multimodal hand hygiene strategy in United States of America health care facilities. *Am J Infect Control* 2014;**42**:224–230.

Chapter 35

National Hand Hygiene Campaigns

Claire Kilpatrick and Julie Storr
Infection Prevention and Control Global Unit, Department of Service Delivery and Safety, World Health Organization, Geneva, Switzerland

KEY MESSAGES

- There has been an explosion in national hand hygiene campaigns in the 10 years from 2005 to 2015. The evaluation of their impact is variable and, in many instances, unknown. National campaigns focused on hand hygiene improvement can inspire action in healthcare facilities across the globe, if adequately funded with a clear mandate.

- Components of national campaigns vary; however, a multimodal approach is common. The influence of World Health Organization guidelines, recommendations, implementation toolkit, and engagement strategy is accepted as being the main driver in the number and nature of national campaigns.

- The sharing of experiences between national campaigns might relieve campaign fatigue and help in analyzing critical success factors. The approach taken and period required for national campaigns to have the greatest impact is unclear, with a range of indicators potentially used in decision making and determining the further evaluation required.

The main objective of a national, health-focused campaign should be to leverage an unprecedented social pressure for participation in a public health topic. If a comparison was to be made between national approaches to public health campaigning, for example for hand hygiene improvement, and political campaigns,

Hand Hygiene: A Handbook for Medical Professionals, First Edition.
Edited by Didier Pittet, John M. Boyce and Benedetta Allegranzi.
© 2017 John Wiley & Sons, Inc. Published 2017 by John Wiley & Sons, Inc.

this quote from the *Huffington Post* might serve to describe the intended direction of travel:

> *Political campaigns are all about one thing and one thing only: results. There's no room in a political campaign for any nonsense like "awareness" or "getting your name out there." Everything is geared to one purpose, and one purpose only: getting prospects to take the desired ACTION (vote). Business owners must think the same way, and focus on directing prospects to take a specific action whenever they do any marketing or advertising.*[1]

World Health Organization (WHO) presents a compelling argument for campaigning as a way of achieving global health improvement and outlines components for success called the 7Cs (*World Health Organization Effective Communications Participant Handbook*, WHO, Geneva 2015). In addition, the Global Public Private Partnership for Handwashing with Soap and the Institute for Healthcare Improvement (IHI) 100K Lives and Five Million Lives Campaigns all employ the fundamental principles of campaigning to effect transformational change.

Campaigning can help build collective will, energy, and momentum. Campaigns tend to be practically focused and aid in the creation of a movement of individuals and groups, united in a common cause.

Key lessons have been learned from existing public health campaigns, including:

1. Knowing and understanding your audience.
2. Having a clear unambiguous message.
3. Using the right media.

But it is interesting to note that in the 150 years since Semmelweis first published incontrovertible evidence on the cause and effect between hand hygiene and patient outcome, there were no recorded national campaigns on this important public health topic. The solution to the problem of hand hygiene omissions as a determinant of poor patient outcome by Semmelweis could be described as outstanding, but no collective action was taken in the intervening years at a national level. However, Professor Didier Pittet and colleagues in Switzerland and leaders in England, Belgium and Australia, then started the journey of campaigning for hand hygiene improvement based on a multimodal strategy. This approach has gathered pace in recent years, and governments have increasingly been convinced that the problem of healthcare-associated infection (HAI), which is well documented and outlined in other chapters of this book, can be addressed in part through campaigning.

WHAT WE KNOW – THE EVIDENCE

In the *WHO Guidelines for Hand Hygiene in Health Care*,[2] recommendations are given for national governments. These are presented in Table 35.1. These recommendations imply that a multifaceted approach and funded national campaign activities should be part of annual infection prevention focused programs.

Table 35.1   WHO Recommendations for National Governments

A. Make improved hand hygiene adherence a national priority and consider provision of a funded, coordinated implementation program, while ensuring monitoring and long-term sustainability
B. Support strengthening of infection control capacities within healthcare settings
C. Promote hand hygiene at the community level to strengthen both self-protection and the protection of others
D. Encourage healthcare settings to use hand hygiene as a quality indicator

---

Early Developments – 2007

The first review of country or area hand hygiene campaigns was undertaken by WHO in 2007 as part of its First Global Patient Safety Challenge program (as it was then named). In August 2007, 20 representatives from such campaigns also attended the first gathering of countries/areas in Geneva. A key objective of the meeting was to explore opportunities for strengthening the global response to HAI through leveraging the solidarity of a formal partnership of campaigning nations. The network would have one common aim – to address HAI through a focus on better hand hygiene (albeit not exclusively).

2009 and Beyond

During early 2009, intense efforts were made through WHO's network to further identify existing and new campaigns. At this time, there were at least 38 active campaigns/programs in nations/subnations. The survey was repeated to gather information from these countries or areas (see Table 35.2).

In 2015, as acknowledged by WHO, over 50 campaigns/programs have been launched in nations/subnations. Their contribution to local, national, and international campaigning, and the associated global knowledge pool in the pursuit of improved hand hygiene, is acknowledged. It includes the WHO's *SAVE LIVES: Clean Your Hands* 5 May global campaign, when efforts to engage and feed-back on progress from a range of countries are paramount in maintaining the global profile on this topic.

Studies of European campaigns in particular have also been published to assess activity and campaign structures, for example using access to existing HAI surveillance national contact points. In summary, Magiorakos et al. concluded that while not all countries surveyed had national campaigns, all but four of them reported some kind of supported hand hygiene activity.[4] Further work by Latham et al., through a review of existing published information on campaigns and a survey conducted in 2012, summarized that there was an upward trend in hand hygiene campaigning, but that they were underevaluated.[5] Reasons for

Table 35.2 Results from a WHO Survey on Hand Hygiene Promotion Campaigns Worldwide (2009).[3]

- Personnel involved in all 38 existing campaigns/programs in 2009 completed the survey. Of these, 29 were active national/subnational-level initiatives, and 22 (75.8%) were initiated after the First Global Patient Safety Challenge launch in October 2005
- Main targets were general, district, and university hospitals with increasing coverage of long-term care facilities and primary care. The scope varied from awareness-raising to formal scaled-up activities with ongoing evaluation
- Most initiatives (20/29) obtained funding from multiple sources, with governments among the main funders; governments also initiated 25/29 (86.2%) programs
- The facilitator role played by the Challenge in initiating and supporting activities with tools and recommendations was clearly identified. The perceived significance of specific barriers varied considerably across initiatives. Those related to commitment (priority and support) and resource availability were important across all regions
- Hand hygiene is being promoted in healthcare in many nations/subnations with clear objectives, strategies, and governmental support through policies and resource allocation. While this is important for sustainability, further action is required to initiate coordinated activities across the world, including countries with limited resources

---

*An online survey using a structured questionnaire was conducted during March to April 2009.
Source: Mathai 2011. Reproduced with permission from Elsevier.

underevaluation were given, and there is no surprise to read that lack of financial and human resources were quoted as predominant.

There are clearly benefits to sharing the wisdom behind campaign activities, as has been demonstrated in part by the publications cited and further information provided by WHO. Collective learning from nations that have adopted a national approach to hand hygiene campaigning enhances the likelihood of achieving a vision for preventing HAI. The evidence for this has been achieved by WHO virtually bringing together official national campaigns, into a group entitled WHO *CleanHandsNet* in order to:

- Establish contact between like-minded individuals and national bodies
- Exchange knowledge
- Participate in developing and implementing innovative approaches to improve hand hygiene globally
- Be part of a global network that can enhance the opportunities for obtaining support from authorities within country.

A snapshot of the critical success factors gathered and presented in relation to campaign learning is presented in Table 35.3.

Most important, work has been published on the approaches used by campaigns and the impact in country including on HAI rates. This information is covered within other chapters of this book, and in particular from Australia, as an example of a nationally funded campaign (see Chapter 36). However,

Table 35.3   A Summary of the Critical Success Factors Emerging from WHO
CleanHandsNet Discussions

1. Starting point – an acknowledgement of the need for culture change
2. Robust planning and long preparation phase critical
3. Central versus local funding is a key consideration
4. Initial pilot in small number of facilities followed by review and scale-up
5. Local teams with resources to aid implementation (capacity building), prevention of wheel reinvention
6. Local adaptation is important
7. Engagement of key stakeholders at the outset
8. Big hospitals can learn from smaller ones
9. Strong infection control infrastructure is a key contributor
10. Hand hygiene improvement can act as a key performance indicator
11. Hand hygiene can be part of accountability/governance framework
12. Cheap, easily available resources, in particular alcohol-based handrub (ABHR), is a critical factor
13. Hand hygiene improvement should be integrated/embedded within broader patient safety and quality agendas

it is clear that the tools used to engage those in-country campaign activities appear to embrace a multimodal approach as recommended by WHO. And as such, economies of scale can be addressed by a national campaigning approach, preventing duplication of poster production, consolidation of ideas, organization of monitoring and evaluation activities, engagement of marketing expertise, and so forth. This social capital brings together the "best," to have the greatest impact across a range of healthcare settings in a country.

Being part of national campaigning, as experienced by the chapter authors, is rewarding and provides an immense opportunity to gain new skills including negotiation, the power of influence, and the opportunity to learn and engage with many different experts and enthusiasts from beyond the specialty of infection prevention and control. Being part of such important work that plays a role in global health is not to be underestimated.

WHAT WE DO NOT KNOW – THE UNCERTAIN

It is clear that there is a slow increase in the number of evaluations of national hand hygiene campaigns. However, many remain under- or unevaluated as noted earlier in this chapter; in some cases, campaigning was conducted for more than 10 years before results were reported in the literature.[6] There is a need to accelerate this evaluation in order to expand our understanding of what works and what does not, in particular in relation to benefits, barriers, and limitations, building on those already stated in the 2009 WHO Guidelines. In addition, countries should consider the return on investment and the contribution of campaigns to patient outcome.

If national campaigns were a universal panacea to the problem of low compliance with hand hygiene, it would be expected that more than 54 of the world's countries would commit to use this vehicle to drive improvement. That many don't is also worthy of study.

Successful political campaigns tend to be very disciplined in sticking to a message to ensure it is amplified. They also aim to engage with the intended audience rather than just make "announcements." How much national campaigns compare with political campaigns, the best evidence we have for engagement of a population, is lacking.

The alternatives to national campaigning are also underexplored. What is the added value from national campaigns in comparison to local/healthcare facility and international campaigning on the same subject? Would both economic and public health impact be greater or less without national campaign direction?

The published evidence, however, does seem to imply that national campaigns have an impact on behavior but this evidence does not in many cases convince the right actors such as policy makers and national funders. In addition, there will inevitably be confounders: hand hygiene campaigns exist alongside a plethora of competing health-related campaigns that occupy the attention of healthcare decision makers. Trade-offs are inevitable, and it is unclear whether campaign overload is detrimental or complementary to hand hygiene improvement efforts.

An alternative therefore is to consider what value would be added if hand hygiene campaigning was embedded within other campaigns such as those related to sepsis, antimicrobial resistance, and so forth, or vice versa. Would this save time and money and have a greater impact on behaviors and outcome?

Campaign fatigue is a real threat, and this further supports the need for closer scrutiny, including evaluation of existing campaigns, to ensure that this work continues to add value.[7]

In conclusion, making improved hand hygiene adherence a national priority and constantly considering the provision of a funded, coordinated implementation program, while ensuring monitoring and long-term sustainability, remains a vital consideration in the prevention of HAI now and in the future. Hand hygiene improvement is not "fixed" despite many efforts, and national campaigns have a role to play in coordinating an efficient approach to improvement. A global campaign can stimulate action, but national campaigns can allow for the development of country- and context-specific messages aligned with national policy. Hand hygiene has been quoted as one of the Top Ten Strategies ready for implementation.[8] Campaigns are critical to making this happen.

RESEARCH AGENDA

There are still a number of unknowns related to national campaigning for hand hygiene.

Proposed research topics are as follows:

- Outcome research on national campaigning, preferably versus local (individual facility) action.
- The impact of hand hygiene campaign integration versus promotion in isolation.
- Which campaign components yield the greatest return on investment.

REFERENCES

1. Sipress S, 7 marketing lessons we can learn from politicians. *Huffington Post*, January 4, 2014. Available at www.huffingtonpost.com/steve-sipress/7-marketing-lessons-we-ca_b_6096114.html. Accessed March 7, 2017.
2. World Health Organization, *WHO Guidelines on Hand Hygiene in Health Care*. Geneva: WHO, 2009.
3. Mathai E, Allegranzi B, Kilpatrick C, et al., Promoting hand hygiene in healthcare through national/subnational campaigns. *J Hosp Infect* 2011;**77**:294–298.
4. Magiorakos AP, Suetens, C, Boydet L, et al., National hand hygiene campaigns in Europe 2000–2009. *Eurosurveillance* 2009;**14**:pii-19191.
5. Latham J, Magiorakos A-P, Monnet, DL, et al., The role and utilisation of public health evaluations in Europe: a case study of national hand hygiene campaigns. *BMC Public Health* 2014;**14**:131.
6. Fonguh S, Uwineza A, Catry B, et al., Belgian hand hygiene campaigns in ICU, 2005–2015. *Arch Public Health* 2016;**74**:47.
7. Seto WH, Yuen SW, Cheung CW, et al., Hand hygiene promotion and the participation of infection control link nurses: an effective innovation to overcome campaign fatigue. *Am J Infect Control* 2013; **41**:1281–1283.
8. Schekelle PG, Pronovost PJ, Wachter RM, et al., The top patient safety strategies that can be encouraged for adoption now. *Ann Intern Med* 2013;**158**:365–368.

Chapter 36

Hand Hygiene Campaigning: From One Hospital to the Entire Country

Philip L. Russo[1] and M. Lindsay Grayson[2]

[1] Hand Hygiene Australia, Melbourne, Australia

[2] Infectious Diseases Department, Austin Hospital and University of Melbourne, Melbourne, Australia

KEY MESSAGES

- A successful national hand hygiene program requires clear support and commitment from both national and state health departments, as well as executive support within all participating hospitals. Without support from these jurisdictional representatives – hospitals' executive staff, clinical leaders, and local champions – any effort to introduce a national program will be wasted.

- A long-term (>5-year) vision and commitment to resources are required from funding bodies. At the height of the National Hand Hygiene Initiative (NHHI) implementation, over 10 full-time staff were employed nationally. Frequent interstate travel, the development of a mobile web application and database, audit tools, and educational resources made up a large part of the expenses.

- As with any data collection system, timely feedback of data is essential to ensure improvement. With the use of the Hand Hygiene Australia (HHA) mobile web application for data collection and submission, immediate feedback on compliance levels was available.[6] At a national level, following submission of hospital-level data and jurisdictional review of data, HHA publishes national data on the website six weeks following the end of a data collection period. This timeframe will be reduced once all participating hospitals use the mobile web application.

WHAT WE KNOW – THE EVIDENCE

The successful introduction of a national hand hygiene campaign can be achieved using a variety of approaches. However, the process undertaken to implement the Australian National Hand Hygiene Initiative (NHHI) appears to provide a reasonable blueprint for other countries that may be considering a national strategy to improve hand hygiene in acute-care hospitals. The following steps were followed:

1. "Proof of concept" study in one large hospital, with outcome measures including both improved hand hygiene compliance and infection-related outcomes (number of *Staphylococcus aureus* clinical isolates and rates of *S. aureus* bacteremia). The intervention was based on previous implementation of the multimodal strategy at the University of Geneva Hospitals.[1] This provided important local data.[2]

2. Multisite (*n* = 6) pilot program – replicating the core elements of single-site study in a number of busy urban and rural hospitals. This confirmed the improvement in both hand hygiene compliance and the significant reduction in rates of *S. aureus* bacteremia observed in the single-site program; in addition, it garnered substantial multisite support for maintenance of the program.[3]

3. Statewide rollout of the hand hygiene program to all public hospitals (86 hospitals in Victoria, Australia) with further confirmation of improved hand hygiene compliance and disease reduction outcomes.[2]

4. Adaptation of the WHO Five Moments[4] to suit Australian conditions and development of a national education and implementation strategy, with central coordination – via Hand Hygiene Australia (HHA) – funding, and provision of educational and implementation materials. This process was funded nationally by the Australian Commission on Safety and Quality in Healthcare (ACSQHC) and included the establishment of a national system of hand hygiene compliance auditor training such that only standardized auditors were eligible to submit data and that all compliance data were comparable nationally (www.hha.org.au).

5. A detailed collaborative communication strategy with each of the states and territories in Australia was developed such that each of these jurisdictions retained overall responsibility for their hand hygiene promotion program (and results), but collaborated with HHA to ensure nationally consistent and timely data collection, analysis, and data release.

6. Establishment of a National Hand Hygiene Advisory Committee, consisting of health department representatives from each state/territory and federally, to review data collected by HHA and to recommend changes and modifications to the NHHI, where appropriate.

7. Establishment of a nationally applicable minimum standard or target for hand hygiene compliance in acute-care hospitals (currently, 2016, 70%), with public reporting of results for all participating hospitals on a government website that was readily accessible by consumers (www .myhospitals.gov.au).

8. Establishment of a standardized pathway of data management – including a timetable for data collection, validation by HHA, review by the Hand Hygiene Advisory Committee, release to each state/territory health department, then public release on a government website.

9. Linkage of participation in the NHHI to hospital funding, both from each state and nationally. In some states, hand hygiene compliance levels became a mandated reporting item for each hospital's board of management and a performance standard for each hospital's chief executive officer – this was implemented to ensure greater executive leadership and focus on the importance of hand hygiene compliance.

10. Consumer education in infection control and hand hygiene via a readily available website – encouraging the concept that *Infection control is everybody's business* and that patients and their families should expect their healthcare workers (HCWs) to have high standards in hand hygiene compliance (www.hha.org.au).

Specific Details Regarding the Australian NHHI

Following a successful statewide hand hygiene program in Victoria, the ACSQHC (www.safetyandquality.gov.au) in 2008 funded the three-year NHHI, to implement a uniform hand hygiene program across public and private acute healthcare facilities in Australia, improve compliance, increase use of alcohol-based handrub (ABHR), reduce the rates of healthcare-associated infection and ultimately make hand hygiene core business for all HCWs (www.hha.org.au). A crucial task prior to implementation was to seek commitment and support of the NHHI from the departments of health in all Australian states and territories (jurisdictions), since some jurisdictions already had existing local hand hygiene programs that were not based on the WHO Five Moments.[4]

Commencing mid-2008, HHA was responsible for implementing the NHHI, with the HHA team comprising a director, national project manager, and a team of project coordinators based in Melbourne, with HHA representatives in most jurisdictions. An HHA implementation toolkit was developed, which included an implementation manual, online learning packages, and educational and audit tools. All resources were made available through the HHA website (www.hha.org.au) and freely accessible to any participating hospital. Initial funding for the NHHI was AUD$3.6M (approx. US$3.4M) over three years.

Commencing late 2008, a staged 18-month roll-out was implemented across Australia. To ensure compliance data quality, approximately 280 training workshops were conducted nationally, which instructed participants on program implementation and data collection methodology. Only accredited HHA auditors who had participated in the workshops and passed assessment were permitted to submit hand hygiene compliance data.[6]

Hand hygiene compliance data were first collected in March 2009 from 105 hospitals, with the overall national compliance level at that time of 63.6% (95%CI, 63.2–64.0).[6] Subsequently, the NHHI has received broad support and uptake across Australia, such that in December 2014, as depicted in Figure 36.1, 828 hospitals (537 publicly funded; 291 privately funded) submitted compliance data (hand hygiene compliance = 81.9%; 95%CI, 81.8–82.0%). In addition, more than 250,000 HCWs had completed a variety of online training packages. Many Australian hospitals now mandate that all HCWs complete a hand hygiene online training package when beginning employment and then annually.

Among HCW groups, levels of compliance vary, with nursing staff consistently demonstrating a 10–15% higher hand hygiene compliance rate than medical staff – nevertheless, both groups have improved steadily since the commencement of the NHHI. When first measured in 2009, the national average compliance among medical staff in public facilities was 51.7% (95%CI, 50.6–52.8%), but by the end of 2014, it had increased to 70.2% (95%CI, 69.9–75.0%). For the same time period, nursing staff compliance increased from 69.3% (95%CI, 68.8–69.8%) to 85.5% (95%CI, 85.4–85.6%).

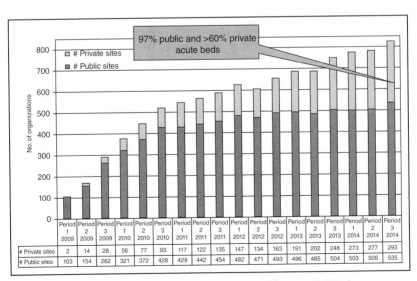

Figure 36.1   Australian NHHI participation, private and public, (2014) 828 sites.

In 2011, HHA summarized the potential effect of the NHHI on national rates of *S. aureus* bacteremia (including MRSA)[6] – a significant decline in hospital-onset and non-hospital-onset MRSA bacteremia rates was observed in the two years following the initial introduction of the NHHI. Although the decrease in nationwide MRSA bacteremia rates cannot be definitively linked to the observed improvements in compliance among HCWs only, the findings are similar to those previously reported with other hand hygiene programs.[1–3]

A number of additional benefits of the NHHI have been anecdotally reported, with many infection prevention staff citing an enhanced relationship with hospital executives and their boards regarding infection control issues, increased profile as a result of frequent auditing, and enhanced opportunities to discuss specific non-hand hygiene infection prevention issues with HCWs.

The NHHI has now become embedded in Australian healthcare and has therefore entered a maintenance phase, whereby hand hygiene compliance data are routinely collected by participating sites and submitted to HHA three times annually for collation and validation before public release. Hospital-level compliance levels are now reported publicly on the MyHospitals website (www .myhospitals.gov.au), and a target of 70% compliance has been promoted by the National Health Performance Authority (www.nhpa.gov.au). Interest in improved hand hygiene compliance has increased significantly in primary care facilities, and educational messages and auditing recommendations have been amended for these settings.

A major challenge for the implementation of the NHHI was engaging those jurisdictions that had existing local hand hygiene campaigns. While every attempt was made to leverage off existing programs, inevitably educational messages and materials needed to be brought into line with the NHHI, and a new rigorous auditing process was introduced. This required HHA to work carefully and collaboratively with jurisdictional representatives and key stakeholders. Another key challenge has been in improving the efficiency of hand hygiene compliance data collection to reduce the time taken in auditing, improve data accuracy, and streamline data analysis. To achieve this, HHA developed an online web application, which can be used on all mobile devices to collect data. It is estimated that this innovation has saved approximately 50% of the time previously required to undertake compliance audits and has markedly improved data accuracy.[5]

WHAT WE DO NOT KNOW AND RESEARCH AGENDA

The Australian NHHI has been highly successful, but a number of issues remain uncertain or require clarification. These include:

What correlation is there between improvements in hand hygiene compliance and observed reductions (if any) in hospital-acquired infections? At what level of compliance should one expect to see significant reductions in disease?. Based on HHA data, most Australian hospitals appeared to experience considerable reductions in methicillin-resistant *S. aureus* (MRSA) bacteremia rates once they regularly achieved hand hygiene compliance levels of at least 55%, with a "power-band" of impact observed between 55% and 75% compliance. However, does this differ for other microorganisms (e.g., multiresistant Gram-negative pathogens)?

Since most hand hygiene compliance auditing is undertaken during daytime care, how representative are these compliance levels of other periods (e.g., night shifts and weekends)? Furthermore, it is known that compliance may be higher during periods of observation (the so-called Hawthorne effect) than at other times, but the quantification of this difference is uncertain.[7] There are few data on these important issues. Levels of hand hygiene compliance vary substantially between HCW groups – especially between nurses and doctors.[8] Should we be surprised by this, given that personality profiling suggests these two groups are somewhat different? Thus, do we need education and promotional strategies that are better targeted to the various types of HCWs if we aim to improve compliance in all sectors? How educational efforts may need to be targeted to certain groups deserves further research (see Chapters 13 and 22).

While it is clear that the current HHA system of hand hygiene compliance auditing has major advantages in terms of data validity and HCW education, it remains time consuming. A key research question is whether new electronic approaches to monitoring compliance may reduce auditing time and improve efficiency, while maintaining the educational advantages of the current auditing system.

What level of auditing should be undertaken in non-acute facilities? While the NHHI is applicable to all healthcare facilities, and emphasis has been placed on larger acute inpatient sites, the quantity and frequency of auditing that should be undertaken in nonacute facilities remains unknown. This includes sites such as dental health, mental health, and primary care settings.

REFERENCES

1. Pittet D, Hugonnet S, Harbarth S, et al., Effectiveness of a hospital-wide programme to improve compliance with hand hygiene. *Lancet* 2000;**356**:1307–1312.
2. Johnson P, Martin R, Burrell LJ, et al., Efficacy of an alcohol/chlorhexidine hand hygiene program in a hospital with high rates of nosocomial methicillin-resistant Staphylococcus aureus (MRSA) infection. *Med J Aust* 2005;**183**:509–514.
3. Grayson ML, Jarvie LJ, Martin R, et al., Significant reductions in methicillin-resistant *Staphylococcus aureus* bacteraemia and clinical isolates associated with a multisite, hand hygiene culture-change program and subsequent successful statewide roll-out. *Med J Aust* 2008;**188**:633–640.
4. Sax H, Allegranzi B, Uçkay I, et al., 'My five moments for hand hygiene': a user-centred design approach to understand, train, monitor and report hand hygiene. *J Hosp Infect* 2007;**67**:9–21.

5. Russo PL, Heard Cruickshank M, Grayson ML, et al., The development of an online database and mobile web application for the collection and analysis of hand hygiene compliance data. International Conference on Prevention and Infection Control, Geneva, 2011.

6. Grayson ML, Russo PL, Cruickshank M, et al., Outcomes from the first 2 years of the Australian National Hand Hygiene Initiative. *Med J Aust* 2011;**195**:615–619.

7. Kwok YL, Juergens CP, McLaws ML, Automated hand hygiene auditing with and without intervention. *Am J Infect Control* 2016;**44**:1475–1480.

8. Grayson ML, Macesic N, Huang GK, et al., Use of an innovative personality-mindset profiling tool to guide culture-change strategies among different healthcare worker groups. *PLoS one* 2015;**10**:e0140509.

Chapter 37

Improving Hand Hygiene through Joint Commission Accreditation and the Joint Commission Center for Transforming Healthcare

Mark R. Chassin, Barbara I. Braun, and Anne Marie Benedicto

The Joint Commission, Oakbrook Terrace, USA

KEY MESSAGES

- As the largest accrediting body in the United States, the Joint Commission has had an important impact on improving hand hygiene in US hospitals and other settings through multiple methods and strategies.

- Healthcare workers and organizations need clear expectations for hand hygiene performance and structured and auditable measurement and improvement processes and tools to achieve and sustain high rates of adherence to hand hygiene guidelines.

- Reasons for noncompliance with hand hygiene guidelines vary across organizations, and solutions must be tailored to individual organizational needs.

Hand Hygiene: A Handbook for Medical Professionals, First Edition.
Edited by Didier Pittet, John M. Boyce and Benedetta Allegranzi.
© 2017 John Wiley & Sons, Inc. Published 2017 by John Wiley & Sons, Inc.

The Joint Commission is an independent, not-for-profit organization founded in 1951 and the oldest and largest healthcare accrediting body in the United States. It seeks to continuously improve healthcare for the public by evaluating healthcare organizations and inspiring them to excel in providing safe and effective care of the highest quality. The Joint Commission accredits or certifies more than 21,000 healthcare organizations and programs in the United States in settings such as hospitals, home care organizations, long-term care facilities, behavioral healthcare organizations, ambulatory care clinics, and clinical laboratories. Joint Commission International (JCI), its international arm, began evaluating organizations in 1999 and currently (May 2016) accredits or certifies 862 healthcare organizations or programs in 64 countries.

Two primary functions associated with accreditation are development of standards and on-site evaluation of compliance with these standards. Joint Commission standards are written with measurable expectations that affect the safety and quality of patient care. Standards address the organization's level of performance in key functional areas such as clinical care, treatment, and services; infection prevention and control; and medication management. Standards set expectations for an organization's performance, while also providing an avenue for assessing the organization's integration of the standards into routine operations.

To earn and maintain accreditation, organizations must undergo an on-site survey by a survey team at least every three years.

WHAT WE KNOW – THE EVIDENCE

Hand hygiene has been an important activity tied to Joint Commission infection prevention and control standards for many years. Most notably, in 2004 the Joint Commission established a National Patient Safety Goal (NPSG) on hand hygiene. NPSGs are high-profile accreditation requirements that address pressing areas of patient safety. The hand hygiene NPSG (07.01.01) requires organizations to comply with the current hand hygiene guidelines from the Centers for Disease Control and Prevention (CDC) or the World Health Organization (WHO). It also asks organizations to set goals for improving compliance with the guidelines and to implement improvements. NPSG 07.01.01 is assessed on site by observing care processes during which opportunities for hand hygiene arise for different types and levels of staff. Healthcare staff are interviewed to assess knowledge of hand hygiene guidelines, perceptions of compliance, and familiarity with organizational processes for improving hand hygiene. Patients and their families may also be interviewed to obtain their perceptions of staff hand hygiene processes.

When surveyors find that hand hygiene practice is not compliant with the standard, organizations are required to submit a correction plan, followed by quantitative evidence showing compliance improvements according to requirements. Initially, the Joint Commission scoring rules set the expected level for post-survey evidence of compliance at 90%. It soon became clear, however, that measurement strategies varied dramatically across healthcare organizations, which resulted in the Joint Commission not receiving reliable information regarding levels of compliance.

To assist hospitals and other healthcare organizations in both compliance with NPSG 07.01.01 and accomplishing meaningful change in hand hygiene practices, the Joint Commission Center for Transforming Healthcare (JCCTH, or "the Center") and eight leading hospitals and health systems came together to work on the problem. The eight participating organizations were located in the following states: California, Colorado, Maryland, Michigan, New Jersey, North Carolina, Texas, and Wisconsin. Using a consistent measurement system based on data collected by well-trained secret observers, aggregate baseline compliance was 47.5%, surprising many participants who had assumed their performance was much higher. Secret observers in Center participating hospitals collected data on the compliance of healthcare workers who were expected to perform hand hygiene upon room entry and exit. Adding to the concern was a published systematic review of 96 studies that reported an overall median compliance rate of 40%.[1] Consequently, revisions were made to the NPSG to focus on setting goals for improvement and achieving those goals, rather than being 90% compliant. The NPSG was revised as follows: "Comply with either the current CDC hand hygiene guidelines or the current WHO hand hygiene guidelines: 1) Implement a program that follows categories IA, IB, and IC of either the current CDC or WHO hand hygiene guidelines; 2) Set goals for improving compliance with hand hygiene guidelines; and 3) Improve compliance with hand hygiene guidelines based on established goals."[2] One lesson learned from this experience is that setting expected levels of performance is best done when standardized, reliable measurement systems exist that can be audited for accuracy.

Having clear expectations for performance – such as WHO guidelines and Joint Commission standards – is a necessary prerequisite for driving change. These expectations spell out what to do and when to do it. However, expectations by themselves do not provide specific guidance on how to improve performance. Translating knowledge into practice and changing behavior both at the individual and organizational level is difficult.[3] The Center was developed through recognition that an effective, systematic approach, together with robust tools and guidance, is needed to help healthcare organizations improve performance.

Interest is growing among healthcare organizations in the high reliability achieved by industries such as nuclear power and commercial aviation and in the tools and methods used by many companies to create processes that sustain high levels of performance.[4,5] These methods – Lean Six Sigma and change management – with their emphasis on data-driven problem solving, analytical tools that identify specific factors that contribute to performance failure, and recognition of the needs and strengths of the people who will implement and sustain the required changes, offer a systematic approach to dissecting complex safety problems and guiding organizations to deploy focused, highly effective solutions. These methods are collectively called Robust Process Improvement™ (RPI) at the Joint Commission.

RPI experts from the Center, along with RPI experts and clinical sponsors from the eight participating hospitals and health systems, used RPI tools to find the most significant causes of hand hygiene failure and to validate these statistically.[6] The teams found 41 different causes of inadequate hand hygiene, with each cause requiring a different intervention or solution. These causes did not occur with equal frequency. Typically, five or six causes were demonstrated to be responsible for the majority of failures at any one hospital. As shown in Table 37.1, the causes differed from hospital to hospital. Each hospital developed a set of interventions that were targeted specifically to its own main causes of hand hygiene failure. Since causes differed by hospital, effective solutions also differed by hospital. A set of solutions that would work for Hospital A, for example, would not necessarily be effective for Hospital H (see Table 37.1). This finding, which has since been validated in subsequent Center projects, has led us to seriously question the viability of typical "best practice" approaches that presuppose one solution or bundle for every problem, without considering varying local circumstances and settings.

After implementing their site-specific solutions, the eight hospitals reported an aggregate hand hygiene rate of 81%, which they sustained for the remaining 11 months of the project.[6] Solutions and methods used were validated in 19 pilot sites and then incorporated into the Targeted Solutions Tool™ (TST).[7] The TST is a web-based application that guides healthcare organizations through a step-by-step process to accurately measure their organization's actual performance and identify the factors that contribute to performance failure. It then directs them to proven solutions customized to address their particular causes of failure. The TST is the primary means of widely sharing the hand hygiene solutions and measurement system developed by the Center and is available to the healthcare organizations the Joint Commission accredits or certifies.

In the five years and eight months since the launch of the TST in September 2010, organizations have entered 3.4 million observations of hand hygiene compliance into the TST. The TST data demonstrate that through accurately measuring compliance, determining the specific factors that contribute to noncompliance, and implementing solutions targeted to address those factors, healthcare organizations are significantly improving their hand hygiene compliance rates throughout the United States. On average, organizations using the TST have improved 44% over their baseline measurements and are sustaining those results. A detailed analysis of the first three full years of TST implementation demonstrated these findings.[8] Across the United States, compliance with NPSG 07.01.01 has improved substantially. In addition, the TST has also been used in an international pilot study within nine hospitals in eight countries, in which rates of improvement similar to those of US TST users were demonstrated.[9] Figure 37.1 shows the baseline and improved rates of hand hygiene compliance in each of these three groups of hospitals.

Table 37.1 Main Causes of Failure to Clean Hands and Potential Solutions Identified by Hospitals Participating in the Center for Transforming Healthcare Hand Hygiene Initiative

| Main Causes | Participating Hospitals | | | | | | | | Solutions |
	A	B	C	D	E	F	G	H	
Ineffective placement of dispensers or sinks		x		x	x		x	x	Provide easy access to hand hygiene equipment and dispensers
Hand hygiene compliance data are not collected or reported accurately or frequently	x	x		x	x			x	Provide data collected locally as a framework for a systematic approach for improvement
									Utilize a sound measurement system to determine the real score in real time
									Scrutinize and question the data
									Measure the specific, high-impact causes of hand hygiene failures in your facility and target solutions to those causes

(*continued*)

Table 37.1 (*Continued*)

Main Causes	Participating Hospitals								Solutions
	A	B	C	D	E	F	G	H	
Lack of accountability and just-in-time coaching		X	X	X	X		X	X	Engage leadership to commit to hand hygiene as an organizational priority and to demonstrate support by role modeling consistent with hand hygiene compliance
									Train leaders as just-in-time coaches to reinforce compliance
									Through just-in-time coaches, intervene to remind healthcare personnel to clean their hands
									Implement employee contracts to be signed by all healthcare personnel to reinforce their commitment to hand hygiene
									Apply progressive disciplinary action against repeat offenders. Expectations should be applied equally to all healthcare personnel
Safety culture does not stress hand hygiene at all levels			X	X	X	X		X	Make hand hygiene a habit – as automatic as looking both ways when you cross the street or fastening your seat belt when you get in your car
									Commitment of leadership to achieve hand hygiene compliance of 90+ percent
									Serve as a role model by practicing proper hand hygiene
									Hold everyone accountable and responsible – doctors, nurses, food service staff, housekeepers, chaplains, technicians, therapists

Barrier					Strategy
Ineffective or insufficient education		x	x	x	x	Provide general education on hand hygiene expectations. Include information on infection prevention, and stress the organization-wide commitment to hand hygiene
						highlighting strategies deployed to reinforce compliance such as posters and visual cues. Some organizations make this part of annual training provided to new and existing employees
						Provide discipline-specific education that puts hand hygiene within the context of an employee's daily work and processes
						Reinforce education with just-in-time coaching
Hands full	x	x	x	x	x	Create a place for everything: for example, a HCW with full hands needs a dedicated space where he or she can place items while performing hand hygiene
Wearing gloves interferes with process	x	x	x	x	x	Locate glove dispensers near handrub dispensers and sinks to facilitate the proper use of gloves
						Provide training on glove use that incorporates hand cleansing and glove use within a specific work flow. Use visual cues to reinforce and remind

(continued)

Table 37.1 (Continued)

Main Causes	Participating Hospitals								Solutions
	A	B	C	D	E	F	G	H	
Perception that hand hygiene is not needed if wearing gloves	x		x	x	x		x	x	Provide discipline-specific education that puts hand hygiene within the context of an employee's daily work and processes Standardize the work processes that involve entry into a patient's room, and specify when and why hand hygiene is required. For instance, standard processes for food tray delivery and room cleanings Provide discipline-specific education and training on glove use
Healthcare workers forget or distractions	x	x		x			x		Identify a code word to be used among HCWs to signal to a peer that they missed an opportunity and need to clean hands Identify new technologies to make it easy for HCWs to remember to clean their hands, such as RFID, automatic reminders, and warning systems Train and deploy just-in-time coaches to provide real-time reinforcement and feedback to HCWs. Just-in-time coaches are critical in creating a change in culture and behavior Use visual cues to reinforce hand hygiene messages and training. These include stickers, colors, and posters. Visual cues need to be changed periodically so that they continue to be effective Apply progressive disciplinary action against repeat offenders. Expectations should be applied equally to all HCWs

Note: An "x" means that the cause was found to be statistically significantly related to hand hygiene noncompliance (a "main cause") by the participating hospital. HCW, healthcare worker

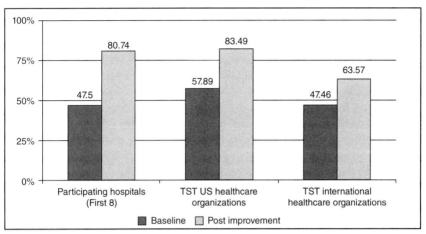

Figure 37.1   Overall hand hygiene compliance: US and international hospitals participating in Center for Transforming Healthcare Hand Hygiene initiatives[1,2] (data as of September 2013). [1]The eight participating organizations included Cedars-Sinai Health System, California; Exempla Lutheran Medical Center, Colorado; Froedtert Hospital, Wisconsin; The Johns Hopkins Hospital and Health System, Maryland; Memorial Hermann Health Care System, Texas; Trinity Health, Michigan; Virtua, New Jersey; and Wake Forest Baptist Health, North Carolina. The nine international hospitals who used the TST are the Medical City in Pasig City, Philippines; Institute Jantung Negara in Kuala Lumpur, Malaysia; Premier Jatinegara Hospital, Jakarta, Indonesia; Azienda Ospedaliero Universitaria (S Maria della Misericordia) di Udine, Udine, Italy; UZ Leuven, Leuven, Belgium; National Center for Cancer Care & Research, Doha, Qatar; King Faisal Specialist Hospital & Research Centre, Jeddah, Saudi Arabia; King Faisal Specialist Hospital & Research Centre, Riyadh, Saudi Arabia; and Sheikh Khalifa Medical City, Abu Dhabi, UAE. [2]Percents shown are averaged over number of units from which data were collected. Each hospital contained one or more units. First eight Participating Hospitals: 95% confidence intervals cannot be calculated because some hospitals submitted rates rather than numerator and denominator data. TST US Health Care Organizations (1) Baseline: lower and upper 95% confidence intervals for average percent = 57.89 are 57.66 and 58.12, respectively, (2) Post Improvement: lower and upper 95% confidence intervals for average percent = 83.49 are 83.39 and 83.60, respectively. TST International Health Care Organizations (1) Baseline: lower and upper 95% confidence intervals for average percent = 47.46 are 46.59 and 48.33, respectively, (2) Post Improvement: lower and upper 95% confidence intervals for average percent = 63.57 are 62.71 and 64.42, respectively.

One hospital system (Memorial Hermann Health System, Houston, TX) thoroughly reported and analyzed its deployment of the TST in all 150 inpatient units in all 12 of its hospitals.[10] Average hand hygiene compliance across all 12 hospitals improved from 58% to 96% and was sustained for two years. Concomitantly, central-line-associated bloodstream infections in all their adult intensive care units (ICUs) fell by 49% (to 0.42 per 1000 line-days), and ventilator associated pneumonia rates in the same ICUs fell by 45% (to 0.57 per 1000 ventilator-days).

At baseline, the rates of both of these infections were well below prevailing national averages.

There are three key findings from the Joint Commission's experience and from US hospitals participating in the Center's hand hygiene project. The first is that without a consistent and rigorous measurement system, healthcare organizations are likely to be overestimating their hand hygiene performance. The second lesson is that hand hygiene compliance is a complex, organization-wide activity, and simple slogans or campaigns are not enough to achieve and sustain high levels of performance. Similarly, demanding that healthcare workers try harder is not the answer. The third lesson is that a one-size-fits-all improvement method, based on the prevailing model of adopting known best practices, is not likely to be as effective as the targeted approach described here.

WHAT WE DO NOT KNOW – THE UNCERTAIN

As stated by Ovretveit, "In quality improvement, nothing ever happens for one reason or cause."[11] The Joint Commission has had an important role in driving improvements in hand hygiene, and it is one driver among many others including initiatives such as the WHO *Clean Care is Safer Care* campaign,[12] changes in technology for product delivery and hand hygiene monitoring, and myriad secular influences over time that have helped improve compliance.

Despite significant advances for hospitals in hand hygiene measurement and improvement methods, many other healthcare settings continue to struggle with standardized approaches for measuring and improving adherence to guidelines. For example, home care and ambulatory care settings are particularly challenging since there is often no third party to observe healthcare workers' use of hand hygiene products during patient encounters. Staff in nursing homes and inpatient behavioral health settings frequently have to contend with inconvenient product availability due to the potential for inappropriate use of hand hygiene products by residents and patients. Due to faulty measurement systems, many healthcare organizations have a false sense of their hand hygiene performance and are not aware of their opportunities for improvement.

The Center participating hospitals practiced "wash in/wash out," which directs healthcare workers to clean their hands upon entry and exit from a patient's room. This allows secret observers to observe two surrogates of the five WHO moments (i.e presumably Moment 1 and Moment 4, or Moment 5, see Chapter 20) – hand hygiene before and after patient contact – while still retaining their anonymity. The use of secret observers and "wash in/wash out" is part of the methodology recommended by the Center's Targeted Solutions Tool (TST). Therefore, all of the healthcare organizations in the United States and internationally that are using the TST are also using this methodology. Secret observers are not able to observe how hand hygiene is practiced in a patient's room and cannot reliably assess compliance with the five moments of the WHO, and in particular cannot assess three of the five WHO moments (i.e. Moment 2, Moment 3, and presumably Moment 4 or 5, see Chapter 20). We recognize that the methodology used by the Center would need further validation, in particular towards the most widely used WHO five moments.

RESEARCH AGENDA

Further research is needed to address the following questions:

- Given limited resources, which indications are essential to assess when measuring hand hygiene compliance? To what extent does measuring compliance with hand hygiene upon room entry and exit serve as an acceptable proxy for measurement of the WHO Five Moments?
- What are the best methods for measuring and improving hand hygiene adherence to guidelines in non-hospital settings such as home care, ambulatory care, nursing homes, and long-term care?
- What is the preferred data collection and measurement strategy for hospitals that can be widely adopted and used to make valid comparisons across organizations?
- How can one best evaluate the relative impact of external policy-level interventions on hand hygiene practice across settings?
- In the absence of standardized measurement approaches across healthcare organizations, how should external evaluators such as accrediting bodies and government regulators best evaluate hand hygiene adherence when on site?

REFERENCES

1. Erasmus V, Daha TJ, Brug H, et al., Systematic review of studies on compliance with hand hygiene guidelines in hospital care. *Infect Control Hosp Epidemiol* 2010;**31**: 283–294.
2. Joint Commission, *Comprehensive Accreditation Manual for Hospitals 2012*. Oakbrook Terrace, IL.
3. Grimshaw JM, Eccles MP, Hill SJ, et al., Knowledge translation of research findings. *Implementation Sci* 2012;**7**:50.
4. Chassin MR, Loeb JM, The ongoing quality improvement journey: next stop, high reliability. *Health Aff (Millwood)* 2011;**30**:559–568.
5. Chassin MR, Loeb JM, High-reliability healthcare: getting there from here. *Milbank Q* 2013;**91**:459–490.
6. Chassin MR, Mayer C, Nether K, Improving hand hygiene at eight hospitals in the United States by targeting specific causes of noncompliance. *Jt Comm J Qual Patient Saf* 2015;**41**:4–12.
7. Joint Commission Center for Transforming Healthcare, Hand hygiene project. Available at www.centerfortransforminghealthcare.org/projects/detail.aspx?Project=3. Accessed March 7, 2017.

8. Chassin MR, Nether K, Mayer C, et al., Beyond the collaborative: spreading effective improvement in hand hygiene compliance. *Jt Comm J Qual Patient Saf* 2015;**41**:13–25.

9. Grand-Clement S, Karam Z, Using robust process improvement to transform hand hygiene culture. APIC 2013 Annual conference poster presentation, June 9, 2013, Fort Lauderdale, FL.

10. Shabot MM, Chassin MR, France A-C, et al., Using the targeted solutions tool® to improve hand hygiene compliance is associated with decreased health care-associated infections. *Jt Comm J Qual Patient Saf* 2016;**42**:6–17.

11. Ovretveit J, Understanding the conditions for improvement: research to discover which context influences affect improvement success. *BMJ Qual Saf* 2011;**20**(Suppl. 1):i18ei23. doi:10.1136/bmjqs.2010.045955.

12. World Health Organization, "Clean Care is Safer Care." Available at www.who.int/gpsc/en/. Accessed March 7, 2017.

Chapter 38

A Worldwide WHO Hand Hygiene in Healthcare Campaign

Claire Kilpatrick,[1] Julie Storr,[1] and Benedetta Allegranzi[2]

[1] *Infection Prevention and Control Global Unit, Department of Service Delivery and Safety, World Health Organization, Geneva, Switzerland*

[2] *Infection Prevention and Control Global Unit, Department of Service Delivery and Safety, World Health Organization, and Faculty of Medicine, University of Geneva, Geneva, Switzerland*

KEY MESSAGES

- A World Health Organization global hand hygiene campaign can reach healthcare settings in all corners of the globe.
- The global approach taken to ensure global engagement can be simple and on the whole virtual in nature, while it clearly requires a dedicated campaign focus, time, planning, and centralized and local commitment, leadership and resources, as well as the availability of tools that promote action.
- Impact can in part be measured through "sign-up" to a campaign, campaign website access and downloads alongside social media reach, and examples of local action; while a clear target and denominator for demonstrating campaign success should be employed.

A health campaign is described as being an effort to persuade a defined public group to engage in activities or behaviors that will improve health or to refrain from unhealthy or harmful behaviors.

A campaign must have strong branding and focus to succeed. Varying messages and activities is essential to engaging target groups, and campaigns must plan to sustain engagement year on year.

The World Health Organization (WHO) *SAVE LIVES: Clean Your Hands* campaign was launched in 2009. This global, annual campaign was conceived as an

Hand Hygiene: A Handbook for Medical Professionals, First Edition.
Edited by Didier Pittet, John M. Boyce and Benedetta Allegranzi.
© 2017 John Wiley & Sons, Inc. Published 2017 by John Wiley & Sons, Inc.

extension of the WHO *Clean Care is Safer Care* program launched in 2005, aimed at ensuring patient safety through infection prevention, with a focus on sustaining hand hygiene improvement and making the topic a priority on national agendas. The campaign is targeted at healthcare facilities and has the overall aim of "*Bringing people together to improve and sustain hand hygiene action*" every fifth of May – the annual day for highlighting the necessity for cleaning hands in healthcare, which is a life-saving action.

The *SAVE LIVES: Clean Your Hands* campaign has the following characteristics:

- A foundation in science and evidence, aiming to inform effective activism and communications;

- Is centered on engagement through coalition building and crowdsourcing, with technical experts driving the development of resources to mobilize the target audience to improve patient outcomes;

- Reflects on its global impact, learning from campaign experiences and adjusts annual strategies.

To protect and effectively care for patients, it takes leadership, commitment, resources, and focused, timely actions. *SAVE LIVES: Clean Your Hands* provides global leadership on the importance of clean hands at the point of patient care. Resources translated from English into other official WHO languages (Arabic, Chinese, French, Russian, Spanish) support action. In 2009, the dedicated team within WHO initiated the campaign.

On May 5, 2009, WHO published the *WHO Guidelines on Hand Hygiene in Health Care* (draft version, 2006)[1] alongside an implementation toolkit, a range of *SAVE LIVES: Clean Your Hands* advocacy resources including dedicated WHO web pages with a campaign brand. The campaign also enabled global sharing of information about local and national campaign activities.

As of June 2016, more than 19,000 healthcare facilities from 177 countries had registered their commitment to the campaign, in part supported by WHO's engagement of more than 140 Ministries of Health who signed a pledge to tackle healthcare-associated infection (HAI). More than 50 national/subnational hand hygiene campaigns had been formed.

WHAT WE KNOW – THE EVIDENCE

Addressing the Global Problem

Published data collated by WHO highlight the importance of a global approach to controlling HAI.[2] This global campaign demonstrates WHO's acknowledgement of hand hygiene as a patient safety priority, key to reducing HAI and combating antimicrobial resistance.

Through national commitment and the *SAVE LIVES: Clean Your Hands* campaign's healthcare facility registrations, an approach of engaging a target audience through sign-up to an official, mandated campaign can instigate global patient safety action. This forms part of what is termed a "social movement." Similarity exists with the Stop TB campaign, which has recognized the importance of international "sign-up" from both developed and developing countries.[3] Another characteristic common to international campaigns is the use of an annual day or event to focus attention and activities on the health issue in question, such as WHO's World Health Day.

Promoting Local Action

The use of improvement resources to stimulate action is key. Since the launch of the campaign, WHO web-based resources are actively promoted for use and adaptation through monthly e-newsletters to all registered facilities and key organizations/others. For developing countries, postal mailing of resources has at times been required to ensure true global engagement.

The concept of cascade messaging to promote local action is at the heart of WHO activities. Media such as WHO Twitter and Facebook accounts and virtual presentation software and podcasts are therefore also part of the campaign. Ultimately, communication is key in campaigning.

Campaign Progress and Actions to Prevent Campaign Fatigue

Healthcare campaigns must have a solid basis in science, a brand, and focus, while messages and activities must vary from year to year to sustain engagement. *SAVE LIVES: Clean Your Hands* has issued a call to action for healthcare facilities each year since its launch. The initial focus was on "sign-up" and a preliminary target of 5,000 health facilities committing to the campaign was made and achieved. In subsequent years, more extensive targets were made, and achieved (10,000 in 2010). Engagement of healthcare facilities in all countries is challenging, and more recently the campaign focus has shifted to areas of the world where uptake has been the lowest. On analyzing the gaps remaining in *SAVE LIVES: Clean Your Hands* campaign registrations, it has been clear that those countries yet to have a facility sign-up are smaller, poorer, often involved in conflict, or more isolated.

To build on the ethos of WHO *Clean Care is Safer Care* and to maintain engagement, two new tools were issued in 2010 to help healthcare facilities move from "demonstrating commitment to taking action." The first was a targeted hand hygiene monitoring tool culminating in a WHO global survey of hand hygiene "Before touching a patient"[4] – the first global survey of its kind. By September 2010 WHO issued a report, allowing for greater understanding of global hand hygiene compliance. A total of 327 healthcare settings from 47 countries submitted results.[5] The innovative WHO Hand Hygiene Self-Assessment Framework (HHSAF) was also launched (see Chapter 34).

The campaign evolved further, and in 2011 WHO invited healthcare facilities around the world to track their progress and submit their HHSAF results online. Global survey results, issued in 2012,[6] provided learning and the opportunity to adjust campaign strategies going forward, with over 2,000 healthcare facilities from 69 countries sharing results.

In 2012, the call to action was "create your action plan, based on your facility's results from the WHO HHSAF with WHO providing example template action plans." In response to requests received, the new WHO Hand Hygiene in Outpatient and Home-based Care and Long-term Care Facilities document aimed at engaging a wider community was also launched.

In 2013, the campaign focus was hand hygiene monitoring and feedback. Additionally, "Tips for Implementing a Successful Patient Participation Program" and "Tips for Patients to Participate in Hand Hygiene Improvement" documents were launched to guide facilities in their progress toward achieving the HHSAF criteria. A survey was again conducted to understand patient participation in facilities around the globe with 260 respondents from 46 countries covering all six WHO regions.

Five years into the campaign, in 2014, hand hygiene was positioned within the context of other HAI issues. To align with the global focus on antimicrobial resistance the theme was "are you ready to prevent the spread of antimicrobial resistant germs?" and a literature review on multidrug-resistant organisms and the relationship with hand hygiene, alongside a number of posters and a screensaver were issued. The call to action also asked for participation in global surveys on multidrug-resistant organisms in healthcare and the use of surgical antibiotic prophylaxis, and "WHO Information for Patients and Consumers on Hand Hygiene and Antimicrobial Resistance" was launched.

In 2015 and 2016, hand hygiene continued to be positioned within the context of other issues including safe surgery, and the HHSAF global survey was repeated. Profile raising was refreshed through the use of social media given its growing position in the field of healthcare information provision. WHO statistics have recognized that *SAVE LIVES: Clean Your Hands* social media reach is on par if not better than other messages issued in support of WHO campaigns.

Outside of May 5 activities, a range of communications are issued to promote sign-up and engagement, including promotion of related scientific publications and through announcing new supporting coalitions. For example, the launch of Private Organizations for Patient Safety (POPS) in 2012; a "social responsibility"-focused collaboration with industry. Prevention of campaign fatigue is a constant feature, as well as aiming to further contribute to the science base for hand hygiene.

Understanding the Impact of the Campaign

Data on a number of process indicators were evaluated for the period December 5, 2008, to May 31, 2010. Information on campaign registrations, website hits and downloads, and healthcare facility activity sharing was collated. Taking web page views as a marker of success has been used by other campaigns. The approach allows campaigns to identify the characteristics, including geographical, of those seeking information as well as confirming that a website is an important tool in campaigning. The impact of e-mail as a strategy in campaign engagement has also been examined including the viral effect this can have; that is, for *SAVE LIVES: Clean Your Hands* facilities hearing about the campaign from colleagues receiving the monthly e-mail newsletter. In addition to the analyses presented, informal reviews and reflections have continued at WHO, to better understand what works and what doesn't in engaging the target audience year after year.

- Campaign registrations:
  - The majority of registrations are achieved in the immediate months leading up to May 5. A gentler registration curve could mean better overall engagement throughout the year, but does not cause the same buzz. Three countries achieved thousands of registrations during the period studied; the United States, France, and the Philippines. It is known that individual commitment and a top-down mandate contributed to success in these countries, albeit the individuals and mandates driving the success were different. In 2014, the WHO Eastern Mediterranean Region was announced as the first to have a healthcare facility signed up in every country.
  - At the end of July 2010, there were 57 Member States with no registered healthcare facilities. However, from these 57, 14 e-enquiries had been received, access to the webpages had occurred, demonstrating some connection with the campaign, with 28 (49%) of the 57 already having signed the WHO pledge to address HAI.
  - In 2010, those registered were asked how they heard about *SAVE LIVES: Clean Your Hands*, with a 30% response rate. The categories can be seen in Figure 38.1.
- Website hits and downloads:
  - WHO hand hygiene tools are frequently accessed and downloaded (see Figure 38.2) and although not yet fully analyzed, could have contributed to campaign success. Besides any publications or scientific presentations that may mention them, this has been the only way WHO has actively promoted the tools.
- Healthcare facility activities shared with WHO:
  - In 2010, it was noted that the volume of information being received, including photographs and videos, could not be hosted by WHO web pages. Web pages were therefore arranged to feature links to organizations and facilities that featured their own May 5 information and a link back to WHO, providing bidirectional promotion. Year after year, it has been evident that a number of organizations feature May 5 information.

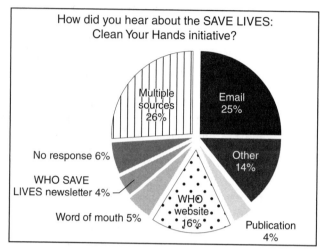

Figure 38.1 Categories associated with how campaign registered healthcare facilities hear about *SAVE LIVES: Clean Your Hands* – 2010. *See plate section for color representation of this figure.*

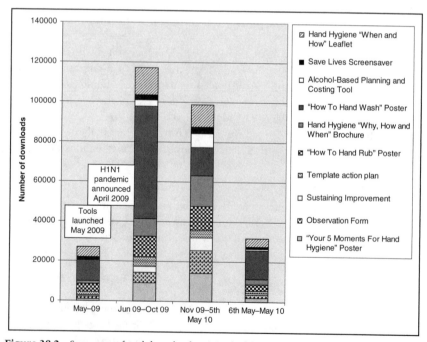

Figure 38.2 Summary of tool download activity for 2009 and 2010 and key events that may have influenced these. *See plate section for color representation of this figure.*

However, the fact that not all facilities are able to have dedicated hand hygiene messaging or web pages limits campaign information sharing, which could be a motivating factor in campaign sustainability.

The WHO resources required to support such a campaign are not covered in this chapter. However, the campaign demonstrates that a small central global resource can stimulate significant global action. Furthermore, the WHO Collaborating Centre on Patient Safety at the University of Geneva Hospitals and Faculty of Medicine (Switzerland), led by Professor Didier Pittet, has been designated to provide continuous technical and motivational support to the campaign.

All information on the campaign can be found at www.who.int/gpsc/5may/en.

WHAT WE DO NOT KNOW – THE UNCERTAIN

What is the Best Way to Evaluate Such a Global Healthcare Campaign?

One challenge faced by WHO is the lack of an accurate estimate of the number of healthcare facilities worldwide, which is necessary to calculate the percent of facilities that have signed up to the campaign. Therefore, being able to use a strong measurable campaign target, similar to that of other campaigns, has not been possible. Awareness of local activities gives some indication of success as well as those arbitrary process indicators described. Hand hygiene publications and awareness of the WHO Five Moments may also be indicators; however, this information is collected opportunistically rather than systematically. Further, being able to judge how far all healthcare facilities have progressed in improving hand hygiene compliance and reducing HAI due to WHO activities is still elusive, while reports on completion of the HHSAF allow for some global understanding (see also Chapter 34). Dissemination of campaign messages to and then within healthcare facilities – the viral effect – contributes to influencing success and has been considered as a vital ingredient for campaigning.[8] This has been observed in part through social media messaging.

While the campaign approach mirrors that of other global campaigns, including Stop TB (Stop TB's model is one of advocacy, communication, and social mobilization – ACSM),[7] it is different from the majority in that it is primarily aimed at HCWs, not the general public. There are and have been a number of national and international campaigns that in some way seek to improve health outcomes, and consideration was given to these when addressing the model for this campaign. How applicable ACSM is for solely a healthcare audience has not been fully evaluated. Another key difference between *SAVE LIVES: Clean Your*

Hands and other campaigns is that many focus on a single health outcome or disease such as TB or polio, which is clearly measurable.

Given the scale of a global campaign, developing collaborations is important. Formalizing relations with key organizations and groups, like the one that has been established with POPS, may enhance its impact and potential for evaluation going forward. Targeting the general public – the consumers of healthcare – in an attempt to capitalize on the power they might have in promoting hand hygiene action in healthcare facilities is yet to be fully explored, although this work has started. Country examples do exist, including the *Germs: wash your hands of them* campaign run by NHS Scotland, which evaluated the changing behaviors of HCWs and the public, and also campaigns targeted at a reduction in antibiotic use.[9]

Can the *SAVE LIVES: Clean Your Hands* Campaign be Considered as a Social Movement Going Forward?

Social movements, and especially health social movements, are not a new phenomenon, and there is a significant body of literature that explains them, including in relation to HIV/AIDS. Some authors have suggested that organizations with a responsibility for initiating and sustaining change in healthcare, such as WHO, could or should seek to create or nurture such movements to assist them in achieving their goals.[8,10,11] Social movements are often described as networks of activists with a common purpose, or at least interest. Although they are often groups of non experts or lay people, professionals and experts can and do get involved and even provide leadership at times. The campaign could be viewed as the latter kind of social movement, similar in some ways to the European Healthy Cities project.[10]

RESEARCH AGENDA

There are still a number of unknowns based on the complexities of global campaigning on such a healthcare topic (Table 38.1).

Proposed research topics are as follows:

- What is the optimum approach and outcome measure for a global healthcare campaign focused on hand hygiene?
- Can hand hygiene compliance and HAI rates be made available reliably and regularly for every healthcare facility in every country, with the aim of driving continuous improvement on a global scale?
- Could consumers/the public drive healthcare improvement if engaged in global campaigning?
- Can healthcare-related organizations around the globe maintain the activities and success of a global WHO campaign?

Table 38.1   The Research Agenda – What is Missing to Ensure a Successful Global Campaign?

What is Missing	The Question Now	Why Needed
Securing reliable data in every country	How could hand hygiene compliance and HAI rates be made available for every healthcare facility in every country?	To further demonstrate the need for and the impact and importance of campaigning on such a topic – every campaign needs data on the problem, facts and figures to drive action
Learning from consumers	How could consumers/the public further drive and keep alive *SAVE LIVES: Clean Your Hands*?	To allow for broadening of campaign coalitions and to understand the power of the public voice in improving hand hygiene
Currency of campaign healthcare collaborations	How effectively can healthcare-related organizations around the globe be activists for *SAVE LIVES: Clean Your Hands*?	To address sustainability and further reach of the campaign, through formally capitalizing on the expertise and activities of professionals working outside of WHO
Understand how campaign evaluation can be undertaken	What is the most appropriate, measurable target for a campaign such as *SAVE LIVES: Clean Your Hands*, which is shaped around a process undertaken by healthcare professionals?	To be able to demonstrate success and seriously engage the pubic and professionals in the campaign's aim year on year
Harnessing the energy created through the first five years of *SAVE LIVES: Clean Your Hands* and the beginnings of a social movement	What is the best approach for a campaign like *SAVE LIVES: Clean Your Hands* in sustaining engagement and ensuring a true global social movement?	To further inform the evidence base around healthcare campaigning and raise the profile of this global hand hygiene in healthcare campaign

REFERENCES

1. World Health Organization, *WHO Guidelines on Hand Hygiene in Health Care*. Geneva: WHO, 2009.
2. Allegranzi B, Bagheri Nejad S, Combescure C, et al., Burden of endemic health-care-associated infection in developing countries: systematic review and meta-analysis. *Lancet* 2011;**377**:228–241.
3. Fanning A, Billo N, Tannenbaum T, et al., Stop TB – Halte à la Tuberculose – Canada: engaging industrialised nations in the challenge to meet global targets. *J Tuberc Lung Dis* 2004;**8**:147–150.

4. Sax H, Allegranzi B, Uçkay I, et al., "My five moments for hand hygiene": a user-centered design approach to understand, train, monitor and report hand hygiene. *J Hosp Infect* 2007;**67**:9–21.

5. World Health Organisation, *WHO Hand Hygiene Moment 1 – Global Observation Survey Summary Report*. Geneva: WHO, 2010.

6. World Health Organization, *WHO Hand Hygiene Self-Assessment Framework Global Survey Summary Report*. Geneva: WHO, 2012.

7. World Health Organization, *WHO Advocacy, Communication and Social Mobilisation: A Handbook for Country Programmes*. Geneva: WHO, 2007.

8. Bate P, Robert G, Bevan H, The next phase of healthcare improvement: what can we learn from social movements? *Qual Saf Health Care* 2004;**13**:62–66.

9. Huttner B, Goossens H, Verheij T, et al., Characteristics and outcomes of public campaigns aimed at improving the use of antibiotics in outpatients in high-income countries. *Lancet Infect Dis* 2010;**10**:17–31.

10. De Leeuw E, Evidence for Healthy Cities: reflections on practice, method and theory. *Health Promot Int* 2009;**24**(Suppl 1):i19–i36.

11. Marmot M, Allen J, Goldblatt P, A social movement, based on evidence, to reduce inequalities in health. *Soc Sci Med* 2010;**71**:1254–1258.

Chapter 39

The Economic Impact of Improved Hand Hygiene

Nicholas Graves

School of Public Health and Institute of Health and Biomedical Innovation, Queensland University of Technology, Brisbane, Australia

KEY MESSAGES

- Cost increases, cost savings, and health benefits of programs to improve hand hygiene compliance should be quantified using the best data and methods available.
- The current evidence about the economics of these programs is uncertain, and it would be sensible to do a high-quality and critical review of the evidence for cost-effectiveness.
- It is possible that when risk of infection is low the extra cost per unit of health benefit gained from further hand hygiene improvement is prohibitive. Of course, it goes both ways, and for settings where baseline infection risks are high, then improving hand hygiene could be excellent value for money.

Programs to improve hand hygiene compliance have three major economic impacts. First is that implementing them uses up people's time and other valuable resources, making them costly to implement. Second is that resources and costs are saved because cases of healthcare-associated infection (HAI) are prevented. Third is that some patients avoid morbidity and higher risks of mortality, meaning there are health benefits. It is important to measure and value these impacts using the best data and methods available. The findings should be presented to decision makers in a form they understand if an economic case for improving hand hygiene compliance is to be made.

Hand Hygiene: A Handbook for Medical Professionals, First Edition.
Edited by Didier Pittet, John M. Boyce and Benedetta Allegranzi.
© 2017 John Wiley & Sons, Inc. Published 2017 by John Wiley & Sons, Inc.

Methods for estimating the cost of infection control programs are presented by Page et al.[1] Ways to accurately identify and then value, in monetary terms, the human and capital inputs of a program are described. They emphasize that considerations of cost should focus not only on accurate data, but also on the quantification of uncertainty in the estimate. Good survey design is stressed, and the reader is reminded that measuring the costs of a program is an essential first step if the cost-effectiveness and economic value of that program are to be understood.

Cost savings from a program will arise from fewer cases of HAI. Resources that would have been used up are hospital bed-days and those required for treatment and making diagnoses. The majority of the cost of an infection is the number of extra-days' stay in hospital for treatment. There are many estimates published in the literature, but most of them are biased upward. Reliable estimates arise from statistical methods that account for the timing of the onset of HAI; for this, state-based models are typically used. The key authors are Jan Beyersmann, Martin Wolkewitz, and Adrian Barnett. Estimates of the extra-hospital-days' stay arising from matching studies or linear regressions that ignore the timing of the important events will mislead decision makers; even worse are unadjusted comparisons of infected versus uninfected patients' lengths of stay. Assigning a monetary value to the bed-days saved is another challenge, and simply applying hospital accounting costs will overstate the real cost.[2] Much better is a contingent valuation approach that elicits decision makers' willingness to pay for bed-days released by an infection prevention and control (IPC) program. This economic valuation of marginal bed-days is superior to an accounting cost estimate that shows nothing more than a summary of the money already spent; importantly, this money cannot be recovered for another use. Stewardson et al.[3] used a contingent valuation method to value bed-days and found it much lower than the accounting value of bed-days released.

The health benefits of a program arise from improving both the quantity and quality of life of patients protected from HAI. The quality-adjusted-life year (QALY) includes both dimensions. The number of QALYs gained from preventing infections in a cohort of patients relies on the effectiveness of the program, the mortality risk given that a patient becomes infected, and the preference-based valuation of the health states they occupy while suffering HAI. Because the duration of morbidity is usually short, the differences between QALYs gained and life-years gained (LYG) is often minuscule, making LYG a reasonable alternate outcome measure for cost-effectiveness studies.

Beware using measures other than LYG or QALYs gained. Despite the concept of disability-adjusted life years rapidly gaining popularity in health policy, their usefulness as measures of a "gross domestic product of health" or a metric to help in "setting priorities in health policy" has been questioned.[4] Anand and Hansen[5] suggest the conceptual and technical basis for disability-adjusted life years (DALYs) is flawed. Intermediate outcome measures such as the number of infections prevented or improved rates of hand hygiene events will only demonstrate how to maximize the specific outcome for a given infection prevention budget. These items tell us nothing about the value of IPC as a service, when held against other health services that demand scarce resources.

The outcome of a cost-effectiveness analysis is an estimate of the monetary cost of gaining one LYG or QALY. This information can be elicited for the whole range of competing healthcare services. Priorities can then be set based on preferring services that deliver cheaper LYG/QALYs and deprioritizing services that deliver LYG/QALYs at greater cost. The constraint is that the budget for healthcare is fixed and society should aim to get as many health benefits as possible from a fixed budget. It will be impossible to continually relax this constraint and spend more and more each year on health services. The time when increases in health spending find a plateau is near, and then the policy relevance of cost-effectiveness work will grow.

In order to investigate the cost-effectiveness of a hand hygiene promotion program, the population it will impact must be defined. The cost savings from the program should be deducted from the cost increases to give a change to total cost, and the health benefits from preventing infections should be expressed by either LYG or QALYs gained. Dividing the "change to costs" by the "change health benefits" reveals the "cost per life year gained" or "cost per QALY gained" from a program to improve hand hygiene compliance. This statistic allows comparison with competing healthcare programs. Some made-up data that show a comparison are presented in Table 39.1. Remember we are trying to get the maximum number of health benefits from a fixed budget. A simple calculation of €100,000 divided by 15 shows the cost per life year gained is €6,250 if the hand hygiene program is chosen. Repeating this calculation shows that the estimate is €9,000 if the two extra nurses were chosen and €16,000 if the magnetic resonance imaging scanner were chosen. Rational and risk-neutral decision makers who aim to maximize health benefits from a fixed health budget should first choose hand hygiene, not because it is the cheapest, but because it offers the greatest health return per €1 invested.

The data from Table 39.1 are illustrated in graph form in Figure 39.1 to show that all programs increase costs and increase health benefits relative to the starting position. You can draw straight lines from the origin of the two axes labeled "Start Position," and each of the three competing programs to confirm the hand hygiene program is the best value for money. If extra health benefits are sought above

Table 39.1   The Value for Money of Three Programs Competing for Healthcare Funds*

Competing Health Program	Total Costs	Health Benefits
Hand hygiene promotion program	€100,000	15 life years
Two extra nurses in the emergency department	€270,000	30 life years
Replacing the Magnetic resonance imaging (MRI) scanner	€400,000	25 life years

*Made up data (data are not real data).

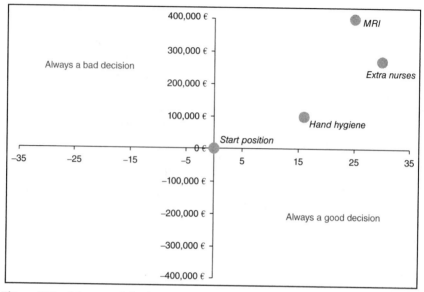

Figure 39.1   A framework for decision making; the *y*-axis shows costs and the *x*-axis shows health benefits in life years gained.

those obtained by hand hygiene, then the incremental cost-effectiveness of the nurses and the MRI relative to hand hygiene must be estimated.

Two other possible outcomes from health decisions are shown in Figure 39.1. If a novel health program increases costs and leads to reduced health benefits, then it occupies a point northwest of the start position. This is always a bad decision, as the health system is worse off by both cost and by health outcomes. Decision makers should be careful not to invest in programs that occupy this part of the graph. Rather they should aim to find health programs that are cost saving and deliver health benefits, and this is southeast of the start position. Smart decision makers will search for these programs. It is possible that effective hand hygiene programs will occupy the bottom right quadrant, but only if the cost savings exceed the cost increases, and also lead to health benefits.

WHAT WE KNOW – THE EVIDENCE

Little research has been published on the cost-effectiveness of hand hygiene promotion programs. Two good systematic reviews of effectiveness data have been published,[6,7] but these only tell part of the story. The change to costs and health benefits also need to be quantified if the economic impact of hand hygiene is to be determined.

A literature search revealed nine papers and opinion pieces on the economic impacts of improved hand hygiene compliance.

Huis et al.[8] performed a cost-effectiveness evaluation of an evidence-based hand hygiene program compared to an "experimental hand hygiene strategy" that added three novel elements. The extra costs and the cost saving from the experimental program were included and valued in the model. Crucially, the years of life gained from preventing HAIs were not counted. Instead, the benefits of the program were expressed by improved hand hygiene compliance, which is only an intermediate measure of benefit. The main finding was that the cost of improving compliance by 9% was on average $5,497 per ward. The shortcoming of this study is that the cost per life year gained was not estimated, and so the value of this novel hand hygiene program cannot be compared to other uses of scarce health resources. Their modeling might be extended to estimate the cost per life year gained. Chen et al.[9] did an economic study of a hospital-wide hand hygiene program that increased compliance from 43% in 2004 to 96% in 2007. They modeled the costs of implementing the program including the extra alcohol-based handrub (ABHR) and the time of staff. They also included the cost savings from avoided cases of HAI. Benefits were expressed as the number of HAIs avoided, rather than the number of life years gained. The cost of preventing one case of infection was US$163, and the overall savings of the program were reported to be US$5,289,364. Because the program was found to be cost saving, there is no need to quantify the health benefits. Decision makers can be confident they are doing the right thing by investing to save costs.

Different conclusions would be drawn from a study of the cost-effectiveness of a national initiative to improve hand hygiene compliance in Australia using the outcome of healthcare-associated *Staphylococcus aureus* bacteremia.[10] The change to costs and health outcomes of this program implemented between 2009 and 2012 were compared to the costs and health outcomes of the local programs in each state and territory that it replaced. It was a large and comprehensive study of 1,294,656 admissions from the 50 largest acute Australian hospitals. Total annual costs increased by $2,851,475 for a return of 96 years of life, giving an incremental cost-effectiveness ratio of $29,700 per life year gained. Among the separate states and territories it was only cost-effective in the Australian Capital Territory, Queensland, and New South Wales. The respective costs per life year saved were $1,030, $8,988, and $33,353 for these jurisdictions. No evidence was found for cost-effectiveness in the remaining states and territories.

Six more studies were found, but none were formal economic evaluations. Instead the authors interpreted information on key economic parameters and made judgments about the cost-effectiveness of hand hygiene programs. Freeman[11] made judgments from information arising in New Zealand about increased compliance and the costs of infection to conclude a hand hygiene program was cost saving and delivered health benefits. Harris et al.[12] reported that improving hand hygiene compliance in a US pediatric intensive care unit improved mortality rates and reduced length of stay, making cost savings of $12 million. They suggested the costs of achieving these gains were modest and concluded the programs represent a significant return on investment.

Cummings et al.[13] simulated patient contacts by US healthcare workers with dirty hands and summed the costs related to methicillin-resistant *S. aureus* (MRSA) infections by synthesizing published information of the costs of infection. They concluded that very small improvements in hand hygiene compliance were required to result in significant cost savings. Nguyen et al.[14] estimated HAI rates in a Vietnamese hospital fell from 13.1% to 2.1% because of hand hygiene, and that the length of patient stay and the costs for antibiotics reduced. Pittet et al.[15] estimated for the period between 1994 and 2001 the costs of extra ABHR, the salaries of staff, and the costs from organizing a hand hygiene promotion campaign. They predicted large cost savings from cases of HAI avoided and found that if only 1% of the cases of infection prevented were due to the hand hygiene campaign, then the program would have paid for itself. A case study of the England and Wales national hand hygiene program[16] made predictions that overall costs would be reduced and infections avoided, generating health benefits.

The authors of these studies and opinion pieces all suggest the hand hygiene programs would occupy some space in the bottom right quadrant of Figure 39.1. This means that expanding hand hygiene would save costs and increase health benefits, and they must be adopted as compared to the start position.

WHAT WE DO NOT KNOW – THE UNCERTAIN

Valuable data are included in these studies, but overall the economic case for hand hygiene remains uncertain. Only one[10] of the three formal economic evaluations included health benefits measured by life years gained. And the evidence for cost-effectiveness was not overwhelming. The remaining literature included economic outcomes somewhat arbitrarily. A rigorous and critical review of all papers would establish whether data were used selectively to build an economic argument to support hand hygiene programs.

RESEARCH AGENDA

One thing to be done is an exhaustive and independent review of cost-effectiveness studies for hand hygiene interventions. There are more studies available than can be included in this chapter. Halton[17] did just such a review of evidence regarding the cost-effectiveness of strategies to prevent catheter-related bloodstream infections. The focus was on the quality and usefulness of the economic evidence for reducing risks of line-related bloodstream infections. It would be a template for a team interested in critically reviewing the economics of hand hygiene programs.

A final issue to consider is the maturity of hand hygiene programs and how the economics evolves as they become routine in health services.[18] The solid black line in Figure 39.2 shows a hypothetical relationship between total costs (*x*-axis) and the proportion of HAIs prevented (*y*-axis). It reveals that improving safety is costly and always effective. Situations where everyone gets HAI and no one gets HAI are excluded, and the region between 20% and 97% of infections prevented is where decision making is likely to be relevant. Most important is that the line between benefit and cost levels off as safety is improved.

The dotted lines show that improving from 20% to 70% changes total costs from €67 to €866; for this change we might describe hand hygiene as "innovative" as each unit on the y-axis only costs €16, and this could be very good value for money. Making further improvements from 70% to 90% changes costs from €866 to €2,983, and each unit on the y-axis costs €106. In this region hand hygiene might be described as "maturing," but could still represent good value for money. Pushing past 90% to 97% requires extra costs of €3,560 (€6,543 less €2,983), and the cost per extra unit of safety is €509 (more than 30-fold the cost when risks were higher). The value for money is diminishing because as risks move toward zero cases, a reservoir of patients will remain such as elderly or immune-suppressed individuals who are so vulnerable that infection becomes much harder to prevent.[19] It may be that in this region hand hygiene becomes too expensive for health services.

Because there are many more demands placed on healthcare budgets than society can afford, there always comes a point where some other health program is better value for money. It is possible that hand hygiene programs suffer diminishing marginal returns, especially when the risks of HAI are close to zero. The information in Table 39.2 summarizes all the points marked by the lines drawn in Figure 39.2.

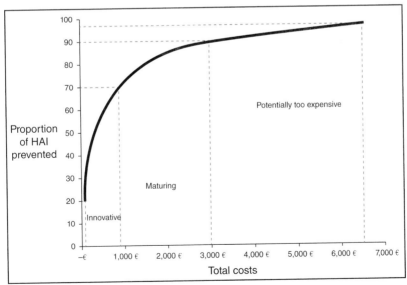

Figure 39.2 Diminishing returns for hand hygiene programs (all data are hypothetical). HAI, health-care associated infections.

Table 39.2   Diminishing Marginal Returns and Improving Patient Safety

Total Costs	Safety	Change to Total Costs	Change to Safety	Cost per Extra Unit of Safety
€ 67	20%	€ 799	50	€ 16 INNOVATIVE
€ 866	70%	€ 2,118	20	€ 106 MATURING
€ 2,983	90%	€ 3,560	7	€ 509 TOO EXPENSIVE

REFERENCES

1. Page K, Graves N, Halton K, et al., Humans, 'things' and space: costing hospital infection control interventions. *J Hosp Infect* 2013;**84**:200–205.
2. Graves N, Harbarth S, Beyersmann J, et al., Estimating the cost of health care-associated infections: mind your p's and q's. *Clin Infect Dis* 2010;**50**:1017–1021.
3. Stewardson AJ, Harbarth S, Graves N, Valuation of hospital bed-days released by infection control programs: a comparison of methods. *Infect Control Hosp Epidemiol* 2014;**35**:1294–1297.
4. Lyttkens H, Time to disable DALYs? *Eur J Health Econ* 2005;**4**:195–202.
5. Anand S, Hanson K, Disability adjusted life years: a critical review. *J Health Econ* 1997;**16**:685–702.
6. Schweizer ML, Reisinger HS, Ohl M, et al., Searching for an optimal hand hygiene bundle: a meta-analysis. *Clin Infect Dis* 2014;**58**:248–259.
7. Luangasanatip N, Hongsuwan M, Limmathurotsakul D, et al., Comparative efficacy of interventions to promote hand hygiene in hospital: systematic review and network meta-analysis. *Br Med J* 2015;**351**:h3728.
8. Huis A, Hulscher M, Adang E, et al., Cost-effectiveness of a team and leaders-directed strategy to improve nurses' adherence to hand hygiene guidelines: a cluster randomised trial. *Int J Nurs Stud* 2013;**50**:518–526.
9. Chen YC, Sheng WH, Wang JT, et al., Effectiveness and limitations of hand hygiene promotion on decreasing healthcare-associated infections. *PLoS ONE* 2011;**6**:e27163.
10. Graves N, Page K, Martin E, et al., Cost-effectiveness of a national initiative to improve hand hygiene compliance using the outcome of healthcare associated *Staphylococcus aureus* bacteraemia. *PLoS ONE* 2016;**11**:e0148190.
11. Freeman J, Sieczkowski C, Anderson T, et al., Improving hand hygiene in New Zealand hospitals to increase patient safety and reduce costs: results from the first hand hygiene national compliance audit for 2012. *NZ Med J* 2012;**125**:178–181.
12. Harris BD, Hanson C, Christy C, et al., Strict hand hygiene and other practices shortened stays and cut costs and mortality in a pediatric intensive care unit. *Health Aff (Project Hope)* 2011;**30**:1751–1761.
13. Cummings KL, Anderson DJ, Kaye KS, Hand hygiene noncompliance and the cost of hospital-acquired methicillin-resistant *Staphylococcus aureus* infection. *Infect Control Hosp Epidemiol* 2010;**31**:357–364.
14. Nguyen KV, Nguyen PT, Jones SL, Effectiveness of an alcohol-based hand hygiene program in reducing nosocomial infections in the Urology Ward of Binh Dan Hospital, Vietnam. *Trop Med Int Health* 2008;**13**:1297–1302.
15. Pittet D, Sax H, Hugonnet S, et al., Cost implications of successful hand hygiene promotion. *Infect Control Hosp Epidemiol* 2004;**25**:264–266.

16. World Health Organization, *WHO Guidelines on Hand Hygiene in Health Care*. Assessing the economic impact of hand hygiene promotion. Geneva: WHO, 2009;168–173.

17. Halton K, Graves N, Economics of preventing catheter-related bloodstream infection? *Emerg Infect Dis* 2007;**13**:815–823.

18. Graves N, Barnett A, White K, et al., Evaluating the economics of the Australian National Hand Hygiene Initiative. *Healthcare Infect* 2012;**17**:5–10.

19. Graves N, McGowan JE, Jr, Nosocomial infection, the Deficit Reduction Act, and incentives for hospitals. *JAMA* 2008;**300**:1577–1579.

Chapter 40

Hand Hygiene: Key Principles for the Manager

Eleanor Murray,[1] Alison Holmes,[2] and Didier Pittet[3]

[1] Saïd Business School, University of Oxford, Oxford, UK
[2] National Institute for Health Research, Health Protection Research Unit in Healthcare Associated Infection and Antimicrobial Resistance, Imperial College London, London, UK
[3] Infection Control Program and WHO Collaborating Centre on Patient Safety, University of Geneva Hospitals and Faculty of Medicine, Geneva, Switzerland

KEY MESSAGES

- Managers exist at multiple levels in the organization and play an important role in hospitals to ensure that hand hygiene guidelines are adhered to.

- The key parameters for managers to influence hand hygiene compliance at institutional level include leadership, recognition of the critical role of systems and behaviors, and achieving the correct balance between individual and collective accountability.

- Although a range of factors can influence institutional hand hygiene compliance, the key challenge for managers is to adapt actions and interventions to fit their organizations. Further research is required to test the efficacy of multiple interventions to sustain levels of hand hygiene compliance.

Hand Hygiene: A Handbook for Medical Professionals, First Edition.
Edited by Didier Pittet, John M. Boyce and Benedetta Allegranzi.
© 2017 John Wiley & Sons, Inc. Published 2017 by John Wiley & Sons, Inc.

WHAT WE KNOW – THE EVIDENCE

Managers (or administrators) play an important role in hospitals to ensure that hand hygiene guidelines are adhered to. Managers exist at multiple levels in the organization as team leaders; departmental or divisional managers; and executive directors, putting them in a position to influence the effectiveness of hand hygiene operationally and strategically in the organization. Promoting and facilitating hand hygiene among healthcare workers are important actions for managers,[1] and there is increasing recognition that an organizational approach to improving hand hygiene, one that addresses systems and behavioral issues, is important owing to the low levels of hand hygiene compliance exhibited by healthcare workers. The short-term impact of most interventions and the existence of a number of reported barriers to effective hand hygiene have contributed to this low level of compliance.[2] This chapter summarizes the key principles of hand hygiene for managers, drawing on recent research to examine the broad range of institutional issues that can improve hand hygiene compliance in the organization.

Leadership

Leadership is a critical factor in achieving effective infection prevention control (IPC) or hand hygiene promotion programs.[3] A recent study identified four key factors associated with successful IPC leaders, which would apply equally well to hand hygiene compliance: (i) nurturing a culture of clinical excellence and effectively communicating it to staff; (ii) overcoming barriers of resistance from people or organizational challenges that prevent effective healthcare-associated infection (HAI) management; (iii) acting as inspirational role models; and (iv) thinking strategically while acting locally, which involves coalition building, leveraging personal reputations to move ideas forward, and influencing committees through politicking.[4] The same study found that IPC leaders could be more effective in improving patient safety activities than senior executives seeking to achieve the same goal. This leadership capacity could be harnessed and more successfully utilized with hand hygiene promotion. Unit leaders will understand their local barriers to resistance and be more aware of cultural issues that need to be addressed. Providing support and incentives locally to assist leaders in promoting a positive culture and safety climate within their ward or division reflects the evidence that safety climate partially mediates the relationship between safety leadership and safety performance.[5]

Two mechanisms for encouraging hand hygiene leadership throughout the organization are the use of role models and the identification/creation of champions. The first mechanism is highlighted in research studies which emphasize the importance of key clinical leaders effectively role-modeling positive behaviors relating to IPC and antibiotic stewardship.[6,7] Role modeling by consultants can be a key influencer of junior doctors' behaviors, particularly in relation to areas such as hand hygiene and aseptic technique; however, all professional groups can benefit from excellent role models in their area of work.[3] A further leadership mechanism is the development of active champions who can influence organizational change through four functions: (i) building organizational support for new practices; (ii) protecting those involved in implementation from organizational rules and systems that may be barriers; (iii) helping to access the use of organizational resources for implementation; and (iv) supporting the growth of organizational coalitions to achieve implementation.[8,9] Most IPC improvements, such as hand hygiene compliance, require organization-wide behavior change and therefore a network of active champions who are skilled at developing interprofessional coalitions is required. This might be achieved through local clinical leadership with an existing ward nurse taking on a champion role or a designated doctor within a clinical team championing hand hygiene compliance.[3]

Systems Design

There is increasing recognition of the influence that systems and behaviors have on hand hygiene compliance and that hand hygiene interventions must consider the importance of understanding individual, group, and institutional levels.[10] Table 40.1 illustrates the range of factors that can influence hand hygiene compliance and identifies associated examples. Some of these factors apply at the individual level – for example, cognitive and behavioral factors – and others at ward or institutional level, such as process, capacity, and cultural factors.

The challenge for the manager is to determine, in collaboration with other stakeholders, the range of interventions that are likely to have the highest impact and most significant return for the amount of effort and resource invested to improve compliance. A good starting point is to address system-wide issues, building on existing infrastructures that are in place in the organization. For example, many hospitals have in place a performance management framework, linked to a balanced scorecard, a mechanism for setting targets and monitoring a range of performance metrics (clinical, finance, human resources, strategic).[11] If local targets and ward-level data for hand hygiene compliance can be built into the balanced scorecard, this provides comparative information for which local leaders can be held accountable, which in turn can precipitate behavioral change owing to peer pressure to perform against targets.

Individual and Collective Accountability

A further issue for managers is achieving the balance between individual and collective accountability. One question is, should the approach be punitive and sanction-driven leveled at individuals or reward-focused and incentive-driven organizationally? The answer is that a positive organizational culture, that is

Table 40.1   Factors that Affect Hand Hygiene Compliance with Associated Examples

Factor	Examples
Environmental	Location of, and sufficient facilities, e.g., sinks, alcohol-based handrub dispensers Sufficient and regularly replenished supplies, e.g., soap, towels, handrub
Capacity	Adequate staffing Optimal occupancy
Capability	Multidisciplinary hand hygiene education and promotion programs Staff trained in standardized hand hygiene audit techniques Availability of toolkits (including audit tools and promotional materials) Interdisciplinary hand hygiene policy
Process	Standardized collection of hand hygiene data Comparative real-time feedback to staff by ward and healthcare worker (HCW) category On-line performance management tools, including targets Evidence-based and accessible guidelines/protocols
Cognitive	Knowledge of guidelines/protocols Increasing awareness of the need for hand hygiene compliance Nudge techniques to regularly prompt staff of the need for compliance Encourage patient challenge to HCW
Behavioral	Positive role models at all levels within the institution Administrative sanctions for noncompliers Rewards and incentives for active leadership Ensuring hand hygiene enhances HCW/patient relationship
Culture	Active participation in hand hygiene compliance at individual and institutional level Creation of a positive safety climate at unit level

HCW, healthcare workers.

reward-focused and incentivized towards positive behaviors, is likely to have more sustainable impact in the longer term, but that sanctions may be required for repeat noncompliers who fail to take personal responsibility for their practice and are unwilling to be held accountable for their actions.

WHAT WE DO NOT KNOW AND RESEARCH AGENDA

There is growing support for adopting institutional-level approaches using systems and behavioral interventions, in conjunction with existing clinical practice changes, to improve hand hygiene compliance. However, the evidence base for these approaches is lacking in healthcare research. Whether actions and interventions supported or promoted by managers have independent positive effects and whether multiple-levels approaches are merely additive or synergistic remain to be determined. Although a range of factors exist that can influence hand hygiene compliance, the key challenge for managers is to adapt these approaches to fit their organizations. Further longitudinal social science research is required to test the efficacy of multiple interventions to sustain levels of hand hygiene compliance.

REFERENCES

1. Pittet D, Hugonnet S, Harbarth S, et al., Effectiveness of a hospital-wide programme to improve compliance with hand hygiene. *Lancet* 2000;**356**:1307–1312.
2. Pittet D, Improving compliance with hand hygiene in hospitals. *Infect Control Hosp Epidemiol* 2000;**21**:381–386.
3. Murray E, Holmes A, Addressing healthcare-associated infections and antimicrobial resistance from an organizational perspective: progress and challenges. *J Antimicrob Chemother* 2012;**67**(Suppl. 1):i29–i36.
4. Saint S, Kowlaski C, Banaszak-Holl J, et al., The importance of leadership in preventing healthcare-associated infection: results of a multisite qualitative study. *Infect Control Hosp Epidemiol* 2010;**31**:901–907.
5. Wu TC, Chen CH, Li CC, A correlation among safety leadership, safety climate and safety performance. *J Loss Prevent Process Indus* 2008;**21**:307–318.
6. Wright SM, Kern DE, Kolodner K, et al., Attributes of excellent attending-physician role models. *N Engl J Med* 1998;**339**:1986–1993.
7. Maudsley R, Role models and the learning environment: essential elements in effective medical education. *Acad Med* 2001;**76**:432–434.
8. Damschroder LJ, Banaszak-Holl J, Kowalski CP, et al., The role of the "champion" in infection prevention: results from a multisite qualitative study. *Qual Saf Health Care* 2009;**18**:434–440.
9. Greenhalgh T, Robert G, Macfarlane F, et al., Diffusion of innovations in service organizations: systematic review and recommendations. *Milbank Q* 2004;**82**:581–629.
10. Pittet D, Boyce JM, Hand hygiene and patient care: pursuing the Semmelweis legacy. *Lancet Infect Dis* 2001;**1**(Suppl. 1):9–20.
11. Kaplan RS, Norton DP, Using the balanced scorecard as a strategic management system. *Harv Bus Rev* 1996;**74**:75–85.

Chapter 41

Effect of Hand Hygiene on Infection Rates

Benedetta Allegranzi,[1] Stephan Harbarth,[2] and Didier Pittet[2]

[1] *Infection Prevention and Control Global Unit, Department of Service Delivery and Safety, World Health Organization, and Faculty of Medicine, University of Geneva, Geneva, Switzerland*
[2] *Infection Control Program and WHO Collaborating Centre on Patient Safety, University of Geneva Hospitals and Faculty of Medicine, Geneva, Switzerland*

KEY MESSAGES

- Evidence demonstrates a temporal association or statistical correlation between interventions leading to significant hand hygiene compliance improvement and healthcare-associated infection (HAI) reduction, especially methicillin-resistant *Staphylococcus aureus* (MRSA) infections. Some studies showed long-term sustainability and cost-effectiveness.

- The large majority of studies showing the successful impact of hand hygiene on HAIs were based on multimodal interventions and included preferred recourse to alcohol-based handrubbing.

- Higher-quality studies – e.g., (cluster) randomized controlled or stepped-wedge designs – are needed to generate stronger evidence and provide answers to unresolved issues.

The literature on the effect of hand hygiene promotion strategies has expanded rapidly over the last decade. The most frequently used indicators of change are hand hygiene compliance, change in infrastructures, including consumption of hand hygiene products, and healthcare workers' (HCWs') knowledge and perceptions. These measures offer important insight to assess the impact on behavioral and mentality change, as well as infrastructure and procurement aspects, which are key factors for feasibility and sustainability. However, the ideal outcome indicator is the burden of healthcare-associated infection (HAI),

Hand Hygiene: A Handbook for Medical Professionals, First Edition.
Edited by Didier Pittet, John M. Boyce and Benedetta Allegranzi.
© 2017 John Wiley & Sons, Inc. Published 2017 by John Wiley & Sons, Inc.

measured in terms of infection rates and associated mortality and costs. In this chapter, we discuss the evidence supporting hand hygiene as an effective measure to reduce HAI and the associated burden.

WHAT WE KNOW – THE EVIDENCE

Research to assess the impact of hand hygiene on HAI rates has been conducted since the 1970s. Even earlier, a pioneer cluster-randomized controlled study comparing handwashing versus no handwashing demonstrated the potential of hand hygiene to reduce the risk of *Staphylococcus* spp. cross-transmission (from 92% to 53%) in newborn infants.[1] In terms of indicators used, studies measuring the effect of interventions on both HCWs' compliance with best hand hygiene practices and infection rates are the most appropriate to answer this research question. More than 100 studies have been published to date on this topic. Despite some limitations, most bring convincing evidence for either a temporal or statistical association between improved hand hygiene practices and reduced infection and cross-transmission rates. A number of narrative reviews have summarized the most recently published studies.[2–5] A Cochrane review was also performed,[6] using stringent criteria for the selection of only randomized controlled trials, controlled clinical trials, controlled before-and-after studies, and interrupted time series analyses. Four studies met the selection criteria. Of these, three evaluated only the impact of hand hygiene promotion on compliance or alcohol-based handrub (ABHR) consumption and not on HAI. Thus, this review brings little added value as a response to the research question regarding the effect of hand hygiene on HAIs. Two systematic reviews, including meta-analyses, published in 2014 and 2015 reported that multimodal hand hygiene improvement strategies were effective to reduce HAIs.[7,8]

Most studies assessing the impact of hand hygiene on reducing HAI are quasi-experimental, before-and-after studies, as more accurate designs are complex to execute and in some cases might even be considered unethical (see also Chapters 6 and 7). However, lessons learned are worth being carefully evaluated. The main features and results of these studies are summarized in Table 41.1.[9–16] Initial interventions focused either on the use of an antimicrobial soap (containing chlorhexidine in most cases) or on improving handwashing behavior through HCWs' education; most showed a reduction of HAI or colonization rates with healthcare-associated pathogens. From the 1990s, a major change in hand hygiene promotion occurred with the replacement of handwashing with soap and water by handrubbing with an alcohol-based formulation. Studies initially assessed their introduction as a single intervention and then within multimodal strategies.

In 2000, Pittet et al. published the first landmark study using a multifaceted and multidisciplinary approach for the promotion of hand hygiene, including the preferred recourse to ABHR, observation of hand hygiene practices, targeted HCW education and training, performance feedback, promotional posters in the workplace, and institutional culture change (Table 41.1).[17] This study and

Table 41.1 Published Studies Assessing the Effect of Hand Hygiene Compliance Improvement on Healthcare-Associated Infections (Selected Studies)*

Year	Authors	Country	Type of Study	Setting	Intervention	Impact on Hand Hygiene Compliance	Impact on HAI	Follow-Up Duration	Reference
1977	Casewell M et al.	United Kingdom	Observational before/after study	Adult ICU	Promotion of HW with a chlorhexidine hand cleanser	NA	Significant reduction in the percentage of patients colonized or infected by *Klebsiella* spp	2 years	Modified from Reference 7
1989	Conly JM et al.	Canada	Observational before/after study	Adult ICU	Education. HH compliance observation, performance feedback	Significant HW compliance increase from 14% to 73% (before patient contact) and from 28% to 81% (after patient contact)	Significant reduction of HAI incidence after HW promotion (from 33% to 12% and from 33% to 10%, after two intervention periods 4 years apart)	6 years	Modified from Reference 7
1990	Simmons B et al.	USA	Observational before/after study	Adult ICU	HW promotion	HH compliance increase from 22% to 29.9% (NS)	No impact on HAI rates	11 months	Modified from Reference 7
1992	Doebbeling BN et al.	USA	Prospective multiple cross-over trial	Adult ICUs	HH with either chlorhexidine soap or HR with 60% isopropyl alcohol rinse with optional HW with plain soap	42% HH compliance with chlorhexidine soap vs 38% with HR and plain soap (RR 1.28, 95% CI, 1.02–1.60)	Significantly lower HAI rates using HW with chlorhexidine soap. No difference in HAI incidence compared to the 8 months before the study	8 months	Modified from Reference 7
1994	Webster J et al.	Australia	Observational before/after study	NICU	Introduction of HW with triclosan 1% wt/vol	NA	Reduction of vancomycin use. Significant reduction of nosocomial BSI (from 2.6% to 1.1%) using triclosan compared to chlorhexidine for HW	9 months	Modified from Reference 7

(continued)

Table 41.1 (*Continued*)

Year	Authors	Country	Type of Study	Setting	Intervention	Impact on Hand Hygiene Compliance	Impact on HAI	Follow-up Duration	Reference
2000	Larson E et al.	USA	Case control study	MICU/NICU	Multiple components intervention designed to change organizational culture in the intervention hospital	NA	Significant (85%) relative reduction of the VRE infection rate at the intervention hospital; NS (44%) reduction at the control hospital; no significant change in MRSA	8 months	Modified from Reference 7
2000	Pittet D et al.	Switzerland	Observational before/after study	Hospital-wide	Introduction of ABHR, HH observation, training, performance feedback, posters, institutional culture change	Significant increase of HH compliance from 48% to 66%	Significant reduction in the annual overall prevalence of HAI (42%) and MRSA* cross-transmission rates (87%). Continuous increase in ABHR use, stable HAI rates, and cost savings, in a follow-up study	8 years (including follow-up study)	Modified from Reference 7
2003	Hilburn J et al.	USA	Observational before/after study	Orthopedic surgical ward	Introduction of ABHR, posters, feedback on HAI rates, patient education	NA	36% reduction of HAI incidence (from 8.2% to 5.3%)**, UTI and SSI in particular	10 months	Modified from Reference 7
2004	MacDonald A et al.	United Kingdom	Observational before/after study	Hospital-wide	Introduction of ABHR, HH observation, posters, performance feedback, informal discussions	NS increase of HH compliance before and after patient contact	Significant reduction in hospital-acquired MRSA cases (from 1.9% to 0.9%)	1 year	Modified from Reference 7
2004	Swoboda SM et al.	USA	Three-phase quasi-experimental study	Adult inter-mediate care unit	HH electronic monitoring at patient room exit, direct observation, and voice prompts	NS increase of compliance detected by electronic monitoring (from	Reduction in HAI rates (NS)	2.5 months	Modified from Reference 7

Year	Author	Country	Study design	Setting	Intervention	Outcome (HH compliance)	Outcome (HAI)	Duration	Source
2004	Lam BCC et al.	Hong Kong SAR (China)	Observational before/after study	NICU	Introduction of ABHR, HH observation, training, hand hygiene protocols, posters	Significant HH compliance increase from 40% to 53% (before patient contact) and from 39% to 59% (after patient contact)	Reduction (NS) in HAI rates (from 11.3/1000 to 6.2/1000 pt-days)	6 months	Modified from Reference 7
2004	Won S-P et al.	China (Taiwan)	Observational before/after study	NICU	Education, written instructions, HH observation, posters, performance feedback, financial incentives	Significant HH compliance increase from 43% to 80%	Significant reduction in HAI rates (from 15.1 to 10.7/1000 pt-days)	2 years	Modified from Reference 7
2005	Zerr DM et al.	USA	Observational before/after study	Hospital-wide	ABHR introduction, HH observation, training, posters	Significant HH compliance increase from 62% to 81%	Significant reduction in hospital-associated rotavirus infections	4 years	Modified from Reference 7
2005	Rosenthal et al.	Argentina	Observational before/after study	Adult ICUs	HW observation, training, guideline dissemination, posters, performance feedback	Significant HH compliance increase from 23% to 65%	Significant reduction in HAI rates (from 47.5/1000 to 27.9/1000 pt-days)	21 months	Modified from Reference 7

(continued)

Table 41.1 (*Continued*)

Year	Authors	Country	Type of Study	Setting	Intervention	Impact on Hand Hygiene Compliance	Impact on HAI	Follow-up Duration	Reference
2005	Johnson et al.	Australia	Observational before/after study	Hospital-wide	ABHR introduction, HH observation, training, posters, promotional gadgets	Significant HH compliance increase from 21% to 42%	Significant reduction (57%) in MRSA bacteremia	36 months	Modified from Reference 7
2007	Le TA et al.	Vietnam	Before/after study with control ward	Neurosurgery ward	ABHR introduction, training, posters	NA	Reduction (54%, NS) of overall incidence of SSI with significantly lower incidence in the intervention ward. Significant reduction of superficial SSI	2 years	Modified from Reference 7
2007	Pessoa-Silva C et al.	Switzerland	Observational before/after study	Neonatal ward	Posters, focus groups, HH observation, HCWs' perception assessment, feedback on performance, perception, and HAI rates	HH compliance increase from 42% to 55%**	Reduction of overall HAI rates (from 11 to 8.2 infections per 1000 pt-days)** and 60% decrease of HAI risk in very low birth weight neonates (from 15.5 to 8.8 episodes/1000 pt-days)	27 months	Modified from Reference 7
2008	Rupp ME et al.	USA	Prospective controlled, cross-over trial in two units	ICU	ABHR introduction, education, posters	NS HH compliance increase from 38–37% to 68–69%	No impact on device-associated infection and infections due to multidrug-resistant pathogens	2 years	Modified from Reference 7

Year	Author	Country	Study design	Setting	Intervention	HH compliance	Outcome	Duration	Source
2008	Grayson ML et al.	Australia	Observational before/after study	1) 6 pilot hospitals; 2) all public hospitals in Victoria (Australia)	ABHR increased use, HH observation, training, posters, promotional gadgets	1) Significant HH compliance increase from 21% to 48% 2) Significant HH compliance increase from 20% to 53%	1) Significant reduction of MRSA bacteremia (from 0.05/100 to 0.02/100 pt-discharges per month) and of clinical MRSA isolates 2) Significant reduction of MRSA bacteremia (from 0.03/100 to 0.01/100 pt-discharges per month) and of clinical MRSA isolates	1) 2 years 2) 1 year	Modified from Reference 7
2008	Capretti MG et al.	Italy	Observational before/after study	NICU	ABHR introduction, training, posters	NA	Significant reduction of HAI incidence (4.1/1000 pt-days vs 1.2/1000 pt-days)	18 months	Modified from Reference 7
2008	Picheansathian W et al.	Thailand	Observational before/after study	NICU	ABHR introduction, HH observation, training, posters, performance feedback, focus groups	Significant HH compliance increase from 6.3% to 81%	No impact on HAI rates (9.7/1000 pt-days vs 13.5/1000 pt-days)	7 months	Modified from Reference 7
2008	Cromer AL et al.	USA	Observational before/after study	Hospital-wide	HH observation, including technique and feedback, in a setting where HH promotion had been implemented during previous years	HH compliance increase from 72% to 90%**	Significant reduction in facility-acquired MRSA from 0.85 to 0.52 per 1000 pt-days	10 months	Modified from Reference 7

(continued)

Table 41.1 (*Continued*)

Year	Authors	Country	Type of Study	Setting	Intervention	Impact on Hand Hygiene Compliance	Impact on HAI	Follow-up Duration	Reference
2008	Nguyen KV et al.	Vietnam	Observational before/after study	Urology ward	Education of staff and patient relatives, posters, introduction of bed-mounted bottles of ABHR, direct HH observation	Baseline HH compliance assumed to be close to 0%. Overall compliance after intervention not reported, but for specific procedures (e.g., after wound care = 68%)	Significant reduction in HAI incidence from 13.1% to 2.1%	6 months	Modified from Reference 7
2008	Marra AR et al.	Brazil	Prospective case-control study	Two adult step-down units	Electronic monitoring of ABHR use and feedback	NS higher number of HH episodes recorded by electronic monitoring in intervention unit	NS difference in BSI, UTI, and pneumonia incidence density between the two units	6 months	Modified from Reference 7
2009	Lederer JW et al.	USA	Observational before/after study	Hospital-wide, 7 acute care facilities	Education, HH observation and performance feedback, posters, memos and poster-board communications, visitor education program, internal marketing campaign	Compliance increase from 49% to 98% with sustained rates greater than 90%	Significant reduction of MRSA rates from 0.52 to 0.24 episodes/1000 pt-days	3 yrs	Modified from Reference 7

Year	Author	Country	Study design	Setting	Intervention	HH compliance	Infection outcome	Duration	Source
2009	McLaws et al.	Australia	Observational before/after study	Hospital-wide in 208 public hospitals (statewide)	ABHR introduction, HH observation, training, performance feedback, posters	Significant HH compliance increase from 47% to 61%	Significant reduction of 6% of overall MRSA infections/10,000 pt-days. Reductions of 16% in MRSA infection in nonsterile sites in ICU and of 25% in sterile sites in non-ICU wards	18 months	Modified from Reference 7
2010	Helder et al.	The Netherlands	Observational before/after study	NICU	HH education program, encouragement of role models, and culture change in favor of better HH	Significant increase in HH compliance before patient contact from 69% to 87% and after patient contact from 69% to 84%	Significant reduction in the incidence of BSI (from 44.5% to 36.1%) and of overall HAI (from 17.3 to 13.5 per 1000 pt-days)	18 months	Modified from Reference 7
2010	Cheng VCC et al.	Hong Kong SAR (China)	Observational, before/after study	Adult ICU	Phase 1: baseline; Phase 2: ICU renovation with introduction of single room isolation; Phase 3: HH campaign with ABHR introduction, briefing and discussion sessions, posters, HH observation	HH compliance increase** from 29% at baseline (2nd quarter of 2006) to 46% (4th quarter of 2006), 54% (4th quarter of 2007), and 64% (3rd quarter of 2008)	Significant reduction of incidence density of ICU onset bacteremic and nonbacteremic MRSA infection in the intervention units between Phase 3 and Phase 2	3 yrs (follow-up from Phase 2)	Modified from Reference 7

(continued)

Table 41.1 (*Continued*)

Year	Authors	Country	Type of Study	Setting	Intervention	Impact on Hand Hygiene Compliance	Impact on HAI	Follow-up Duration	Reference
2011	Yeung WK et al.	Hong Kong SAR (China)	Clustered randomized controlled trial, within a before/after observational study	7 LTCFs	ABHR introduction in pocket bottles, education, reminders (intervention LTCFs) vs basic life support education (control LTCFs)	Significant HH compliance increase from 26% to 33% in the intervention LTCFs	In the intervention LTCFs, significant reduction of incidence of serious infections (from 1.42 cases to 0.65 cases/1000 resident-days) and significant reduction of mortality due to infection. In the control LTCFs, significant increase of infection incidence and no change in mortality	7 months	Modified from Reference 7
2011	Barrera L et al.	Colombia	Prospective cohort study	6 ICUs	ABHR introduction in dispensers at each bed, education, practical training	NA: ABHR consumption monitoring documenting increase	Significant reduction of CLABSI incidence over time (−12.7% per year)	3.5 yrs	Modified from Reference 7
2011	Chen Y-C et al.	China (Taiwan)	Observational, before/after study	Hospital-wide	ABHR introduction in dispensers at point of care, education, knowledge test, reminders, HH observation and feedback, incentives (US$160.00 to unit and department level), target setting	Significant HH compliance increase from 43% in April 2004 to 96% in 2007 (P<0.001)	8.9% decrease in HAIs. Significant decrease of BSI (P<0.001), UTI (trend, P=0.03), and skin and soft tissue infections (trend, P<0.001). Every US$1 spent on HH could result in a US$23.7 benefit	3.5 yrs	Modified from Reference 7

Year	Author	Country	Study type	Setting	Intervention	Compliance result	HAI result	Duration	Reference
2011	García-Vázquez E et al.	Spain	Observational before/after study	ICU	ABHR introduction at point of care (product not spec), education, reminders, HH observation	Significant compliance increase (before patient: 35% vs 45%; after patient care: 52% vs 63%)	Significant HAI reduction from 13.7% and 8.3%	6 months	Modified from Reference 7
2011	Koff MD et al.	Lebanon	Observational before/after study	ICU	New ABHR deployed by squeezing device, education, HH observation (before entering the room and after leaving), device use monitoring and feedback	Significant improvement from 44–63% (mean 53%) to 67–90% (mean 75%)	Significant reduction of VAP (3.7 vs 6.9/1000 ventilation-days)	12 months	Modified from Reference 7
2011	Grayson ML et al.	Australia	Observational before/after study with interrupted time-series segmented regression analysis	Nationwide (521 hospitals)	HH observation, training, performance feedback, posters, safety climate	In sites not previously exposed to the campaign, significant compliance increase from 44% to 68%	Significant reduction of overall MRSA BSI ($P = 0.008$) but not of hospital-onset MRSA BSI	2 years	Modified from Reference 7
2012	Kirkland KB et al.	USA	Observational before/after study with interrupted time-series analysis	Hospital-wide	HH observation, performance feedback, ABHR availability, training, marketing and communication, leadership, accountability	Significant compliance increase from 41% to 91%	Significant reduction of HAI density from 4.8 to 3.3/1000 pt-days	1 year	8

(continued)

Table 41.1 (*Continued*)

Year	Authors	Country	Type of Study	Setting	Intervention	Impact on Hand Hygiene Compliance	Impact on HAI	Follow-up Duration	Reference
2012	Ho M et al.	Hong Kong SAR (China)	Clustered randomized controlled trial, before/after	18 LTCFs	ABHR introduction, HH observation, performance feedback, training, HH posters and reminders, a health talk, video clips	Significant increase of HH compliance in intervention arms (27% to 61% and 22% to 49%)	Significant decrease of respiratory outbreaks (IRR, 0.12; 95% CI, 0.01–0.93) and MRSA infections requiring hospital admission (IRR, 0.61; 95% CI, 0.38–0.97)	4 months	9
2012	Ling M et al.	Singapore	Observational before/after study	Hospital-wide	ABHR increased availability, HH observation, performance feedback, training, reminders; institutional safety climate	Significant increase of HH compliance from 20% to 61%	Significant reduction of MRSA infections (from 0.6 to 0.3/1000 pt-days)**	4 years	10
2012	Monistrol O et al.	Spain	Observational before/after study	3 internal medicine wards	ABHR increased availability, HH observation, performance feedback, training, reminders; institutional safety climate	Significant 25% HH compliance increase (from 54% to 76%)	Significant reduction of UTI (5.5 vs 3.5/1000 catheter-days); CLA-BSI unchanged. Significant increase of pneumonia and *C. difficile* diarrhoea	1 year	11
2013	Al-Tawfiq AA et al.	Saudi Arabia	Observational time-series analysis	Hospital-wide	HH observation, performance feedback, training, communication campaign, ABHR availability, pins promoting HH, leadership commitment	Significant compliance increase from 38% in 2006 to 83% in 2011	Significant reduction of MRSA infections (from 0.42 to 0.08), VAP (from 6.1 to 0.8), CLA-BSI (from 8.2 to 4.8), catheter-associated UTI (from 7.1 to 3.5)	5 years	12

Year	Author	Country	Study design	Setting	Intervention	HH compliance outcome	Infection outcome	Duration	Ref
2013	Salama MF et al.	Kuwait	Observational before/after study	ICU	HH observation, performance feedback, education, posters, focused group sessions	Significant increase of HH compliance from 43% to 61%	Significant reduction of CLA-BSI (from 18.6 to 3.4/1000 catheter-days), and lower respiratory tract infections (from 17.6 to 5.2/1000 ventilator-days	3 months	13
2013	Mestre G et al.	Spain	Observational before/after study	Hospital-wide	Phase 1: ABHR increased availability, HH observation, performance feedback, training, reminders; institutional safety climate Phase 2: continuous quality improvement approach	Significant 25% HH compliance increase (from 57% to 85%)	Significant reduction of MRSA infections/colonization/10,000 pt-days**	2 years	14
2013	Talbot TR et al	USA	Time-series study design	Hospital-wide	Comprehensive hand hygiene initiative including extensive project planning, leadership buy-in and goal setting, financial incentives linked to performance, and use of a system-wide shared accountability model	Significant increase (p <.001) of HH compliance between April 2009 and January 2011, up to 85%	Hand hygiene adherence rates were inversely correlated with device-associated standardized infection ratios (R(@) = 0.70)	18 months	15
2014	Johnson L et al	USA	Observational before/after study	Hospital-wide	Multimodal quality improvement project including staff education, staff accountability, product selection and accessibility, and organizational culture	From 58% in April 2006 to 98% in September 2012**	CLABSI rates decreased from 4.08 per 1000 device-days to 0.42 per 1000 device-days% between April 2006 and September 2012**	6 years	16

ABHR, alcohol-based handrub; BSI, bloodstream infection; CLA-BSI, central line-associated BSI; HAI, healthcare-associated infection; HH, hand hygiene; HR, handrubbing; HW, handwashing; ICU, intensive care unit; LTCFs, long-term care facilities; MICU, medical intensive care unit; MRSA, methicillin-presistant *Staphylococcus aureus*; NA, not available; NICU, neonatal intensive care unit; pt, patient; SSI, surgical site infection; UTI, urinary tract infection; VAP, ventilator-associated pneumonia; VRE, vancomycin-resistant enterococci.

*Systematic search conducted in PubMed using the following key words: hand hygiene MeSH, handwashing, hand washing, handrubbing, hand rubbing, alcohol-based hand rub, hand disinfection, hand hygiene compliance, cross infection MeSH, healthcare-associated infection, hospital-acquired infection, nosocomial infection, effect, effectiveness, impact, reduction, decrease, improvement.

**Statistics not reported.

long-term follow-up reports by the same research group showed significant and sustained improvement of hand hygiene compliance hospital-wide associated with reduction of overall HAI prevalence and methicillin-resistant *Staphylococcus aureus* (MRSA) cross-transmission. Since the publication of this paper and the demonstration of the strategy's cost-effectiveness, all but two interventions targeting hand hygiene improvement have been based on similar multimodal promotion strategies with adaptations of some components (Table 41.1). Main implemented strategy components were the introduction of ABHR or improvement of its availability and location, compliance observation and data feedback, and HCWs' training. Some interventions included specific methods to stimulate team discussions on hand hygiene (e.g., focus groups), use of gadgets, patient participation, and elements aimed at changing the organizational culture and creating a patient safety climate (Table 41.1). Interventions were implemented either in single wards (22/43; 51%) (mostly intensive care units, 18/43; 42%), several wards (3/43; 7%), or hospital-wide (18/43; 42%) (Table 41.1). Seven studies (16%) reported the implementation of hand hygiene promotion on a larger scale, such as in multiple hospitals, a state/region. Many of these studies had a relatively long follow-up (ranging from 2.5 months to 8 years) for the evaluation of multiple indicators, including hand hygiene compliance and HAI rates. Reduction of either overall HAI rates or specific infection types (mainly bacteremia) or infections due to specific pathogens (mostly MRSA, vancomycin-resistant enterococci [VRE], and rotavirus) was demonstrated by all but four (4/43, 9%) studies implementing hand hygiene as a single intervention (Table 41.1). In three of the four studies failing to show infection reduction, hand hygiene compliance improvement was not significant, thus indicating the absence of any substantial practice change and possibly explaining the lack of impact on outcome.

Over the past decade, an increasing number of studies have investigated the temporal association between hand hygiene product consumption and HAI with a particular focus on ABHR use and MRSA bacteremia. Several reports have demonstrated that an increase in ABHR consumption correlated significantly with a reduction of MRSA bacteremia or the incidence of MRSA clinical isolates, as summarized by Sroka et al. in their review and data pooling (see also Chapter 44A).[20]

On a larger scale, two reports from Australia[9] (see also Chapter 36) and England[21] showed a temporal association of hand hygiene national campaigns with the reduction of MRSA or *S. aureus* bacteremia nationwide. An association between ABHR use and local MRSA rates was also reported by a European ecologic study, after adjustment for multiple confounding factors.[22] Conversely, in another ecologic study from Ontario, improved hand hygiene compliance had no significant effect on the incidence of MRSA bacteremia.[23]

Finally, new technologies are emerging to enable electronic monitoring of hand hygiene practices. In some studies based on automated hand hygiene compliance detection at entry/exit from patient rooms and associated with voice prompts, the introduction of the technology was associated with a significant increase in compliance and a parallel reduction of HAI and VRE infections.[9,24]

WHAT WE DO NOT KNOW – THE UNCERTAIN

Although many studies demonstrated a temporal association or statistical correlation between hand hygiene improvement (proven through an increase of either compliance or ABHR consumption) and reduction of HAI, these have methodological limitations. Despite the fact that these studies focused mainly on hand hygiene promotion, it is not always clear whether other infection-control interventions were implemented at the same time or during some study periods, including their role in determining the observed impact on the outcome measure. In addition, as shown in Table 41.1, many studies monitoring specific pathogens observed an effect of hand hygiene on infections due to MRSA or VRE (14/43, 33%). However, data are quite limited on its role to reduce healthcare-associated transmission and infections due to Gram-negative bacteria.

Most studies assessing hand hygiene impact on HAI are quasi-experimental studies comparing time periods before and after the intervention with potential bias related to temporal and seasonal effects. Furthermore, ecological bias could be another threat to validity, since most studies used aggregate instead of individual patient-level data.

Ideally, (cluster) randomized, controlled studies could provide a stronger evidence of the role of hand hygiene in reducing HAI (see Chapters 6 and 7). This study design could help clarify more accurately the relation between hand hygiene improvement and HAI rates or the spread of antimicrobial resistance. Such studies could also provide responses to unresolved issues, such as time delay and minimum compliance improvement required to achieve HAI reduction following hand hygiene promotion. These and other issues are articulated in the research questions listed below. However, such studies are confronted with numerous difficulties. For example, if conducted within a single facility with randomization occurring at the ward level, the fragmentation of the hospital into groups of wards involves the risk of cross-contamination between control and intervention wards (i.e., movement of staff between wards, workplace reminders, leadership, etc.). In addition, this approach impedes the development of an institutional safety climate, an essential component for the success of implementation strategies.

An alternative study design is the stepped-wedge design, which offers a higher-quality level when compared with before-and-after studies and allows the evaluation of different interventions introduced at different times. One major gap in the research published so far is the lack of data about the specific contribution of each element within multimodal strategies to their effect on change of practices and/or HAI reduction; in these regards, it would be important to understand whether any element is more effective than others. Additionally, mathematical models addressing some of the research questions discussed are still scanty; if based on good-quality data, these could bring added value and help direct clinical studies (see Chapter 5).

Qualitative research should be expanded also to help interpret the results of interventions aimed at reducing HAI through hand hygiene improvement.

In particular, more studies using behavioral theories could help understand the determinants of HCWs' behavioral change and their impact on pathogen transmission and outcome improvement. These approaches should help also to understand why an intervention worked or did not work. This would be particularly useful when a significant impact on the outcome has been shown. Typical approaches of qualitative research are transcripts of focus groups, in-depth interviews, and extended field observations (see Chapters 7 and 18).

Cost-effectiveness studies are of great value to estimate the return on investment from HAI prevention and to inform decision making on priority areas for infection control or argue for sustainment of interventions. Only a few studies assessed cost-effectiveness of hand hygiene interventions aiming at HAI reduction (see Chapter 39). They show that successful improvement requires limited financial investments compared to costs associated with HAI. More data are needed to provide additional support. Accurate estimates should include calculation of the cost of implementing all components of a hand hygiene campaign, including human resources and products, costs of HAI likely to be prevented while taking into account diagnostic and treatment costs, as well as increased length of stay and other complications associated with HAI (see Chapter 39).

Another area in which more data would be of great value is the estimation of any impact of hand hygiene promotion on mortality attributable to HAI as well as other burdens of illness measures, such as disability-adjusted life years. A few studies report data on HAI mortality, and all refer to excess mortality rates compared to nonaffected patients. Mathematical models might help estimate important figures, such as lives saved or disability complications prevented through hand hygiene.

Finally, it is important to note that most (34/43, 79%, Table 41.1) interventions exploring the impact of hand hygiene on HAI were conducted in high-income countries. Only nine (9/43, 21%) were conducted in low-/middle-income countries. Of these, five reported a reduction of HAI following practice improvement, whereas two did not report any effect on practices or infection rates. Hand hygiene compliance is particularly low in settings with limited resources, and HAI rates are usually from 2 to 20 times higher than in high-income countries (see Chapter 1). For this reason, documenting the effect of a simple measure, such as hand hygiene, to reduce the HAI burden would be extremely important. Given that many other gaps and lapses in infection control exist in these settings, these studies would help also to understand whether hand hygiene improvement alone can actually determine substantial change in HAI rates. Furthermore, it would be crucial to gather data on the cost-effectiveness of hand hygiene promotion in these settings as well, because the cost input in the calculations might differ somewhat compared to advanced and high-resource settings. Demonstrating cost-effectiveness of hand hygiene interventions would certainly help executive decision making on key priorities and appropriate resource allocation.

RESEARCH AGENDA

Further research related to the impact of hand hygiene on HAI is necessary to elucidate a number of unresolved issues. Key research questions are:

- Which measure of hand hygiene is best correlated with outcomes (e.g., compliance measured by either direct observation or electronic monitoring, or ABHR consumption)?

- What is the time span between the implementation of the intervention aiming at hand hygiene improvement and the detection of a demonstrable impact on HAI reduction? More time series analyses would help answer this question.

- What is the minimum or ideal target for hand hygiene compliance percentage improvement to have a significant impact on outcomes (if such a level exists)?

- What is the effect of hand hygiene promotion on different types of HAI? Does it vary? Are there infections that are more likely to be prevented through hand hygiene improvement?

- What is the relative importance of the specific elements of multimodal hand hygiene improvement strategies to induce behavioral change and determine outcome improvement?

- What is the impact of hand hygiene promotion on lives saved and the HAI burden reduction (i.e., quality-adjusted life years or disability-adjusted life years)?

REFERENCES

1. Mortimer EA, Lipsitz PJ, Wolinsky E, et al., Transmission of staphylococci between new-borns: the importance of the hands of personnel. *Am J Dis Child* 1962;**104**:289–295.
2. World Health Organization, *WHO Guidelines on Hand Hygiene in Health Care*. Geneva: WHO, 2009. Part I.22. Impact of improved hand hygiene. Available at whqlibdoc.who.int/publications/2009/9789241597906_eng.pdf. Accessed March 7, 2017.
3. Allegranzi B, Pittet D, Role of hand hygiene in healthcare-associated infection prevention. *J Hosp Infect* 2009;**73**:305–315.
4. Backman C, Taylor G, Sales A, et al., An integrative review of infection prevention and control programs for multidrug-resistant organisms in acute care hospitals: a socio-ecological perspective. *Am J Infect Control* 2011;**39**:368–378.
5. Pincock T, Bernstein P, Warthman S, et al., Bundling hand hygiene interventions and mea-surement to decrease healthcare-associated infections. *Am J Infect Control* 2012;**40**:S18–S27.
6. Gould DJ, Moralejo D, Drey N, et al., Interventions to improve hand hygiene compliance in patient care. *Cochrane Database Syst Rev* 2010;**9**:CD005186.
7. Schweizer ML, Reisinger HS, Ohl M, et al., Searching for an optimal hand hygiene bundle: a meta-analysis. *Clin Infect Dis* 2014;**58**:248–259.

8. Luangasanatip N, Hongsuwan M, Limmathurotsakul D, et al., Comparative efficacy of interventions to promote hand hygiene in hospital: systematic review and network meta-analysis. *Br Med J* 2015;**351**:h3728.

9. Pittet D, Allegranzi B, Sax H, Hand hygiene. In: Jarvis WR, ed. *Bennett and Brachmann's Hospital Infections*, 6th edn. Philadelphia: Lippincott Williams and Wilkins, 2013;26–40.

10. Kirkland KB, Homa KA, Lasky RA, et al., Impact of a hospital-wide hand hygiene initiative on healthcare-associated infections: results of an interrupted time series. *BMJ Qual Saf* 2012;**21**:1019–1026.

11. Ho M, Seto W, Wong L, et al., Effectiveness of multifaceted hand hygiene interventions in long-term care facilities in Hong Kong: a cluster-randomized controlled trial. *Infect Control Hosp Epidemiol* 2012;**33**:761–767.

12. Ling ML, How KB, Impact of a hospital-wide hand hygiene promotion strategy on healthcare-associated infections. *Antimicrob Resist Infect Control* 2012;**1**:13.

13. Monistrol O, Calbo E, Riera M, et al., Impact of a hand hygiene educational programme on hospital-acquired infections in medical wards. *Clin Microbiol Infect* 2012;**18**:1212–1218.

14. Al-Tawfiq JA, Abed MS, Al-Yami N, et al., Promoting and sustaining a hospital-wide, multifaceted hand hygiene program resulted in significant reduction in health care-associated infections. *Am J Infect Control* 2013;**41**:482–486.

15. Talbot TR, Johnson JG, Fergus C, et al., Sustained improvement in hand hygiene adherence: utilizing shared accountability and financial incentives. *Infect Control Hosp Epidemiol* 2013;**34**:1129–1136.

16. Johnson L, Grueber S, Schlotzhauer C, et al., A multifactorial action plan improves hand hygiene adherence and significantly reduces central line-associated bloodstream infections. *Am J Infect Control* 2014;**42**:1146–1151.

17. Salama MF, Jamal WY, Al Mousa H, et al., The effect of hand hygiene compliance on hospital-acquired infections in an ICU setting in a Kuwaiti teaching hospital. *J Infect Public Health* 2013;**6**:27–34.

18. Mestre G, Berbel C, Tortajada P, et al., "The 3/3 strategy": a successful multifaceted hospital wide hand hygiene intervention based on WHO and continuous quality improvement methodology. *PLoS ONE* 2012;**7**:e47200.

19. Pittet D, Hugonnet S, Harbarth S, et al., Effectiveness of a hospital-wide programme to improve compliance with hand hygiene. *Lancet* 2000;**356**:1307–1312.

20. Sroka S, Gastmeier P, Meyer E, Impact of alcohol hand-rub use on meticillin-resistant *Staphylococcus aureus*: an analysis of the literature. *J Hosp Infect* 2010;**74**:204–211.

21. Stone SP, Fuller C, Savage J, et al., Evaluation of the national CleanYourHands campaign to reduce *Staphylococcus aureus* bacteraemia and *Clostridium difficile* infection in hospitals in England and Wales by improved hand hygiene: four year, prospective, ecological, interrupted time series study. *Br Med J* 2012;**344**:e3005.

22. MacKenzie FM, Bruce J, Struelens MJ, et al., Antimicrobial drug use and infection control practices associated with the prevalence of methicillin-resistant *Staphylococcus aureus* in European hospitals. *Clin Microbiol Infect* 2007;**13**:269–276.

23. DiDiodato G, Has improved hand hygiene compliance reduced the risk of hospital-acquired infections among hospitalized patients in Ontario? Analysis of publicly reported patient safety data from 2008 to 2011. *Infect Control Hosp Epidemiol* 2013;**34**:605–610.

24. Swoboda SM, Earsing K, Strauss K, et al., Electronic monitoring and voice prompts improve hand hygiene and decrease nosocomial infections in an intermediate care unit. *Crit Care Med.* 2004;**32**:358–363.

Chapter 42A

Hand Hygiene in Specific Patient Populations and Situations: Critically Ill Patients

Caroline Landelle,[1] Jean-Christophe Lucet,[2] and Didier Pittet[3]

[1] Infection Control Unit, Centre Hospitalier Universitaire Grenoble Alpes and University Grenoble Alpes/CNRS, ThEMAS TIM-C UMR 5525, Grenoble, France

[2] Infection Control Unit, Bichat-Claude Bernard Hospital, Paris, France

[3] Infection Control Program and WHO Collaborating Centre on Patient Safety, University of Geneva Hospitals and Faculty of Medicine, Geneva, Switzerland

KEY MESSAGES

- Patients' underlying conditions, immunosuppressive medication, at-risk medical and surgical interventions, and insertion of devices are responsible for higher healthcare-associated infections (HAIs) rates in the critically ill. Hand hygiene is the most important infection control measure, but healthcare workers' compliance remains universally low worldwide in intensive-care units and usually does not exceed 40%.

- Several risk factors for low hand hygiene compliance coexist in this setting, such as high workload, understaffing, composition of the patient zone and intensive-care unit room design, and an erroneous perception of risk transmission and hand hygiene compliance by healthcare workers.

- Multimodal promotion strategies, in particular when the increased recourse to alcohol-based handrub is endorsed, are associated with increased compliance and, when assessed, HAI rate reduction.

Hand Hygiene: A Handbook for Medical Professionals, First Edition.
Edited by Didier Pittet, John M. Boyce and Benedetta Allegranzi.
© 2017 John Wiley & Sons, Inc. Published 2017 by John Wiley & Sons, Inc.

In developed countries, healthcare-associated infections (HAIs) affect about 30% of patients admitted to intensive care units (ICUs), and crude mortality rates vary from 12% to 80%.[1-3] The burden of HAIs is even higher in developing countries.[4] The lower respiratory tract is the most common site of infection in all types of ICUs. High rates of pulmonary infections are unique to adult ICUs where patients are frequently admitted because of respiratory distress and require mechanical ventilation. Although primary bacteremia and infections associated with the use of vascular devices are less frequent, the morbidity and mortality associated with these infections are particularly high.

WHAT WE KNOW – THE EVIDENCE

Risk Factors for ICU-Acquired HAI

Patients' underlying conditions play a key role in the high rates of ICU-acquired HAI (ICU-HAI). Another reason for these high rates is the selective pressure induced by the large amount of antimicrobial use that facilitates colonization and infection by resistant organisms. Importantly, almost all ICU patients are equipped with at least one vascular access or device breaking the normal skin barrier, thus enabling direct connection with the external environment. Therefore, all unnecessary devices should be avoided or removed as quickly as possible. A great deal of equipment surrounds the patient in the ICU, and almost every item of equipment is a source of ICU-HAI. Furthermore, new devices are constantly introduced into ICUs, which increases workload and opportunities for cross-transmission. Cleaning and reprocessing protocols for these devices should be provided, and healthcare workers (HCWs) should be trained in their proper use.

The most important vehicle of cross-transmission remains HCWs' hands. Lack of, or inadequate, hand hygiene is the direct cause of transmission in many endemic and epidemic situations. Based on isolates obtained from clinical cultures, 13% to 35% of infecting isolates originate from another patient, probably through cross-transmission via HCWs' hands.[5]

Risk Factors for Noncompliance with Hand Hygiene Practices

Critically ill patients are often responsible for a high workload. One predictor of poor adherence to hand hygiene is the intensity of care defined as the number of opportunities for hand hygiene per hour of patient care. Not surprisingly, a high demand for hand hygiene is inversely correlated with the number of opportunities per hour of care and the systematic recourse to handrubbing can bypass this time constraint (Figure 42A.1).[6] HCW understaffing is another well-identified risk factor for outbreaks and excess endemic rates of ICU-HAI. In the presence

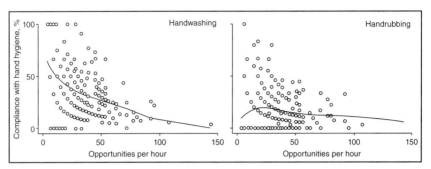

Figure 42A.1   Association between workload and compliance with handwashing and alcohol-based handrubbing. *Source*: Hugonnet 2002. Reproduced with permission from the American Medical Association.

of overcrowding, staphylococcal outbreaks periodically resulted when serious understaffing made frequent handwashing between patient contacts difficult. Importantly, not only the number of staff, but also their level of training, affects outcomes. Furthermore, the emergency nature of care provided could also compromise hand hygiene practices.

A major difficulty explaining the lack of adherence with hand hygiene in ICUs is the uncertain composition of the patient zone in comparison with a standard room in surgical or medical wards (see also Chapter 20). For example, it is unclear how daily surveillance charts (whether paper or computer) are to be considered: should they be included or excluded from the patient zone? The contribution of the ICU design to infection control is difficult to evaluate, and several well-conducted studies failed to demonstrate improvement after the wards were transferred into modern structures. Some studies demonstrated the importance of a single ICU room to reduce the transmission of multidrug-resistant bacteria. It seems prudent to consider some issues when remodeling or designing new wards. Implementation of a single room policy in ICUs often goes together with other improvements, such as human engineering (location of sinks or dispensers), general hygiene conditions (room ventilation, improved privacy), and a better demarcation between patients and patient zones. Adequate space around beds is also important. Clean activities and storage of clean items should be physically separated from dirty activities and waste disposal, and sinks and rub dispensers should be located in convenient locations.

Several studies observed that HCWs have an erroneous evaluation of risk transmission, including the grading of potentially dangerous patient care activities. Furthermore, perceived compliance with hand hygiene is universally higher than actual compliance. Barriers to hand hygiene compliance are described in Chapter 12. An additional explanation for low hand hygiene compliance in ICUs is the perceived lower priority over other patient needs.

Hand Hygiene Improvement

Despite difficulties linked to the particular specificities of both critical care and ICU patient populations, hand hygiene improvement is feasible. A number of studies in ICUs implemented hand hygiene multimodal promotion strategies, including the introduction of alcohol-based handrub (ABHR), and showed a temporal association between improved hand hygiene practices and reduced HAI rates (Table 42A.1).[7] The WHO Multimodal Hand Hygiene Improvement Strategy was pilot tested for Europe in a network of 41 Italian ICUs. Overall, a significant improvement in hand hygiene compliance (from 55% to 69%) was observed.[8] The most recent large improvement in this setting was observed in 13 European ICUs. This 26-month intervention study led to an improvement of hand hygiene compliance from 52% to 77% and demonstrated that chlorhexidine body washing, combined with a hand hygiene improvement strategy adapted from the WHO approach, reduced methicillin-resistant *Staphylococcus aureus* (MRSA) acquisition by 3.6% per week.[9]

WHAT WE DO NOT KNOW – THE UNCERTAIN

As ICU patients are bedridden, pathogen transmission occurs usually by HCWs' hands, inappropriate application of infection control practices, clinical equipment that is poorly cleaned or not cleaned at all, or visitors. ICU patients are also likely to be cared for by many consultants exterior to the ICU team, such as surgeons, physicians, dietitians, physiotherapists, and so on, and are often moved outside the unit for further care (operating room, postanesthesia care unit, radiology unit, etc.). The exact contribution of external consultants and care in areas other than the ICU for the acquisition of HAI is not well evaluated. In addition, the intensity and frequency of care varies greatly between staff members and according to patients' case-mix. Nurses and nurse assistants have the highest number of care opportunities, but other itinerant HCWs may represent a higher risk of cross-transmission, despite a lower intensity of care in case of low hand hygiene compliance rates.[10]

The relation between glove use and compliance with hand hygiene is not completely clear. Universal glove and gown use increased hand hygiene on room exit and decreased HCW patient visits. But the use of gloves and gowns for all patient contact (fewer visits with better hand hygiene on room exit) compared with usual care did not decrease the acquisition of MRSA or vancomycin-resistant enterococci.[11]

One possible explanation for low hand hygiene compliance in ICUs is the inconvenient placement of hand cleansing facilities. To our knowledge, no study has explored the optimal locations for dispensers, such as wall-mounted, bed-mounted, HCW pocket carriage, or clip-on dispensers, but a higher density of available dispensers was associated with higher compliance with hand hygiene.

Table 42A.1   Association Between Hand Hygiene Improvement and Healthcare-Associated Infection Rates in Intensive Care Units (Excluding Pediatric and Neonatal Intensive Care Units): 1975–2013

Year	Authors	Significant Results	Duration of Follow-Up
1977	Casewell & Phillips[12]	Significant reduction in the percentage of patients colonized or infected by *Klebsiella* spp.	2 years
1989	Conly et al.[13]	Significant reduction in HAI rates immediately after hand hygiene promotion (from 33% to 12% and from 33% to 10%, after two intervention periods 4 years apart, respectively)	6 years
1990	Simmons et al.[14]	No impact on HAI rates (no statistically significant improvement of hand hygiene adherence)	11 months
1992	Doebbeling et al.[15]	Significant difference between rates of HAI using two different hand hygiene agents	8 months
2000	Larson et al.[16]	Significant (85%) relative reduction of VRE rate in the intervention hospital; statistically insignificant (44%) relative reduction in the control hospital; no significant change in MRSA	8 months
2005	Rosenthal et al.[17]	Significant reduction in HAI rates (from 47.5/1000 patient-days to 27.9/1000 patient-days)	21 months
2008	Rupp et al.[18]	No impact on device-associated infection and infections due to multidrug-resistant pathogens	2 years
2010	Cheng et al.[19]	Significant reduction of incidence density of ICU onset bacteremic and non-bacteremic MRSA infection in the intervention units	3 years
2011	Garcia-Vazquez et al.[20]	Significant HAI reduction from 13.7% and 8.3%.	6 months
2011	Koff et al.[21]	Significant reduction of VAP (from 6.9 to 3.7 episodes/1000 ventilation-days)	1 year
2011	Barrera et al.[22]	Significant reduction of CLABSI incidence over time (−12.7% per year)	3.5 years
2013	Salama et al.[23]	Significant reduction in HAI rates (from 37.2/1000 patient-days to 15.1/1000 patient-days)	7 months
2013	Marra et al.[24]	Significant reduction in device-associated infection rates (from 13.2/1000 patient-days to 7.5/1000 patient-days)	1 year

Source: Pittet 2006. Reproduced with permission from Elsevier.
HAI, healthcare-associated infection; MICU, medical intensive care unit; VRE, vancomycin-resistant *Enterococcus* spp.; MRSA, methicillin-resistant *Staphylococcus aureus;* CLABSI, central line-associated bloodstream infection; VAP, ventilator-associated pneumonia.

The most appropriate density of dispensers available for ICU patients remains to be defined. The importance of strict adherence to the correct hand hygiene technique (duration and coverage of the entire hand surface, see also Chapter 10) is also not well known in ICUs.

Infection control in ICUs is based on a number of procedures and strategies, some specifically directed to a specific infection site. Hand hygiene is part of almost all care procedures (e.g., bloodstream infection bundles, ventilator-associated prevention bundles, urinary catheter infection prevention), and its relative importance among all the recommendations is not defined precisely.

RESEARCH AGENDA

- Evaluate the relative importance of hand hygiene compliance during high-risk procedures compared with its importance during low-risk procedures.
- Analyze the role of staff members in cross-transmission, depending on their function, workload, and compliance with hand hygiene.
- Assess the effect of improving the ergonomics of hand hygiene products and practices in critical care.
- Evaluate the impact of hand hygiene compliance on mortality attributable to ICU-HAI.

REFERENCES

1. Vincent JL. Nosocomial infections in adult intensive-care units. *Lancet* 2003;**361**:2068–2077.
2. Vincent JL, Bihari DJ, Suter PM, et al., The prevalence of nosocomial infection in intensive care units in Europe. Results of the European Prevalence of Infection in Intensive Care (EPIC) Study. EPIC International Advisory Committee. *JAMA* 1995;**274**:639–644.
3. Vincent JL, Rello J, Marshall J, et al., International study of the prevalence and outcomes of infection in intensive care units. *JAMA* 2009;**302**:2323–2329.
4. Allegranzi B, Bagheri Nejad S, Combescure C, et al., Burden of endemic health-care-associated infection in developing countries: systematic review and meta-analysis. *Lancet* 2011;**377**:228–241.
5. Weist K, Pollege K, Schulz I, et al., How many nosocomial infections are associated with cross-transmission? A prospective cohort study in a surgical intensive care unit. *Infect Control Hosp Epidemiol* 2002;**23**:127–132.
6. Hugonnet S, Perneger TV, Pittet D, Alcohol-based handrub improves compliance with hand hygiene in intensive care units. *Arch Intern Med* 2002;**162**:1037–1043.
7. Pittet D, Allegranzi B, Sax H, et al., Evidence-based model for hand transmission during patient care and the role of improved practices. *Lancet Infect Dis* 2006;**6**:641–652.
8. Allegranzi B, Gayet-Ageron A, Damani N, et al., Global implementation of WHO's multimodal strategy for improvement of hand hygiene: a quasi-experimental study. *Lancet Infect Dis* 2013;**13**:843–851.

9. Derde LP, Cooper BS, Goossens H, et al., Interventions to reduce colonisation and transmission of antimicrobial-resistant bacteria in intensive care units: an interrupted time series study and cluster randomised trial. *Lancet Infect Dis* 2014;**14**:31–39.

10. Hornbeck T, Naylor D, Segre AM, et al., Using sensor networks to study the effect of peripatetic healthcare workers on the spread of hospital-associated infections. *J Infect Dis* 2012;**206**:1549–1557.

11. Harris AD, Pineles L, Belton B, et al., Universal glove and gown use and acquisition of antibiotic-resistant bacteria in the ICU: a randomized trial. *JAMA* 2013;**310**:1571–1580.

12. Casewell M, Phillips I, Hands as route of transmission for *Klebsiella* species. *Br Med J* 1977;**2**:1315–1317.

13. Conly JM, Hill S, Ross J, et al., Handwashing practices in an intensive care unit: the effects of an educational program and its relationship to infection rates. *Am J Infect Control* 1989;**17**:330–339.

14. Simmons B, Bryant J, Neiman K, et al., The role of handwashing in prevention of endemic intensive care unit infections. *Infect Control Hosp Epidemiol* 1990;**11**:589–594.

15. Doebbeling BN, Stanley GL, Sheetz CT, et al., Comparative efficacy of alternative hand-washing agents in reducing nosocomial infections in intensive care units. *N Engl J Med* 1992;**327**:88–93.

16. Larson EL, Early E, Cloonan P, et al., An organizational climate intervention associated with increased handwashing and decreased nosocomial infections. *Behav Med* 2000;**26**:14–22.

17. Rosenthal VD, Guzman S, Safdar N, Reduction in nosocomial infection with improved hand hygiene in intensive care units of a tertiary care hospital in Argentina. *Am J Infect Control* 2005;**33**:392–397.

18. Rupp ME, Fitzgerald T, Puumala S, et al., Prospective, controlled, cross-over trial of alcohol-based hand gel in critical care units. *Infect Control Hosp Epidemiol* 2008;**29**:8–15.

19. Cheng VC, Tai JW, Chan WM, et al., Sequential introduction of single room isolation and hand hygiene campaign in the control of methicillin-resistant *Staphylococcus aureus* in intensive care unit. *BMC Infect Dis* 2010;**10**:263.

20. Garcia-Vazquez E, Murcia-Paya J, Canteras M, et al., Influence of a hygiene promotion programme on infection control in an intensive-care unit. *Clin Microbiol Infect* 2011;**17**:894–900.

21. Koff MD, Corwin HL, Beach ML, et al., Reduction in ventilator associated pneumonia in a mixed intensive care unit after initiation of a novel hand hygiene program. *J Crit Care* 2011;**26**:489–495.

22. Barrera L, Zingg W, Mendez F, et al., Effectiveness of a hand hygiene promotion strategy using alcohol-based handrub in 6 intensive care units in Colombia. *Am J Infect Control* 2011;**39**:633–639.

23. Salama MF, Jamal WY, Mousa HA, et al., The effect of hand hygiene compliance on hospital-acquired infections in an ICU setting in a Kuwaiti teaching hospital. *J Infect Public Health* 2013;**6**:27–34.

24. Marra AR, Noritomi DT, Westheimer Cavalcante AJ, et al., A multicenter study using positive deviance for improving hand hygiene compliance. *Am J Infect Control* 2013;**41**:984–988.

Chapter 42B

Hand Hygiene in Specific Patient Populations and Situations: Neonates and Pediatrics

Walter Zingg[1] and Hanan H. Balkhy[2]

[1] *Infection Control Program and WHO Collaborating Centre on Patient Safety, University of Geneva Hospitals and Faculty of Medicine, Geneva, Switzerland*

[2] *Infection Prevention and Control Department, King Saud bin Abdulaziz University for Health Sciences, Riyadh, Saudi Arabia*

KEY MESSAGES

- Neonates are at particular risk for healthcare-associated infections (HAIs), and hand hygiene is the most important preventive measure.

- Hand hygiene is the most critical measure in outbreak management – not only for viral gastroenteritis, but also for respiratory viruses and (multidrug-resistant) bacteria.

- Families, as care team partners, must be encouraged to comply with hand hygiene; they may also be engaged in reminding healthcare workers to perform hand hygiene.

Hand Hygiene: A Handbook for Medical Professionals, First Edition.
Edited by Didier Pittet, John M. Boyce and Benedetta Allegranzi.
© 2017 John Wiley & Sons, Inc. Published 2017 by John Wiley & Sons, Inc.

WHAT WE KNOW – THE EVIDENCE

The history of hand hygiene is closely linked to the pediatric population. In 1847, Ignácz Semmelweis not only made the association between hand hygiene and puerperal fever among women (see also Chapter 2), but also noted its relation with perinatal infection rates.[1]

Neonates are at high risk for HAIs due to an immature immune system, low levels of transplacentally acquired antibodies, and breaches in natural barriers such as a gastrointestinal tract lacking acidity, a fragile skin, and the absence of a protective microflora.[2] The incidence of catheter-associated bloodstream infection and clinical sepsis is inversely proportional to birth weight. This is not only due to the above-mentioned intrinsic risk factors, but also to the frequent use of invasive devices in preterm infants. On the other hand, the risk for HAI among school-aged children is similar to young adults, unless they suffer from any kind of immune suppression.

Hand Hygiene in the Neonatal Intensive Care Unit (NICU)

Hand hygiene in children has been studied most often in the neonatal intensive care unit (NICU). As compared to adult settings, hand hygiene compliance is often better, but continues to remain a challenge in many hospitals worldwide. HAI rates were reduced from 11.3/1000 patient-days to 6.2/1000 patient-days in one study following a multimodal intervention strategy using problem-based and task-orientated hand hygiene education, enhancement of minimal handling protocols, clustering nursing care, liberal provision of alcohol-based handrub (ABHR), improvement of hand hygiene facilities, ongoing regular hand hygiene audits, and implementation of HAI surveillance.[7]

One of the practical concerns when caring for neonates is that, due to the small size of the infant, healthcare workers (HCWs) have difficulties in performing hand hygiene between two different body sites; thus, their hands can touch "dirty" and "clean" regions at the same time, resulting in cross-contamination.[8] As a consequence, work flow must be adjusted (moving from clean to dirty sites) and hand hygiene opportunities reduced to effectively improve compliance. This was achieved within the context of at least two multimodal hand hygiene promotion strategies in neonates, and resulted in HAI prevention.[9,10] Hand hygiene not only prevents HAI as part of aseptic technique; it also reduces cross-transmission of microorganisms between patients. This is particularly important when multidrug-resistant pathogens are involved. The improvement of hand hygiene from 50% to 84% substantially reduced methicillin-resistant *Staphylococcus aureus* (MRSA)-acquisition in a NICU that had suffered from an outbreak and was not able to control the situation despite establishing other MRSA prevention measures.[10] A different NICU controlled an outbreak due to extended-spectrum beta-lactamase-producing *Klebsiella pneumoniae* by applying a multidisciplinary intervention based on standard infection prevention practices in which hand hygiene was an integral part.[11]

Families

The general principles of hand hygiene in child care beyond the neonatal period follow largely what is known from adults with one major difference: the presence of family. Family-centered care has become standard in most pediatric institutions. It is based on the belief that a partnership between healthcare providers and families is the best way to meet children's needs. Parents and caregivers take over the responsibility for many duties in daily care. As part of the care team, they need to be engaged in hand hygiene. In most countries, it is currently recommended to promote education via leaflets, posters, and direct information by HCWs.[1]

Outbreaks

Outbreaks are more common in children's hospitals than in adult settings. Seasonal outbreaks of rotavirus, norovirus, respiratory syncytial virus, and other respiratory viruses occur frequently and are a challenge for most institutions. Hand hygiene plays a predominant role in managing such outbreaks. This was shown for viral gastroenteritis[12] and respiratory viruses.[13] The latter may seem unexpected, but neonates and small infants do not produce droplets as do adults and thus, transmission is less likely to occur by droplets, but more by contact. For bacteria, hands were identified as the predominant source of outbreaks due to *Pseudomonas aeruginosa*,[14] and most, if not all, outbreaks with *Serratia* spp. MRSA eradication was achieved by improving hand hygiene compliance in one study, after the widespread use of mupirocine in staff and patients did not control the outbreak.[15]

WHAT WE DO NOT KNOW – THE UNCERTAIN

Children would be poorly cared for if the family or close relatives were not available to help HCWs in daily routine. However, the presence of family members in the hospital is a challenge due to overcrowded emergency and patient rooms; insufficient facilities (sinks, showers, toilets) for family members; short distance between ill children, siblings, and families; children playing with each other; and caregivers participating in the care of other children sharing the same room. Most hospitals were not built to host a caregiver for every hospitalized child, and thus situations in patient rooms can be somewhat chaotic. There are insufficient data about families' behavior in pathogen cross-contamination, and the transmission of pathogens in childcare. We should know how to engage caregivers to become better partners in HAI prevention and in particular in further improving hand hygiene, among both families and HCWs. And while education of HCWs and caregivers alike seems obvious and simple, it requires dedication and manpower as well as an understanding of cultural barriers for the adoption of a new behavior.

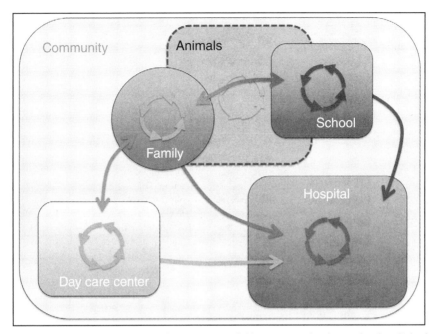

Figure 42B.1   The introduction of pathogens to childcare is complex due to the close link of children's hospitals with families, day care centers and schools, where microorganisms circulate easily.

RESEARCH AGENDA

Behavioral factors associated with better compliance in childcare as compared to adult care should be explored and tested. Although parents usually act as the child's advocate, their active contribution to improve hand hygiene among HCWs often is low. Further research is needed to better understand the role of hand hygiene in the context of the caregiver-HCW relationship.[16] The dynamics of pathogen transmission in the context of families, day care centers, schools, and hospitals and the role of animal exposure and seasonal variations should be better understood to protect hospitalized children but also avoid overreaction, since children and families are closer to the community than to healthcare settings (Figure 42B.1).

REFERENCES

1. Posfay-Barbe KM, Zerr DM, Pittet D, Infection control in paediatrics. *Lancet Infect Dis* 2008;**8**:19–31.
2. Zingg W, Posfay-Barbe KM, Pittet D, Healthcare-associated infections in neonates. *Curr Opin Infect Dis* 2008;**21**:228–234.

3. Zingg W, Posfay-Barbe KM, Pfister RE, et al., Individualized catheter surveillance among neonates: a prospective, 8-year, single-center experience. *Infect Control Hosp Epidemiol* 2011;**32**:42–49.

4. Graham PL, Simple strategies to reduce healthcare associated infections in the neonatal intensive care unit: line, tube, and hand hygiene. *Clin Perinatol* 2010;**37**:645–653.

5. Rosenthal VD, Pawar M, Leblebicioglu H, et al., Impact of the International Nosocomial Infection Control Consortium (INICC) multidimensional hand hygiene approach over 13 years in 51 cities of 19 limited-resource countries from Latin America, Asia, the Middle East, and Europe. *Infect Control Hosp Epidemiol* 2013;**34**:415–423.

6. Pittet D, Simon A, Hugonnet S, et al., Hand hygiene among physicians: performance, beliefs, and perceptions. *Ann Intern Med* 2004;**141**:1–8.

7. Lam BC, Lee J, Lau YL, Hand hygiene practices in a neonatal intensive care unit: a multimodal intervention and impact on nosocomial infection. *Pediatrics* 2004;**114**:e565–e571.

8. Pessoa-Silva CL, Dharan S, Hugonnet S, et al., Dynamics of bacterial hand contamination during routine neonatal care. *Infect Control Hosp Epidemiol* 2004;**25**:192–197.

9. Pessoa-Silva CL, Hugonnet S, Pfister R, et al., Reduction of health care associated infection risk in neonates by successful hand hygiene promotion. *Pediatrics* 2007;**120**:e382–e390.

10. Song X, Stockwell DC, Floyd T, et al., Improving hand hygiene compliance in health care workers: strategies and impact on patient outcomes. *Am J Infect Control* 2013;**41**:e101–e105.

11. Cantey JB, Sreeramoju P, Jaleel M, et al., Prompt control of an outbreak caused by extended-spectrum beta-lactamase-producing *Klebsiella pneumoniae* in a neonatal intensive care unit. *J Pediatr* 2013;**163**:672–679.

12. Zerr DM, Allpress AL, Heath J, et al., Decreasing hospital-associated rotavirus infection: a multidisciplinary hand hygiene campaign in a children's hospital. *Pediatr Infect Dis J* 2005;**24**:397–403.

13. Thomas Y, Boquete-Suter P, Koch D, et al., Survival of influenza virus on human fingers. *Clin Microbiol Infect* 2014;**20**:O58–O64.

14. Foca M, Jakob K, Whittier S, et al. Endemic *Pseudomonas aeruginosa* infection in a neonatal intensive care unit. *N Engl J Med* 2000;**343**:695–700.

15. Lepelletier D, Corvec S, Caillon J, et al., Eradication of methicillin-resistant *Staphylococcus aureus* in a neonatal intensive care unit: which measures for which success? *Am J Infect Control* 2009;**37**:195–200.

16. Bellissimo-Rodrigues F, Pires D, Zingg W, et al., Role of parents in the promotion of hand hygiene in the paediatric setting: a systematic literature review. *J Hosp Infect* 2016;**93**:159–163.

Chapter 42C

Hand Hygiene in Long-Term Care Facilities and Home Care

Maria Luisa Moro,[1] Marie-Noëlle Chraïti,[2] and Benedetta Allegranzi[3]

[1] Health and Social Agency Emilia-Romagna Region, Bologna, Italy

[2] Infection Control Program and WHO Collaborating Centre on Patient Safety, University of Geneva Hospitals and Faculty of Medicine, Geneva, Switzerland

[3] Infection Prevention and Control Global Unit, Department of Service Delivery and Safety, World Health Organization, and Faculty of Medicine, University of Geneva, Geneva, Switzerland

KEY MESSAGES

- Healthcare workers' (HCWs') hands in long-term care facilities (LTCFs) are contaminated and likely to spread germs. Hence, best hand hygiene practices are necessary when and where care is delivered.

- As in acute care settings, system change is a prerequisite to expect further improvement in hand hygiene.

- Results of studies based on multimodal interventions to improve hand hygiene in LTCFs are positive and encouraging. Innovative and adapted strategies could help to overcome resource constraints and other specific issues.

In the past decades, health service systems in industrialized countries have undergone significant transformation, mainly due to the aging of the population, which has resulted in a larger demand for long-term care. *Long-term care* is a term that refers to a wide range of medical and social services, provided at a patient's home, in the community, in residential facilities, in nursing homes, or in other settings. The type of care provided in long-term care facilities (LTCFs) may be very heterogeneous, ranging from only minimal support for daily activities to full 24-hour skilled nursing care.

Hand Hygiene: A Handbook for Medical Professionals, First Edition.
Edited by Didier Pittet, John M. Boyce and Benedetta Allegranzi.
© 2017 John Wiley & Sons, Inc. Published 2017 by John Wiley & Sons, Inc.

The burden of healthcare-associated infections in LTCFs is considerable: in some settings endemic infection rates are comparable to those in acute care hospitals, while outbreaks are more frequent. In addition, high rates of colonization of residents with antimicrobial-resistant microorganisms have been reported, as well as inappropriate antimicrobial prescribing. Compared to acute care hospitals, infection control activities, including hand hygiene promotion, appear more difficult to implement in these settings for the following reasons: LTCFs are the permanent domicile for most of the residents, there are scarce resources, such as personnel, expertise, and diagnostic and supportive services, and no or poor coordination of medical care.

WHAT WE KNOW – THE EVIDENCE

Hand Contamination of Healthcare Workers in LTCFs

Due to the level of dependency, daily contacts between healthcare or social workers and residents of LTCFs are numerous; however, few studies have addressed the frequency of Healthcare workers' (HCWs') hand colonization. In a 162-bed LTCF in Michigan, Mody et al. found that HCWs' hands were frequently colonized at baseline with Gram-negative bacteria (66%), *Candida* spp. (41%), *Staphylococcus aureus* (20%), and vancomycin-resistant enterococci (9%). In a small study in a LTCF in Hong Kong, Ho et al. reported contamination of HCW hands and enteral feeding tubes.

Compliance with Hand Hygiene

Studies in different countries have shown that hand hygiene compliance in LTCFs is on average quite low in the absence of ad hoc interventions, ranging from 9.3% in Taiwan[1] to 14.7% in Canada and 17.5% in Italy, to 19.0% and 25.8% in two studies in Hong Kong.[2,3] Similarly, knowledge of hand hygiene principles has been reported to be inadequate among LTCFs' staff.[1,4]

Knowledge, perceptions, and beliefs influence infection control practice among HCWs in LTCFs: participants with a better perception of hand hygiene were more likely to appropriately use gloves, and the probability of reporting good fingernail traits was positively associated with a stronger belief that fingernails played a role in infection transmission.[5] Likewise, increased knowledge has been positively associated with increased hand hygiene compliance.[1]

Hand hygiene compliance can be effectively improved in LTCFs, through multimodal interventions and national campaigns. In Norway, a national campaign conducted both in acute care hospitals and nursing homes, using the same methodology (pre- and post-campaign surveys, an advertising campaign, focus groups, internet resources, and a hand hygiene package for local use), resulted in a significant increase in the consumption of hand antisepsis agents: among the

45 participating nursing homes, a relative increase of 451% in the use of those products was observed, compared with only 38% in hospitals.[6] A study based on multidisciplinary teams' visits to all LTCFs for elderly persons in Central Finland ($n = 123$) resulted in a significant increase in the mean amount of alcohol-based handrubs (ABHRs) used.[7]

The most frequently used components of multimodal campaigns effective in improving hand hygiene in LTCFs (Table 42C.1) include system change (easy access to ABHRs), educational programs with feedback of local hand hygiene compliance data, reminders in the workplace, and involvement of hand hygiene champions. Compliance significantly improved after these multimodal campaigns, but no study reported compliance rates higher than 60%.

Hand Hygiene and Infection Rates

The positive impact of increased hand hygiene compliance on infection rates in LTCFs has been reported both in observational and cluster-randomized controlled studies (Table 42C.1).[1–3,8,9] In particular, increased hand hygiene compliance had a significant effect on respiratory infections and on those caused by methicillin-resistant *S. aureus*.

Application of the WHO Multimodal Hand Hygiene Improvement Strategy

To achieve better compliance with hand hygiene in outpatient care, the WHO recommendations have been adapted to these particular settings,[10] providing adaptations of the "patient zone" concept and the WHO My Five Moments for Hand Hygiene approach in LTCFs and home care (see also Chapters 20 and 24).

In LTCFs, the application of the "patient zone" concept is particularly challenging. In specialized nursing homes where residents are mentally or physically disabled and mainly cared for in a dedicated space with dedicated equipment, these concepts and recommendations should be applied in the same way as for acute care hospitals. In the case of residential facilities where residents are semi-autonomous and live in a community, the hand hygiene recommendations are related only to situations where healthcare is delivered to residents (e.g., rehabilitation sessions, vital signs check) at the point of care.

The components for the effective multimodal strategies recommended by WHO in acute care hospitals are the same in LTCFs, including evaluation and feedback. However, monitoring ABHR or soap consumption may need to be adapted to the available resources and expertise, thus focusing on the most frequent and relevant hand hygiene opportunities occurring in these settings.[10]

Table 42C.1 Hand Hygiene Compliance and Healthcare-associated Infections Rates in LTCFs; Selected Studies

Author, Publication Year (Ref.)	Study Design	Study Population	Intervention Components	Hand Hygiene Compliance (% of Observed Opportunities)	Infection Rates
Loeb M, 2003[8]	Prospective study	50 LTCFs (Canada and USA), 9156 residents	The effect of increased staffing, antibacterial soap use, number of sinks among LTCFs was studied		Reduced risk of MRSA Reduced risk of TMP-SMX R Enterobacteriaceae
Huang TT, 2008[1]	Before/after study	3 LTCFs (Taiwan)	Staff education (lectures, hands-on training, written manual); feedback; engineering controls and reminders (verbal and posters)	9.3% (pre-intervention), 30.4% (postintervention)	From 1.74% (December 2004 to February 2005) and 2.04% (June 2005 to August 2005) to 1.52% (December 2005 to February 2006) ($P<0.001$)
Schweon SJ, 2012[9]	Before/after study	1 skilled nursing facility (USA)	Touch-free dispensers throughout the facility; alcohol-based sanitizing wipes in resident common areas; educational program for all HCPs; posters promoting hand hygiene; a champion identified each month among HCPs to advocate hand hygiene; educational information to residents; monthly hand hygiene compliance monitoring	54% (during the intervention only)	From 0.97 to 0.53 infections per 1000 resident days ($P=0.01$)

| Yeung WK, 2011[2] | Cluster RCT | 6 LTCFs, recruited via snowball sampling, 3 intervention and 3 control (Hong Kong) | The treatment group received a multifaceted hand hygiene intervention program, including a free supply of pocket-sized containers of ABHR, a 2-hour seminar on hand hygiene, posters, and specially designed ballpoint pens that served as reminders. LTCFs in the control group received a basic life support program, including 3 identical workshops on resuscitation knowledge and skills | Intervention group: handrubbing: from 1.5% to 15.9% ($P=0.001$) Handwashing: from 24.3% to 17.4% ($P<0.001$). Hand hygiene overall: from 25.8% to 33.3% ($P<0.01$) Control group: Handwashing: from 25.8% to 30% (ns) | Serious infections decreased from 1.42 cases to 0.65 cases per 1000 resident-days in the intervention group ($P=0.002$), compared to 0.49 cases pre- to 1.05 cases per 1000 resident-days post-in the control group ($P=0.004$). In the treatment group, reduction of pneumonia and death rate attributable to infection (not in the control group) |

(continued)

Table 42C.1 (*Continued*)

Author, Publication Year (Ref.)	Study Design	Study Population	Intervention Components	Hand Hygiene Compliance (% of Observed Opportunities)	Infection Rates
Ho ML, 2012[3]	Cluster RCT	18 LTCFs randomly allocated to 2 intervention arms and a control arm (Hong Kong)	Both intervention arms: 100-mL pocket-size and 500-mL pump-size ABHR; posters and reminders; 2-hour health talk; video clips tailormade; hand inspection cabinet and fluorescent dye as training aids; train-the-trainer approach and provided training materials to each intervention home; immediate feedback to HCPs; performance reports. Intervention arm 1: slightly powdered gloves. Intervention arm 2: powder-less gloves. Control arm: A different 2-hour health talk was delivered by trained infection control nurses to HCWs of each control home	Intervention arm 1: from 27.0% to 60.6% ($P<0.001$) Intervention arm 2: from 22.2% to 48.6% ($P<0.001$) Control arm: from 19.5% to 21.6%	Respiratory outbreaks (IRR, 0.12; 95% CI, 0.01–0.93; $P=0.04$) and MRSA infections requiring hospital admission (IRR, 0.61; 95% CI, 0.38–0.97; $P=0.04$) were reduced after intervention

Abbreviations used: LTCFs, long-term care facilities; HCP, healthcare practitioner; RCT, randomized controlled trial; ABHR, alcohol-based handrub; MRSA, methicillin-resistant *Staphylococcus aureus*; TMP-SMX R, trimetoprim-sulfamethoxazole resistant.

WHAT WE DO NOT KNOW – THE UNCERTAIN

In recent years, studies have focused on healthcare-associated infections and hand hygiene in LTCFs; however, available evidence remains limited to selected countries, and studies in home care are scanty.

Determinants of hand hygiene behavior in LTCFs and home care have been unevenly studied; more data on perception, attitudes, and beliefs affecting hand hygiene behavior in these settings would be useful to develop effective interventions.

Data available on effective interventions in LTCFs are encouraging; however, evidence is still scarce on the applicability of these interventions to other countries and settings, where LTCFs have different cultural, environmental, organizational, socioeconomic characteristics, and specific regional or national policies.

Similarly, interventions shown to be effective so far are quite resource-demanding, including education, reminders, and direct observation and feedback; given the lack of resources in LTCFs, innovative strategies should be developed and tested to promote hand hygiene compliance in all LTCFs and to sustain it over time.

RESEARCH AGENDA

Further well-designed studies are required, both in LTCFs and home care, to better elucidate:

- The burden of infections;
- The role of hand contamination on infection cross-transmission;
- The determinants of hand hygiene behavior and the best approaches to behavioral change;
- The cost-effectiveness of hand hygiene programs;
- The effectiveness of hand hygiene interventions in home care;
- The applicability of multifaceted intervention programs.

REFERENCES

1. Huang TT, Wu SC, Evaluation of a training programme on knowledge and compliance of nurse assistants' hand hygiene in nursing homes. *J Hosp Infect* 2008;**68**:164–170.
2. Yeung WK, Tam WS, Wong TW, Clustered randomized controlled trial of a hand hygiene intervention involving pocket-sized containers of alcohol-based handrub for the control of infections in long-term care facilities. *Infect Control Hosp Epidemiol* 2011;**32**:67–76.
3. Ho ML, Seto WH, Wong LC, et al., Effectiveness of multifaceted hand hygiene interventions in long-term care facilities in Hong Kong: a cluster-randomized controlled trial. *Infect Control Hosp Epidemiol* 2012;**33**:761–767.

4. Ashraf MS, Hussain SW, Agarwal N, et al., Hand hygiene in long-term care facilities: a multicenter study of knowledge, attitudes, practices, and barriers. *Infect Control Hosp Epidemiol* 2010;**31**:758–762.

5. Aiello AE, Malinis M, Knapp JK, et al., The influence of knowledge, perceptions, and beliefs, on hand hygiene practices in nursing homes. *Am J Infect Control* 2009;**37**:164–167.

6. Kacelnik O, Førland OJ, Iversen B, Evaluation of the national campaign to improve hand hygiene in nursing homes in Norway. *J Hosp Infect* 2011;**77**:359–360.

7. Rummukainen M, Jakobsson A, Karppi P, et al., Promoting hand hygiene and prudent use of antimicrobials in long-term care facilities. *Am J Infect Control* 2009;**37**:168–171.

8. Loeb MB, Craven S, McGeer AJ, et al., Risk factors for resistance to antimicrobial agents among nursing home residents. *Am J Epidemiol* 2003;**157**:40–47.

9. Schweon SJ, Edmonds SL, Kirk J, et al., Effectiveness of a comprehensive hand hygiene program for reduction of infection rates in a long-term care facility. *Am J Infect Control* 2013;**41**:39–44.

10. World Health Organization, *WHO Hand Hygiene in Outpatient and Home-based Care and Long-Term Care Facilities: a Guide to the Application of the WHO Multimodal Hand Hygiene Improvement.* Geneva: WHO, 2012.

ADDITIONAL REFERENCES

11. Montoya A, Mody L, Common infections in nursing homes: a review of current issues and challenges. *Aging Health* 2011;**7**:889–899.

12. Moro ML, Gagliotti C, Antimicrobial resistance and stewardship in long-term care settings. *Future Microbiol* 2013;**8**:1011–1025.

13. Mody L, McNeil SA, Sun R, et al., Introduction of a waterless alcohol-based handrub in a long-term-care facility. *Infect Control Hosp Epidemiol* 2003;**24**:165–171.

14. Ho SS, Tse MM, Boost MV, Effect of an infection control programme on bacterial contamination of enteral feed in nursing homes. *J Hosp Infect* 2012;**82**:49–55.

15. Smith A, Carusone SC, Loeb M, Hand hygiene practices of health care workers in long-term care facilities. *Am J Infect Control* 2008;**36**:492–494.

16. Pan A, Domenighini F, Signorini L, et al., Adherence to hand hygiene in an Italian long-term care facility. *Am J Infect Control* 2008;**36**:495–497.

Chapter 42D

Hand Hygiene in Ambulatory Care

Marie-Noëlle Chraïti,[1] Sepideh Bagheri Nejad,[2] and Benedetta Allegranzi[3]

[1] *Infection Control Program and WHO Collaborating Centre on Patient Safety, University of Geneva Hospitals, Geneva, Switzerland*
[2] *Department of Service Delivery and Safety, World Health Organization, Geneva, Switzerland*
[3] *Infection Prevention and Control Global Unit, Department of Service Delivery and Safety, World Health Organization, and Faculty of Medicine, University of Geneva, Geneva, Switzerland*

KEY MESSAGES

- Although the transmission risk may vary in different situations, hand hygiene is as important in ambulatory care as in hospital care to prevent microbial cross-transmission and healthcare-associated infection (HAI).

- The WHO concept of My Five Moments for Hand Hygiene addresses most of the needs for hand hygiene in ambulatory care.

- Adaptations to implement multimodal approaches to improve hand hygiene in ambulatory care are necessary; however, key principles applied in the acute care hospital settings remain essential, and their application leads to successful improvements.

The majority of patients seeking healthcare are cared for in ambulatory settings, which are usually the first level of contact with the health system. Ambulatory settings include specialized settings such as hospital outpatient departments, polyclinics, general practitioners' offices, physical therapy and rehabilitation centers, as well as a large variety of settings and clinics. The risk of HAI in ambulatory care is commonly estimated to be low. However, the magnitude of the problem is not well understood, due to the lack of data. There are few reports, in particular of outbreaks, suggesting that HAIs also have to be addressed in ambulatory

Hand Hygiene: A Handbook for Medical Professionals, First Edition.
Edited by Didier Pittet, John M. Boyce and Benedetta Allegranzi.
© 2017 John Wiley & Sons, Inc. Published 2017 by John Wiley & Sons, Inc.

care. It has been demonstrated that healthcare workers' (HCWs') hands play an important role in the genesis of outbreaks.[1] Therefore, hand hygiene appears to be as important as in inpatient settings to prevent cross-transmission of pathogens.

WHAT WE KNOW – THE EVIDENCE

Practitioners' and other HCWs' hands have been shown to be contaminated by potential pathogens in various outpatient settings such as ophthalmologic, pediatric, hemodialysis, or dermatology clinics, as reported in the World Health Organization (WHO) guidance document on hand hygiene in outpatient care.[2] Moreover, several studies showed that hand hygiene compliance in ambulatory care is poor, sometimes well below 50%.[3,4] In a recent study conducted in the United States,[5] the assessment of infection control practices in ambulatory surgical centers highlighted important lapses, including poor hand hygiene and low use of personal protective equipment. However, it has been recently demonstrated that improvement can be achieved.

Significant increase in hand hygiene compliance was observed in two outpatient clinics following the introduction of alcohol-based handrub (ABHR) and informational posters; improvement was maintained in the follow-up period.[4] A Spanish study performed in primary care also showed the positive impact of a multimodal strategy; hand hygiene compliance improved from 8% to 21%.[3] Another study demonstrated enhanced compliance by medical doctors in an otolaryngology outpatient department following education and the increased availability of ABHR in the patient care area.[6] While pointing out low baseline hand hygiene compliance in ambulatory care, the interventional studies cited above demonstrate that multifaceted approaches are required to improve hand hygiene in the ambulatory care context.

To achieve practices improvement, WHO recommends an evidence-based multimodal strategy that includes the following components: system change; education and training; evaluation and performance feedback; reminders in the workplace; and an institutional safety climate (see also Chapter 33). With adaptation to the peculiarities of ambulatory care settings, this approach can be used in outpatient facilities, and the concept of My Five Moments for Hand Hygiene (see also Chapter 20) remains at the core of the strategy to change HCWs' behavior. Specific adaptations have been identified by WHO; for instance, in most ambulatory care settings, the understanding of *patient zone, healthcare area*, and *critical sites* might be slightly different, which in turn affects the application of the My Five Moments for Hand Hygiene approach. In this perspective, WHO has developed a range of practical examples and visuals (Figures 42D.1 and 42D.2) of care situations to show how the My Five Moments for Hand Hygiene approach can be practiced in specific situations typically occurring in outpatient care.[3] There are situations where a large number of patients undergo a care procedure one after the other, and thus hand hygiene indications occur with very high frequency in a short time period. In other

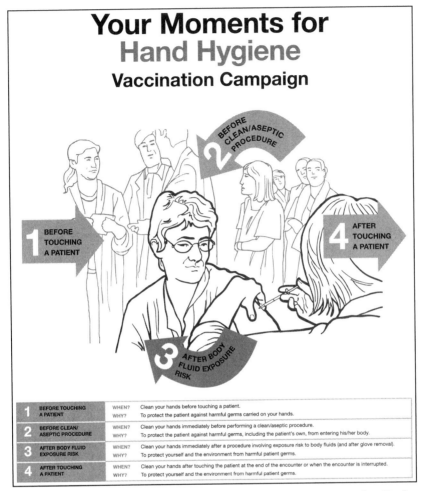

Figure 42D.1   Hand hygiene indications in the context of a vaccination campaign. Hand Hygiene in Outpatient and Home-Based Care and Long-Term Care Facilities: A Guide to the Application of the WHO Multimodal Hand Hygiene Improvement Strategy and the "My Five Moments for Hand Hygiene" Approach. WHO, 2012. *Source*: Reproduced with permission from the World Health Organization.
Additional figures illustrating other care situations in outpatient settings are available in the guidance document cited above. *See plate section for color representation of this figure.*

examples, the care situation is very similar to the hospital setting (e.g., dialysis, childbirth delivery in remote areas in low- or middle-income dispensaries). These examples form a basis for acquiring the skills to identify the patient zone and the point of care, as well as hand hygiene indications and opportunities encountered.

The principles of hand hygiene and broader infection prevention and control measures (including standard precautions) must be followed to ensure safe care in

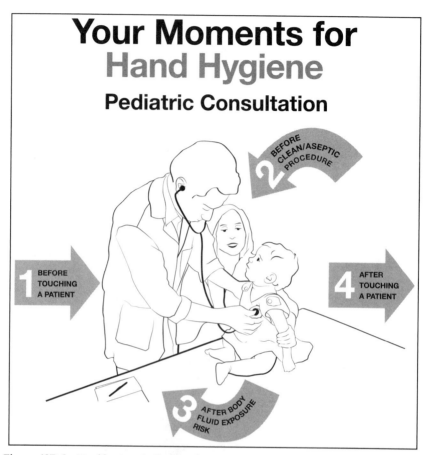

Figure 42D.2 Hand hygiene indications during a pediatric consultation. Hand Hygiene in Outpatient and Home-Based Care and Long-Term Care Facilities: A Guide to the Application of the WHO Multimodal Hand Hygiene Improvement Strategy and the "My Five Moments for Hand Hygiene" Approach. WHO, 2012. *Source*: Reproduced with permission from the World Health Organization.
Additional figures illustrating other care situations in outpatient settings are available in the guidance document cited above. *See plate section for color representation of this figure.*

ambulatory care settings. The US Centers for Disease Control and Prevention (CDC) recently issued a guide to infection prevention in outpatient settings accompanied by an implementation checklist.[7,8] Japanese specialized guidelines in urology also emphasize infection prevention in both ambulatory and hospital practice.[9]

WHAT WE DO NOT KNOW – THE UNCERTAIN

First of all, the main challenge remains to measure the importance of hands and other means of microbial transmission in ambulatory settings, especially beyond outbreak situations. Surveillance of HAI is difficult in ambulatory settings, due to the patient's short stay in this type of setting and to the difficulties in distinguishing healthcare-associated from community-acquired infections. Furthermore, a few studies have reported hand hygiene compliance data using standardized methods. This assessment is usually not performed in outpatient settings due to a range of difficulties (e.g., lack of human resources, expertise, and time) in undertaking direct observations. Therefore, the best methodology to monitor hand hygiene in outpatient settings has not been clearly identified yet, although WHO proposes simplified monitoring approaches.[2] However, the adaptability of the WHO standardized method remains to be piloted in outpatient care. As a consequence of these limitations in the monitoring of outcomes and practices, limited data are available on the impact of poor hand hygiene on HAI rates in ambulatory care.

Environmental contamination plays a relevant role in microbial cross-transmission. In outpatient care, patients are potentially exposed to contaminated surfaces, be it because of suboptimal environmental hygiene, or of medical devices and items not discarded or decontaminated after use. In such a context, the risk of germ cross-transmission by contact is high, regardless of HCWs' compliance with hand hygiene. Therefore, hand hygiene improvement efforts need to be synergized with improved environmental cleaning. A recent overview of infections due to methicillin-resistant *Staphylococcus aureus* related to manual therapy (i.e. physical therapy chiropractic) highlights the basic necessity of hand hygiene and environmental cleaning to prevent cross-contamination and spread from one person to another.[10]

Empowerment of patients and relatives could have a critical effect on hand hygiene improvement strategies; education on hand transmission prevention should be part of the essential information provided to limit microbial spread (see also Chapter 30). Indeed, the boundaries between ambulatory care and community life are very loose, and this can influence infection spread in both settings. However, limited data are available on effective strategies to involve patients and families in hand hygiene improvement and implementation of additional infection prevention measures.

The diversity of ambulatory care settings around the world, providing primary to tertiary care as well as preventive to invasive care, is another challenge to overcome. The risk of cross-transmission can vary significantly due to diversity in infrastructures, type and intensity of care, patient populations, and the education level of care providers. Hence, it is not obvious to implement hand hygiene improvement multimodal strategies without adapting them to the particular contexts. It is also difficult to develop standard methods to measure the impact of hand hygiene. Hand hygiene improvement in ambulatory care may also depend on the structure of the health system and how the ambulatory care settings are embedded into the national system, as some centers are quite isolated from nationally coordinated healthcarel systems.

RESEARCH AGENDA

Further research is needed in the following areas:

- The impact of hand hygiene improvement on HAI. Some of the critical points are to develop suitable and validated approaches and protocols for both hand hygiene monitoring and HAI surveillance with definition criteria specific to ambulatory care. Moreover, these should be adaptable to fit a broad range of settings and type of care.

- The importance of hand hygiene versus environmental hygiene versus the level of patient personal hygiene on microbial transmission should be further defined. Each of these aspects should be studied to explore their respective and combined impact.

- The patient's role in hand hygiene promotion and improvement in ambulatory care, both as a trigger for improving HCWs' hand hygiene and as an action for the patient's own protection, deserves further research.

- The importance of policies and political decisions targeted to ambulatory care systems to influence implementation and sustainability of hand hygiene programs needs to be assessed.

REFERENCES

1. Greeley RD, Semple S, Thompson ND, et al., Hepatitis B outbreak associated with hemato-oncology office practice in New Jersey, 2009. *Am J Infect Control* 2011;**39**:663–670.
2. World Health Organization, *WHO Hand Hygiene in Outpatient and Home-Based Care and Long-Term Care Facilities: a Guide to the Application of the WHO Multimodal Hand Hygiene Improvement Strategy and the "My Five Moments for Hand Hygiene" Approach.* Geneva: WHO, 2012. Available at www.who.int/gpsc/5may/en/index.html. Accessed March 7, 2017.
3. Martin-Madrazo C, Soto-Díaz S, Cañada-Dorado A, et al., Cluster randomized trial to evaluate the effect of a multimodal hand hygiene improvement strategy in primary care. *Infect Control Hosp Epidemiol* 2012;**33**:681–688.
4. Kukanich KS, Kaur R, Freeman LC, et al., Evaluation of a hand hygiene campaign in outpatient healthcare clinics. *Am J Nurs* 2013;**113**:36–42.
5. Schaefer MK, Jhung M, Dahl M, et al., Infection control assessment of ambulatory surgical centers. *JAMA* 2010;**303**:2273–2279.
6. Robertson G, Hathorn I, Ryan K, et al., Hand hygiene compliance in otolaryngology outpatients: how we do it. *Clin Otolaryngol* 2009;**34**:250–253.
7. Centers for Disease Control and Prevention, *CDC Guide to Infection Prevention in Outpatient Settings: Minimum Expectations for Safe Care.* 2011. Available at www.cdc.gov/HAI/settings/outpatient/outpatient-care-guidelines.html. Accessed March 7, 2017.

8. Centers for Disease Control and Prevention, *Infection Prevention Checklist for Outpatient Settings: Minimum Expectations for Safe Care*. Available at www.cdc.gov/HAI/settings/outpatient/outpatient-care-guidelines.html, Accessed March 7, 2017.

9. Hamasuna R, Takahashi S, Yamamoto S, et al., Guideline for the prevention of healthcare-associated infection in urological practice in Japan. *Int J Urol*, 2011;**18**:495–502.

10. Green BN, Johnson CD, Egan JT , et al., Methicillin-resistant *Staphylococcus aureus*: an overview for manual therapists. *J Chiropr Med* 2012;**11**:64–76.

Chapter 42E

Hand Hygiene in Hemodialysis

Marie-Noëlle Chraïti,[1] Sepideh Bagheri Nejad,[2] and Benedetta Allegranzi[3]

[1] Infection Control Program and WHO Collaborating Centre on Patient Safety, University of Geneva Hospitals, Geneva, Switzerland

[2] Department of Service Delivery and Safety, World Health Organization, Geneva, Switzerland

[3] Infection Prevention and Control Global Unit, Department of Service Delivery and Safety, World Health Organization, and Faculty of Medicine, University of Geneva, Geneva, Switzerland

KEY MESSAGES

- Hand hygiene is an important measure to prevent the transmission of viral and bacterial infections, and to limit the spread of multidrug-resistant organisms in hemodialysis facilities.

- The World Health Organization (WHO) My Five Moments for Hand Hygiene approach fully applies in hemodialysis settings and is recommended as part of Standard Operating Procedures related to hemodialysis.

- Glove use is essential in hemodialysis care and should be carefully managed considering hand hygiene requirements.

Viral hepatitis and bloodstream infections are the most frequent infectious complications of hemodialysis, mostly due to contaminated blood or associated with endovascular access. Another issue in hemodialysis settings is the spread of multidrug-resistant organisms as a consequence of the widespread use of antibiotics. Numerous outbreaks have been reported in hemodialysis facilities, frequently due to hepatitis viruses or multidrug-resistant bacteria, as recently illustrated by the Middle-East Respiratory Syndrome Coronavirus (MERS-CoV) infection confirmed in nine hemodialysis patients in a hospital in the Kingdom of Saudi Arabia. Hemodialysis is a multistep, complex, and invasive procedure

Hand Hygiene: A Handbook for Medical Professionals, First Edition.
Edited by Didier Pittet, John M. Boyce and Benedetta Allegranzi.
© 2017 John Wiley & Sons, Inc. Published 2017 by John Wiley & Sons, Inc.

that patients with acute or chronic renal failure undergo repeatedly. Under such conditions, the risk of exposure to blood is high both for the patient and the healthcare worker (HCW). Therefore, the requirements for equipment and asepsis are very strict in order to manage and prevent this risk.

WHAT WE KNOW – THE EVIDENCE

The recommendations of the US Centers for Disease Control and Prevention (CDC) for the prevention of cross-transmission among chronic hemodialysis patients[1] are based on several decades of hemodialysis-associated infection surveillance demonstrating that viral or bacterial pathogens are essentially transmitted by contact. Consequently, most of the risk can be prevented by applying standard precautions, including hand hygiene, in addition to environmental cleaning, clean water supply, and equipment management.

The risk of pathogen transmission in hemodialysis settings has been demonstrated in several outbreaks. For instance, artificial fingernails were proven to be the source of a cluster of Gram-negative bacteremia in five hemodialysis patients.[2] A more recent study showed the increased risk of hepatitis C virus infection in an outpatient hemodialysis center where patients shared a limited space, equipment, and staff, with the latter being the identified source.[3] In this study, several infection control breaches, including hand hygiene and glove use, were identified during care preparation and delivery. Additionally, low compliance with hand hygiene was observed using a modified version of the World Health Organization (WHO) hand hygiene observation method.[4] These findings led to the same conclusions shown in a mathematical model to estimate the nontransfusion, nosocomial transmission of hepatitis C virus, based on contact transmission.[5]

Due to the high exposure risk to blood in hemodialysis, the CDC guidelines emphasized the use of gloves when delivering care to the patient and touching patient equipment, followed by hand hygiene after their removal. This recommendation is certainly appropriate to achieve maximum HCW protection, but can also lead to hand hygiene lapses. An observational multicenter study in 2005 reported poor hand hygiene compliance in all steps of hemodialysis sessions while compliance with glove use was greater than 80%.[6] Recently, an investigation of knowledge, attitudes, and practices of HCWs in hemodialysis units revealed that inappropriate reliance on glove use can jeopardize compliance with hand hygiene and may thus lead to cross-transmission of infectious agents.[7]

The importance of hand hygiene as the single most effective measure to prevent healthcare-associated infections has been emphasized in the WHO guidelines. The WHO concept of My Five Moments for Hand Hygiene (see Chapter 20) fully applies to hemodialysis (Figure 42E.1). It is important to highlight that hand hygiene indications exist regardless of glove use (see Chapter 23).

As in other in- and outpatient settings, there is a need for a sustainable multimodal approach to improve hand hygiene in hemodialysis. Scheithauer

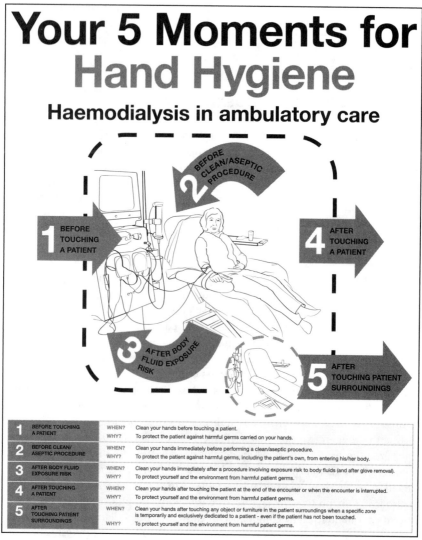

Figure 42E.1   Hand hygiene indications in the context of haemodialysis. WHO Hand Hygiene in Outpatient and Home-Based Care and Long-Term Care Facilities: a Guide to the Application of the WHO Multimodal Hand Hygiene Improvement Strategy and the My Five Moments for Hand Hygiene Approach 2012. *Source*: Reproduced with permission from the World Health Organization. *See plate section for color representation of this figure.*

et al. applied a multimodal strategy including individual and group training on hand hygiene, direct observations with feedback, and implementation of standard operating procedures for dialysis connections and disconnections; this intervention led to a significant increase in hand hygiene compliance.[4] In particular, standard operating procedures allowed a better organization and streamlining of the workflow, which subsequently led to a decrease in the number of hand hygiene opportunities and improvement in compliance, especially regarding the indication "before a clean/aseptic task," when HCWs have critical and high infectious risk contacts with patients.

WHO has developed a number of tools to support the implementation of hand hygiene promotion programs in outpatient care and to help HCWs adopt the "My Five Moments for Hand Hygiene" approach in these settings. In hemodialysis, the WHO approach to hand hygiene best practices takes the hemodialysis sequence into account[8] and proposes specific moments for hand hygiene action within the

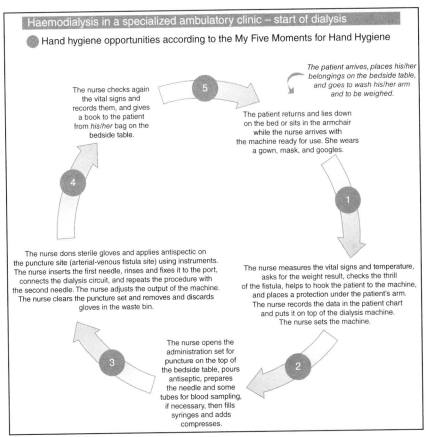

Figure 42E.2   Hand hygiene opportunities in the context of haemodialysis. WHO hand hygiene in outpatient and home-based care and long-term care facilities: a guide to the application of the WHO Multimodal Hand Hygiene Improvement Strategy and the My Five Moments for Hand Hygiene approach 2012. *Source*: Reproduced with permission from the World Health Organization. Figures illustrating the other sessions of hemodialysis are available in the guidance document cited above.

usual workflow of a dialysis session. Some of these steps (Figure 42E.2), that is, start of dialysis, during dialysis, end of dialysis, after dialysis, include the critical access to the endovascular system either through a graft or a catheter. The specific cross-transmission risk related to the percutaneous procedure can be prevented by implementing and applying an infection-control bundle including appropriate hand hygiene.[9,10] Participation in an infection-control collaborative program has been shown to reduce infections.[9,10]

WHAT WE DO NOT KNOW – THE UNCERTAIN

The impact of hand hygiene performance on dialysis-associated infections remains unknown, as well as the level of compliance needed to decrease infection rates. Currently, most infection-prevention measures in dialysis are bundled on the basis of CDC recommendations,[1] and hand hygiene is one of the process indicators evaluated. The study conducted by Scheithauer is a rare example of an intervention focusing on hand hygiene improvement only.[4] Given the paucity of such studies, further research regarding the impact of hand hygiene on dialysis-associated infections is needed. Moreover, considering the risk of transmission by contact, environmental contamination plays an important role in hemodialysis. However, no investigation so far has focused on the relative impact of hand hygiene and environmental cleaning on infections transmitted in these settings.

RESEARCH AGENDA

Further research is needed in the following areas:

- The impact of hand hygiene improvement on dialysis-associated infections.
- The importance of hand hygiene versus environmental hygiene on microbial transmission.
- The most successful strategies to achieve hand hygiene improvement and embed it in the workflow of a dialysis session.
- The role of patient empowerment in achieving best hand hygiene practices in hemodialysis.

REFERENCES

1. Centers for Disease Control and Prevention. CDC, Recommendations for preventing transmission of infections among chronic hemodialysis patients. *Morb Mortal Wkly Rep* 2001;**50**(RR-5):1–43.
2. Gordin FM, Schultz ME, Huber R, et al., A cluster of hemodialysis-related bacteremia linked to artificial fingernails. *Infect Control Hosp Epidemiol* 2007;**28**:743–744.

3. Rao AK, Luckman E, Wise ME, et al., Outbreak of hepatitis C virus infections at an outpatient hemodialysis facility: the importance of infection control competencies. *Nephrol Nurs J* 2013;**40**:101–110.

4. Scheithauer S, Eitner F, Mankartz J, et al., Improving hand hygiene compliance rates in the hemodialysis setting: more than just more hand rubs. *Nephrol Dialysis Transpl* 2012;**27**:766–770.

5. Laporte F, Tap G, Jaafar A, et al., Mathematical modeling of hepatitis C virus transmission in hemodialysis. *Am J Infect Control* 2009;**37**:403–407.

6. Arenas MD, Sanchez-Paya J, Barril G, et al., A multicentric survey of the practice of hand hygiene in haemodialysis units: factors affecting compliance. *Nephrol Dialysis Transpl* 2005;**20**:1164–1171.

7. Bianco A, Bova F, Nobile CG, et al., Healthcare workers and prevention of hepatits C virus transmission: exploring knowledge and evidence-based practices in hemodialysis units in Italy. *BMC Infect Dis* 2013;**13**:76.

8. World Health Organization, *WHO Hand Hygiene in Outpatient and Home-Based Care and Long-Term Care Facilities: A Guide to the Application of the WHO Multimodal Hand Hygiene Improvement Strategy and the "My Five Moments for Hand Hygiene" Approach.* Geneva: WHO, 2012. Available at www.who.int/gpsc/5may/en/index.html. Accessed March 7, 2017.

9. CDC, Reducing BSI in outpatient hemodialysis center. *Morb Mortal Wkly Rep* 2012;**61**:169–173.

10. Lindberg C, Downham G, Buscell P, et al., Embracing collaboration: a novel strategy for reducing bloodstream infections in outpatient hemodialysis centers. *Am J Infect Control* 2013;**41**;513–519.

Hand Hygiene in Specific Patient Populations and Situations: Anesthesiology

François Stéphan

Réanimation adulte, Centre Chirurgical Marie Lannelongue, Le Plessis Robinson, France

KEY MESSAGES

- Hand hygiene compliance is almost universally low among anesthesia providers.
- Studies have demonstrated that anesthesia providers are implicated in cross-contamination.
- Use of point-of-care alcohol-based handrubs significantly facilitates hand hygiene performance and could reduce cross-transmission.

Anesthesiologists play a central role in the perioperative management of patients in the operating room (OR), in the post-anesthesia care unit (PACU), and often in surgical wards. The risk of infection related to the anesthesia act itself is poorly understood, and few studies have been published on this topic.

WHAT WE KNOW – THE EVIDENCE

Perception of Hygiene by Anesthesiologists

Medical television programs do not help to understand the importance of hygiene recommendations. Even in the highly popular television program *Emergency Room*,

Hand Hygiene: A Handbook for Medical Professionals, First Edition.
Edited by Didier Pittet, John M. Boyce and Benedetta Allegranzi.
© 2017 John Wiley & Sons, Inc. Published 2017 by John Wiley & Sons, Inc.

Table 42F.1   Indications for Hand Hygiene (Adapted from ASA/ASA Committees/Recommendations for Infection Control for the Practice of Anesthesiology)

Indications for Hand Hygiene	The Five Moments (M) for Hand Hygiene (according to WHO)
Before and after direct contact with patients	M1–M4
Before donning sterile gloves	M1–M2
After contact with body fluids, nonintact skin, mucous membranes, wound dressings	M3
When hands that have contacted a contaminated body area will subsequently contact a clean site	M3
After contact with high-touch environmental surfaces in the vicinity of the patients	M5
After removal of gloves	M3
Before eating	
After using restroom	*Does not correspond to any of M1 to M5 of WHO*

REMEMBER:

- Spore-forming organisms such as *Clostridium difficile* and *Bacillus anthracis* are poorly inactivated by alcohol-based hand rub
- Gloves should be worn whenever any contact with blood, body fluids, mucous membranes, nonintact skin, or other potentially infectious material is anticipated

Source: Adapted from Stackhouse 2010 with permission.

only 0.20% of opportunities for hand hygiene were actually taken into account! Few data exist on the perception of hygiene measures by anesthesiologists. On a scale of 10, the average rate was 4.7 ± 0.12 for North American anesthesiologists, while the median was 3 (interquartile range 2–6) for English anesthesiologists. How to explain this observation? Anesthesiologists only rarely witness healthcare-associated infections (HAIs) in direct relation to their practice. Moreover, by applying their usual procedures – good or bad – anesthesiologists do not have the feeling of jeopardizing patients' prognosis. Finally, the recommendations of several anesthesia societies on hygiene measures are known by less than 50% of anesthesia providers (Table 42F.1 and Figure 42F.1).

The Risk Does Exist in the Operating Room (OR) and Post-Anesthesia Care Unit (PACU)

On a few occasions, anesthesiology personnel have been identified as the source of infections acquired in the OR. For example, an anesthesia physician with lesions on his hand and skin that harbored a T28 strain of *Streptococcus pyogenes*

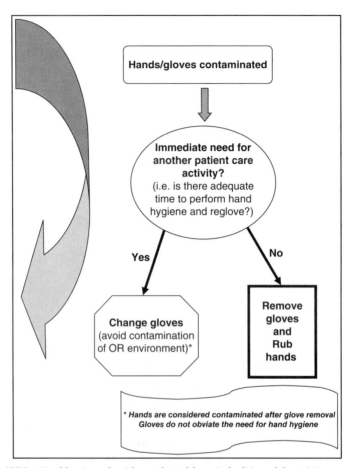

Figure 42F.1   Hand hygiene algorithm (adapted from 3rd edition of the ASA's Recommendations for Infection Control for the Practice of Anesthesiology. *Source*: Adapted from Stackhouse 2010 with permission.

was identified as the source of streptococcal pelvic infections in parturient women.[1] Anesthesiology personnel who had asymptomatic anal, vaginal, or throat carriage or skin lesions due to *S. pyogenes* have also been the source of a number of other outbreaks of streptococcal infections acquired in the OR.[2] In addition, anesthesia personnel whose aseptic technique was suboptimal have been epidemiologically implicated in outbreaks of infections related to contaminated propofol administered in the OR.[3]

Hajjar et al. conducted a study to determine the incidence and risk factors for nosocomial infections related to anesthesia.[4] They reported an incidence of 3.4 infections per 1000 in a group of 7,339 patients. This study provides confirmation of the reality of the infectious risk in relation to anesthesia practice. Loftus et al.

Table 42F.2   Potentially Contaminated Environmental Surfaces and Elements Considered as Possible Sources of Cross-Transmission in the Operating Room

Anesthesia machine

- Adjustable pressure-limiting valve
- Agent dial

Patients' files
Patients' hands, body and devices
Personal in-hospital mobile phone
Fixed phone
Computer keyboard

demonstrated that the anesthesia environmental work area becomes significantly contaminated with potential pathogens in as little as 4 min (Table 42F.2).[5] Moreover, peripheral intravenous tubing (stopcock sets) became contaminated with potentially pathologic bacteria in 23% to 32% of cases. As the bacterial burden increased, so did the probability of obtaining a positive stopcock.

The PACU represents a potential setting for bacterial cross-contamination.[6] Rogues et al. studied the risk of nosocomial transmission linked to a stay in the PACU.[7] During 3 weeks, 75 patients were studied. Potentially pathogenic bacteria were identified in 25 patients on admission and 31 patients at PACU discharge. In 13 patients, bacteria were thought to have been acquired in the PACU. It is important to note that none was the cause of HAI. This work demonstrates that the PACU could be a link in the chain of cross-transmission.[7]

Compliance with Hand Hygiene is Very Poor

Although hand hygiene is the primary measure for the prevention of HAI,[8] anesthesia providers fail to perform hand hygiene properly. In a study published in 2004, Pittet et al. documented a low compliance rate among anesthesiologists (23.3%) compared with physicians belonging to other disciplines (in whom compliance rate reached as high as 80%). In a recent study from Germany,[9] the observed baseline hand hygiene compliance was 10%, but significantly increased to 30% after implementation of a standard operating procedure. Likewise, in another study, hand hygiene application was 2% upon OR entrance and 8.4% upon leaving the OR. Another recent study reported that the rate of baseline hand hygiene events were extremely low (0.15–0.38 hourly hand cleansing).[10]

A study conducted in 2003 focused on hand hygiene in the PACU.[11] The results showed a particularly low compliance with hand hygiene both at time of patient admission (19.6%) and during stay (12.5%). Interestingly, a close relation between workload and the number of indications for hand cleansing was observed. Predictors independently associated with noncompliance at admission were older patients (>65 yrs), recovery from clean/clean-contaminated surgery, and high workload.[11]

Our Hands Are Not as Clean as We Think

In the study of Rogues,[7] 19% of anesthesiologists' hands were colonized with potentially pathogenic bacteria. Loftus et al. obtained samples from the hands of anesthesia providers as they entered the OR but before patient contact. Overall, 66% of provider hands were contaminated with one or more major pathogens (methicillin-resistant *Staphylococcus aureus*, vancomycin-resistant enterococci, Enterobacteriaceae). The increase in the duration of care was linearly associated with the bacterial contamination of nongloved hands.[8]

Hand Hygiene and the Risk for Cross-Contamination

Anesthesia providers were identified as the origin of bacterial transmission to the intraoperative environment in 12% of cases.[12] Specifically, anesthesia providers are implicated in 47% of cases of stopcock contamination. The environment was a source of stopcock contamination in about 50% of cases, while providers' hands were the source in 30%. Reflecting the efficacy of decontamination practices, contamination of the environment before a new case occurred in 7%.[12] When the provider source was excluded, independent predictors of environmental contamination included surgery involving the first case of the day, anesthesiologist supervision of more than one room, increasing patient age, and discharge to the ICU from the OR.[12]

Compliance Improvement Leads to Decreased Bacterial Contamination in the OR

Based on standard operating procedure implementation, a recent study demonstrated that by improving workflow practices in combination with direct observation and feedback at an individual level, compliance can be significantly improved by both decreasing the number of hand hygiene opportunities and increasing hand hygiene actions.[9] Hand hygiene compliance markedly improved (from 10% to 54%) during the study duration.[9] Moreover, this study also showed that hand hygiene compliance would have increased to 76% if all avoidable mistakes had been avoided.[9]

In a well-conducted before-and-after study, Koff et al. reported that baseline hand hygiene decontamination events were extremely low (0.15–0.38 per hour).[10] When the use of a point-of-care alcohol-based handrub (ABHR) dispenser was implemented, the hourly hand hygiene action events increased to 7.1–8.7. In other words, anesthesia providers improved compliance by approximately 6.9 to 8.3 times more per hour. As a consequence, use of the dispenser significantly reduced contamination of the anesthesia machine with an associated reduction in contamination of peripheral intravenous tubing.[10]

WHAT WE DO NOT KNOW – THE UNCERTAIN

The clinical research group at Dartmouth-Hitchcock Medical Center in Lebanon, New Hampshire, United States, found a significant association between the increasing magnitude of anesthesia work area contamination and contamination of peripheral intravenous tubing, likely due to the common denominator of variable aseptic practices of anesthesia providers.[13] Therefore, contaminated intravenous tubing was associated with a trend toward an increase in the incidence of HAI paralleled with an increased mortality. Again, HAI rates were reduced when point-of-care ABHRs were implemented. However, a direct link between the bacteria in contaminated stopcocks and the causative organisms associated with subsequent infections was not demonstrated. Moreover, the occurrence of hospital-acquired infections was not the primary endpoint of these studies.

RESEARCH AGENDA

Education and Promotion:
- Provide anesthesiologists with better education regarding the risk of hand contamination and subsequent cross-transmission.
- Assess the key determinants of hand hygiene among anesthesia providers.
- Implement different components of multimodal hand hygiene promotion programs in anesthesiology.
- Offer the possibility to promote the use of point-of-care alcohol-based handrub and research for the best options.
- Adapt the concept of the My Five Moments for Hand Hygiene to the practice of anaesthesiology within the OR.

Epidemiological Research and Development:
- Develop models (both clinical and experimental) to study cross-contamination from patient to patient and from environment to patients.
- Demonstrate that anesthesiologists could be directly implicated as the cause of surgical and nonsurgical infections.
- Identify the possible source of bacterial cross-transmission in the OR and PACU.

- Study the role of the bacterial "cloud" (spread by large droplets or airborne) in the development of healthcare-associated infections.
- Generate more definitive evidence for the impact of improved compliance with hand hygiene on infection rates.

REFERENCES

1. Jewitt JF, Reid DE, Safon LE, et al., Childbed fever – a continuing entity. *JAMA* 1968;**206**:344–350.
2. Kolmos HJ, Svendsen RN, Nielsen SV, The surgical team as a source of postoperative wound infections caused by *Streptococcus pyogenes*. *J Hosp Infect* 1997;**35**:207–214.
3. Bennett SN, McNeil MM, Bland LA, et al., Postoperative infections traced to contamination of an intravenous anesthetic, propofol. *N Engl J Med* 1995;**333**:147–154.
4. Hajjar J, Girard R, Surveillance des infections nosocomiales liées à l'anesthésie. Etude multicentrique. *Ann Fr Anesth Réanim* 2000;**19**:47–53.
5. Loftus RW, Koff MD, Burchman CC, et al., Transmission of pathogenic bacterial organisms in the anesthesia work area. *Anesthesiology* 2008;**109**:399–407.
6. Stackhouse RA, Beers R, Brown D et al., Recommendations for Infection Control for the Practice of Anesthesiology. Available at www.asahq.org/~/media/sites/asahq/files/public/resources/asa%20committees/recommendations%20for%20infection%20control%20for%20the%20practice%20of%20anesthesiology.pdf. Accessed March 7, 2017.
7. Rogues AM, Forestier J-F, Valentin M-L, et al., Le séjour en salle de surveillance postinterventionnelle peut-il être à l'origine de transmissions croisées? *Ann Fr Anesth Réanim* 2002;**21**:643–647.
8. Pittet D, Allegranzi B, Sax H, et al., Evidence-based model for hand transmission during patient care and the role of improved practices. *Lancet Infect Dis* 2006;**6**:641–652.
9. Scheithauer S, Rosarius A, Rex S, et al., Improving hand hygiene compliance in the anesthesia working room area: more than just more hand rubs. *Am J Infect Control* 2013;**41**:1001–1006.
10. Koff MD, Loftus RW, Burchman CC, et al., Reduction in intraoperative bacterial contamination of peripheral intravenous tubing through the use of a novel device. *Anesthesiology* 2009;**110**:978–985.
11. Pittet D, Stéphan S, Hugonnet S, et al., Hand-cleansing during postanesthesia care. *Anesthesiology* 2003;**99**:530–535.
12. Loftus RW, Muffly MK, Brown JR, et al., Hand contamination of anesthesia providers is an important risk factor for intra-operative bacterial transmission. *Anesth Analg* 2011;**112**:98–105.
13. Loftus RW, Brown JR, Koff MD, et al., Multiple reservoirs contribute to intraoperative bacterial transmission. *Anesth Analg* 2012;**114**:1236–1248.

Chapter 43

Hand Hygiene in Resource-Poor Settings

Nizam Damani,[1] Shaheen Mehtar,[2] and Benedetta Allegranzi[3]

[1] Infection Prevention and Control, Southern Health and Social Care Trust, Portadown, and Queen's University, Belfast, UK

[2] Unit for Infection Prevention and Control, Division of Community Health, Stellenbosch University, Cape Town, South Africa

[3] Infection Prevention and Control Global Unit, Department of Service Delivery and Safety, World Health Organization, and Faculty of Medicine, University of Geneva, Geneva, Switzerland

KEY MESSAGES

- Implementation of hand hygiene is a challenging task, especially in low- and middle-income countries where compliance is particularly low. Lack of infection prevention and control infrastructure and basic knowledge hampers implementation and sustainability of hand hygiene promotion. Better education and training are first key steps for improvement.

- In resource-poor settings, the availability of water and hand hygiene products is a continual challenge that requires health system strengthening and can be overcome by innovative solutions. Unavailability and the high cost of alcohol-based handrubs can be overcome by local production based on the WHO formulations. This will improve compliance and help to overcome the need and availability of wash basins, soap, water, and drying materials.

- Recent studies have demonstrated that the effective implementation of hand hygiene improvement strategies is possible and sustainable, even in resource-poor settings, and has led to significant compliance and knowledge improvement among healthcare workers and to healthcare-associated infection reduction in some cases.

Hand Hygiene: A Handbook for Medical Professionals, First Edition.
Edited by Didier Pittet, John M. Boyce and Benedetta Allegranzi.
© 2017 John Wiley & Sons, Inc. Published 2017 by John Wiley & Sons, Inc.

The risk of acquiring healthcare-associated infections (HAIs) in low- and middle-income (LMI) countries is reported as being 2 to 20 times greater than in high-income countries, especially in vulnerable populations such as neonates and patients admitted to intensive care units.[1] However, the full magnitude of HAI in LMI countries is unknown due to the lack of good-quality surveillance data and publications. Acquiring infections is not only confined to healthcare facilities – each day it is estimated that thousands of patients (especially children ≤5 years) become ill and die from preventable communicable diseases in the community, particularly diarrhea and pneumonia. Three-quarters of these deaths occur in sub-Saharan Africa and South Asian countries and are attributed to lack of basic sanitation and clean water. Evidence supports the fact that improvement of handwashing practices leads to a substantial reduction of these and other infections, in the community setting.[2]

In this chapter, we address hand hygiene practices in resource-poor settings, describe the most frequent constraints and challenges, and summarize successful examples of interventions leading to improvement in hand hygiene.

WHAT WE KNOW – THE EVIDENCE

Despite irrefutable evidence demonstrating the importance of hand contacts in the transmission of pathogens, healthcare workers (HCWs) worldwide usually fail to comply with hand hygiene recommendations in more than 50% of opportunities during care delivery.[3] In healthcare facilities in LMI countries, compliance is reportedly much lower. Patterns of noncompliance with hand hygiene recommendations are similar to those identified in high-income countries, such as higher adherence to indications that protect the HCWs rather than the patient (see Chapter 11). However, while usually nurses are more compliant with best practices, some studies conducted in LMI countries reported higher compliance among doctors than nurses. Some determinants of poor hand hygiene practices in LMI are similar to those identified in high-income countries such as overcrowding, work overload, and understaffing.

Additional challenges in settings with limited resources include:

- Lack of basic infrastructure, such as continuous supply of clean water and erratic availability of hand hygiene products – soap, water, hand-drying material, and alcohol-based handrub (ABHR) – due to cost constraints and archaic bureaucratic procurement systems.

- Lack of trained/qualified infection prevention and control (IPC) practitioners to provide education and training, and reinforcement of basic IPC practices including the importance of hand hygiene.

- Very serious problems of staff shortages and heavy clinical workload, resulting in failure to implement best IPC practices and to attend education and training sessions even when available.

- Clinical care provided by nonclinical staff such as family members or care givers, who are neither advised nor trained in IPC and hand hygiene.
- Lack of basic surveillance and audit systems resulting in failure to provide evidence that improved hand hygiene practices can reduce cross-infection and HAIs, and thus leading to lack of political and financial support by senior managers.
- Lack of locally adapted policies and implementation tools, including translations in local languages.

Several studies have documented these challenges and proposed approaches and practical solutions to overcome them. In countries where knowledge transfer takes place using oral or verbal communication, written documentation is often lacking. Constant verbal reminders by senior staff are more effective than written documents, which are usually ignored since there is little time to read them and sometimes limited capacity to understand them. To improve the understanding of all HCWs, the use of pictorial displays in local language is more effective.

In addition, practical demonstration and training are effective means of teaching. Basic concepts need to be fostered; for instance, demonstration that gloves are inappropriately used to replace hand hygiene leading to high transmission risk (see Chapter 23). Therefore, it is essential that education and training be provided based on the My Five Moments for Hand Hygiene concept (see Chapter 20) and be conveyed using WHO and other standardized tools to provide clear and consistent information. Regular reinforcement and continuous education are essential for sustainability.[3]

Lack of hand hygiene facilities and products is mainly due to cost issues and the need for allocating resources to other priorities. In addition, unavailability of products on the local market and lack of communication between procurement and the IPC practitioners create further significant barriers. During designing or renovating of healthcare facilities, infection prevention and control teams are not consulted in the planning stages, and, therefore, the location and/or the number of sinks or handrub dispensers are not conducive to facilitating hand hygiene performance. Equally, due to lack of availability of dedicated decontamination rooms, and the inadequate availability of handwash basins in clinical areas, they are often also used for the cleaning and decontamination of medical items and equipment, as well as disposal of patient-related liquid waste (Nizam Damani, personal observation).

In resource-poor settings, the use of Tippy Taps is a simple, economical, and effective way of providing handwashing facilities where there is a lack of access to both piped and non-piped water supplies (Figures 43.1 and 43.2).[4] In addition, there are other handwashing systems which represent simple innovative solution to infrastructure problems. In some African countries (e.g., South Africa and Senegal) mobile hand hygiene units have been used, which carry their own water supply and can be set up anywhere including schools and mobile clinics. These

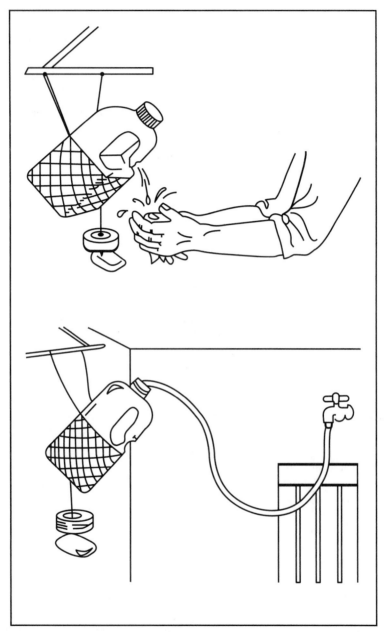

Figure 43.1 Tippy Taps are designed for simple, economical, and effective hand washing stations in countries with resource-poor settings with a lack of access to a piped water supply. *Source*: Reproduced with permission from the Centers for Disease Control and Prevention, www.cdc.gov.

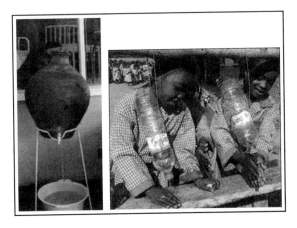

Figure 43.2   Examples of using various types of hand washing facilities in LMI countries where there is a lack of access to a piped water supply. *Source*: Reproduced with permission from the Centers for Disease Control and Prevention, www.cdc .gov. *See plate section for color representation of this figure.*

have had a huge success, especially in rural areas, township schools, and clinical areas.

The microbial quality of tap water is usually poor in LMI countries where the water supply is constantly interrupted. The lack of maintenance of water supply systems results in seepage and contamination of clean water with sewage. Guidelines have been developed to provide safe water systems for hand hygiene in healthcare in developing countries[5] and have been field-tested in Kenya and adapted in other countries in Africa and Asia.[6] According to these and WHO recommendations,[3] water of drinking quality should be used for handwashing. Another major issue in LMI countries after handwashing with soap and water is drying of hands using a single-use disposable towel (paper or cloth), which is not always affordable. Consequently, multi-use cloth towels are used, leading to possible cross-transmission.

Many of the challenges can be resolved by replacing handwashing with the use of alcohol-based handrubs (ABHRs) whenever possible for appropriate indications. ABHRs are currently the preferred method for hand hygiene, as they offer a broad antimicrobial spectrum, high efficacy, good skin tolerance, and can be made available at the point of care.[3,7] However, availability of these products on the market in LMI countries is still limited, often at higher prices than in high-income countries, and hampered by procurement and distribution limitations. As one of the consequences, in order to save money and to get the maximum number of hand hygiene actions per bottle, HCWs often use less than the recommended amount (2–3 mL) of ABHR (Nizam Damani, personal observation). To overcome some of these constraints, WHO developed and tested two alcohol-based formulations for local production at the healthcare facility level (see Chapter 8).[3] These have been shown to be much cheaper to produce than commercially available products and to be associated with good acceptability and tolerability. A e-learning module has been created at the University of Geneva Hospitals to support the local production of ABHR (accessible at pharmacie.g2hp.net/courses/hand-hygiene/). It describes in detail all steps for the production and quality control of locally prepared ABHR. Table 43.1 summarizes the advantages and potential barriers to the local production of ABHRs.

Current evidence clearly indicates that effective implementation of hand hygiene improvement is possible on a global level, including in settings with

Table 43.1   Advantages and Potential Barriers to the Local Production of Alcohol-Based HandRubs

Advantages and Barriers	No. of Sites/Total That Provided Data (%)	Countries (No. of Sites)
Advantages		
Less expensive than marketed alcohol-based handrubs	7/9 (78)	Brazil (1), Cambodia (3), Iran (1), Mongolia (1), Pakistan (1)
Excellent tolerance and acceptability	31/38 (82)	Argentina (1), Bangladesh (1), Brazil (2), Cambodia (3), China (Province of Taiwan) (1), Colombia (1), Ethiopia (1), Indonesia (2), Italy (1), Japan (1), Jordan (1), Kenya (1), Lebanon (1), Malawi (1), Mali (1), Mongolia (1), Nigeria (3), Oman (1), Pakistan (1), Saudi Arabia (1), Senegal (1), Sudan (1), Thailand (1), Tunisia (1), Turkey (1)
Used in health facility as part of a multimodal approach to improve hand hygiene	30/34 (88)	Argentina (1), Brazil (1), Cambodia (6), Colombia (1), Ethiopia (1), Indonesia (2), Islamic Republic of Iran (1), Italy (1), Japan (1), Kenya (1), Lebanon (1), Malawi (1), Mali (1), Mongolia (1), Nigeria (1), Pakistan (1), Philippines (1), Saudi Arabia (1), Senegal (1), Sudan (2), Tunisia (1), Turkey (1), Uganda (1)
Manufactured from locally sourced alcohol[a]	28/39 (72)	Argentina (1), Brazil (2), Cambodia (6), China (Province of Taiwan) (1), Colombia (1), Ethiopia (1), Indonesia (2), Italy (1), Japan (1), Kenya (1), Lebanon (1), Malawi (1), Mali (1), Nigeria (2), Philippines (1), Saudi Arabia (1), Sudan (1), Tunisia (1), Turkey (1), Uganda (1)

Table 43.1   (*Continued*)

Advantages and Barriers	No. of Sites/Total That Provided Data (%)	Countries (No. of Sites)
Barriers to production		
Staff needed training in the production process	29/39 (74)	Argentina (1), Bangladesh (1), Belgium (1), Brazil (1), Cambodia (6), Colombia (1), Ethiopia (1), Indonesia (1), Iran (1), Italy (1), Jordan (1), Kenya (1), Lebanon (1), Malawi (1), Mali (1), Mongolia (1), Nigeria (2), Oman (1), Pakistan (1), Saudi Arabia (1), Sudan (1), Tunisia (1), Turkey (1)
Occasional difficulty in procuring ingredients locally	20/39 (51)	Brazil (1), Cambodia (6), China (Taiwan) (1), Colombia (1), Ethiopia (1), Indonesia (1), Japan (1), Kenya (1), Malawi (1), Mali (1), Mongolia (1), Nigeria (1), Senegal (1), Sudan (1), Turkey (1)
Difficulty in procuring appropriate dispensers[b]	19/37 (51)	Brazil (2), Cambodia (4), Ethiopia (1), Indonesia (1), Kenya (1), Malawi (1), Mali (1), Mongolia (1), Nigeria (2), Pakistan (1), Philippines (1), Saudi Arabia (1), Senegal (1), Uganda (1)
Barriers to quality control		
Suboptimal reprocessing of dispensers	11/24 (46)	Brazil (2), Cambodia (4), Colombia (1), Ethiopia (1), Nigeria (1), Saudi Arabia (1), Sudan (1)
Quality control not performed on site (mainly due to lack of equipment)	11/24 (46)	Argentina (1), Ethiopia (1), Iran (1), Japan (1), Lebanon (1), Malawi (1), Nigeria (2), Pakistan (1), Sudan (1), Turkey (1)
Barriers to acceptability		
Unpleasant smell	4/38 (11)	Belgium (1), Cambodia (1), Philippines (1), Uganda (1)

[a] Alcohol produced from sugar cane, maize, manioc, mahogany or walnut.
[b] The simple washing of used dispensers, with no attempt at disinfection or sterilization.
Source: Adapted from Bauer-Savage 2013. Reproduced with permission from the World Health Organization.

limited resources.[7-9] The WHO multimodal strategy has been successfully implemented and has led to significant compliance and knowledge improvement among HCWs. Importantly, it is also both feasible and sustainable across a range of healthcare settings in different countries.[8] While the reasons for this success have varied geographically, widespread staff education and regular procurement of hand hygiene products, including local production, and performance monitoring and feedback have been the pillars of these programs. In addition, campaigns based on the WHO approach and implementation strategy have been promoted by regional and global organizations such as the Infection Control Africa Network, Asia-Pacific IPC Society, and the International Federation of Infection Control, contributing to their sustainability.

WHAT WE DO NOT KNOW – THE UNCERTAIN

Although there are an increasing number of publications and projects showing that hand hygiene promotion in LMI countries is feasible and can lead to successful improvement of infrastructures, practices, and knowledge, several areas require further research and better evidence.

Long-term sustainability is a common problem, especially in LMI countries. This is mainly due to discontinuation of financial and leadership support to hand hygiene promotion. Therefore, demonstration of successful models to integrate hand hygiene and IPC improvement efforts into regular action plans and budgets, both at the local and national levels, would be highly beneficial. Another constraint leading to lack of sustainability and contributing to poor personal accountability is the lack of conviction and understanding among HCWs that hand hygiene can really reduce transmission risk and HAI. Better evidence is necessary to demonstrate the impact of hand hygiene improvement on HAI reduction in LMI countries. In addition, cost-effectiveness evaluations associated with these studies would be invaluable in helping to convince managers to support and provide resources to help initiate and sustain hand hygiene efforts. An interesting approach has been recently proposed at Stellenbosch University (South Africa) where IPC postgraduate students from African countries have been using local data on HAI incidence and hand hygiene compliance collected at their facilities and applied these findings to a business case towards cost-effective hand hygiene improvement. The impact of this exercise and its translation into practice at the facility level has been noticeable and measurable (Shaheen Mehtar, personal communication).

Senior members of medical and nursing staff are crucial for successful implementation of hand hygiene as they could act as role models; however, they do not frequently consider themselves in this role. A thought-provoking paper by Jang et al. reported that in a survey among medical students, senior staff members were perceived as role models, although the physicians did not see themselves in this role.[10] Effective approaches to induce a change of mentality and behavior among physicians and senior staff should be identified and promoted using evidence with which they can identify.

While the relationship between religion and culture and hand hygiene has been discussed in detail elsewhere (see Chapter 31), the impact of these factors, especially in LMI countries, cannot be underestimated and should be better investigated and used to understand best approaches, to facilitate improved attitudes and behavioral changes, and support improvement.

Caregivers, family members, and patients themselves heavily contribute to care delivery in LMI countries where understaffing is a very serious problem. However, very little evidence is available to identify the best approaches to provide basic training, including IPC issues, and to involve these categories in patient safety and hand hygiene improvement efforts.

Availability of supplies, in particular ABHRs, is essential to enable appropriate hand hygiene performance. Little information is available about market coverage and prices of ABHRs in LMI countries. In addition, the lack of regular availability of basic ingredients and dispensers is an obstacle to continuous local production of the WHO formulations (see Table 43.1). Therefore, better strategies should be investigated for the production and procurement of ABHRs so that supplies are easier to source and less costly to procure.

RESEARCH AGENDA

- Development of simple yet reliable methods for HAIs surveillance and standardized monitoring of hand hygiene compliance for both local evaluation and international benchmarking to establish the link between reduction of HAIs and hand hygiene.

- Evaluation of the impact of culture and social structures and identification of unique methods of promoting hand hygiene and improving HCWs' personal accountability while taking these and other factors into account in settings with limited resources.

- Identification of best approaches to educate and involve patients and family members in hand hygiene improvement efforts, while taking social and cultural dynamics into account in LMI countries.

- Identification of the best methods for assessing the large-scale feasibility and the cost-effectiveness of hand hygiene programs in LMI countries.

REFERENCES

1. World Health Organization, *WHO report on the burden of endemic health care-associated infection worldwide*. Geneva: WHO, 2011.
2. Luby SP, Agboatwalla M, Feikin DR, et al., Effect of handwashing on child health: a randomised controlled trial. *Lancet* 2005; **366**:225–233.

3. World Health Organization, *WHO Guidelines on Hand Hygiene in Health Care*. Geneva: WHO, 2009.

4. Centers for Disease Control and Prevention, *Information on How to Make Tippy Taps*. Available at https://www.cdc.gov/safewater/publications_pages/tippy-tap.pdf. Accessed on March 7, 2017.

5. Centers for Disease Control and Prevention, *Safe water system and handwashing guide for health care workers*, 4th edn. Atlanta, GA: CDC, 2005.

6. Parker AA, Stephenson R, Riley PL et al., Sustained high levels of stored drinking water treatment and retention of hand-washing knowledge in rural Kenyan households following a clinic based intervention. *Epidemiol Infect* 2006;**134**:1029–1036.

7. Allegranzi B, Sax H, Bengaly L, et al., Successful implementation of the World Health Organization hand hygiene improvement strategy in a referral hospital in Mali, Africa. *Infect Control Hosp Epidemiol* 2010;**31**:133–141.

8. Rosenthal VD, Pawar M, Leblebicioglu H, et al., Impact of the International Nosocomial Infection Control Consortium (INICC) multidimensional hand hygiene approach over 13 years in 51 cities of 19 limited-resource countries from Latin America, Asia, the Middle East, and Europe. *Infect Control Hosp Epidemiol* 2013;**34**:415–423.

9. Allegranzi B, Gayet-Ageron A, Damani N, et al., Global implementation of WHO's multimodal strategy for improvement of hand hygiene: a quasi-experimental study. *Lancet Infect Dis* 2013;**13**:843–851.

10. Jang JH, Wu S, Kirzner D, et al., Focus group study of hand hygiene practice among healthcare workers in a teaching hospital in Toronto, Canada. *Infect Control Hosp Epidemiol* 2010;**31**:144–150.

Chapter 44A

Role of Hand Hygiene in MRSA Control

Stephan Harbarth

Infection Control Program and WHO Collaborating Centre on Patient Safety, University of Geneva Hospitals and Faculty of Medicine, Geneva, Switzerland

KEY MESSAGES

- Appropriate hand hygiene during patient care is the primary means of reducing the spread of methicillin-resistant *Staphylococcus aureus* (MRSA).
- The use of gloves during routine care has no proven benefit over regular hand hygiene in controlling MRSA.
- The effectiveness of hand hygiene promotion to reduce MRSA infections may depend on baseline MRSA rates and compliance levels.

Methicillin-resistant *Staphylococcus aureus* (MRSA) was first described in 1961, and in the following decades it became an important cause of healthcare-associated infections (HAIs) worldwide. It is a versatile bacterial pathogen, combining virulence, antibiotic resistance, and survival fitness. Clonal spread is facilitated by cross-transmission via the hands of healthcare workers (HCWs) and the selection pressure exerted by broad-spectrum antibiotic treatment.[1] Control of endemic MRSA relies on several complementary strategies frequently mentioned in the infection control literature (Figure 44A.1). In this short overview, we will

Hand Hygiene: A Handbook for Medical Professionals, First Edition.
Edited by Didier Pittet, John M. Boyce and Benedetta Allegranzi.
© 2017 John Wiley & Sons, Inc. Published 2017 by John Wiley & Sons, Inc.

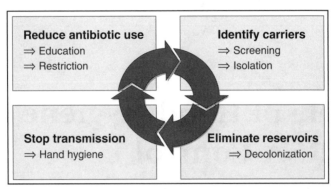

Figure 44A.1   Standard Approaches to the Control of Endemic Methicillin-Resistant *Staphylococcus aureus*. *Source*: Harbarth 2010. Reproduced with permission from John Wiley & Sons, Ltd.

summarize the role of hand hygiene in MRSA control and focus in particular on the question whether improved compliance with hand hygiene may decrease MRSA transmission.

WHAT WE KNOW – THE EVIDENCE

MRSA mostly spreads from patient to patient via the transiently colonised hands of HCWs during patient contact or after handling contaminated materials. Therefore, hand hygiene is an integral part of standard measures in the prevention of MRSA transmission. Most experts would agree that the practice of hand hygiene during patient care at the right time with the correct technique is an important means of reducing the spread of MRSA in the healthcare setting.[2]

Many large-scale studies have shown that promotion of alcohol-based handrubs (ABHRs) can improve compliance and reduce episodes of MRSA cross-infection (see also Chapter 41). Two reports from Australia have shown that improved MRSA control can be achieved through a multimodal culture-change campaign including promotion of ABHR, which does not need to be costly.[3,4] A pan-European ecologic study suggested an association between use of ABHR and local MRSA rates, after adjustment for multiple confounders.[5] The recently published *CleanYourHands* campaign to reduce *S. aureus* bacteraemia in hospitals in England and Wales by improved hand hygiene demonstrated that MRSA bacteraemia rates fell from 1.88 to 0.91 cases per 10,000 bed days.[6] Interestingly, increased procurement of ABHRs was independently associated with reduced MRSA bacteraemia, but only in the last four quarters of the study.

A systematic review has summarized the available literature until 2009 on the impact of ABHR use on MRSA rates.[7] Among 12 included studies, an increase

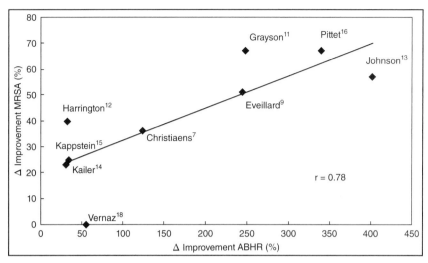

Figure 44A.2   Difference in the improvement of alcohol-based hand rub (ABHR) use and the change in MRSA rates in nine epidemiological studies. *Source*: Sroka 2010. Reproduced with permission from Elsevier.

in ABHR use correlated significantly with an improvement in the MRSA situation (r = 0.78) and was associated with a significant reduction of MRSA rates (Figure 44A.2), whereas there was no such correlation between compliance level and MRSA. This latter observation was confirmed by a recently published prospective, observational study from Ontario, Canada, which failed to demonstrate a positive ecological impact of improved hand hygiene compliance rates and the incidence of MRSA bacteremia, despite significant improvements in rates of compliance among healthcare personnel.[8]

The use of gloves during routine care has no benefit over regular hand hygiene in controlling MRSA infections. In addition, the routine use of gloves may encourage healthcare workers to use gloves as a substitute for good hand hygiene practices if they do not remove or change gloves between patients and perform hand hygiene after glove removal (see also Chapter 23). This has been shown during the epidemic of Severe Acute Respiratory Syndrome (SARS) in Hong Kong, during which universal glove use was performed, contributing to a hospital-wide MRSA outbreak due to low compliance with hand hygiene recommendations.

WHAT WE DO NOT KNOW – THE UNCERTAIN

Several issues related to the impact of improved hand hygiene compliance on MRSA rates remain controversial. First, the delay between improved hand hygiene compliance, increased ABHR use, and decreased MRSA cross-infection rates has not been well defined. Some time-series studies showed an immediate impact with lag times between 0 and 4 months;[9] others like the *CleanYourHands* campaign in the UK, had a substantial delay before an effect was observed. Hand hygiene campaigns involve education and behavior change and are therefore unlikely to have a short-term effect on MRSA rates. Several other studies have shown that they may only be beneficial if activity is sustained over years.

Second, the effectiveness of the promotion of ABHRs on postoperative surgical site infections due to MRSA may be smaller than previously hypothesized. In a recent European multicenter, controlled trial that compared two strategies to reduce MRSA rates in surgical patients, hand hygiene promotion for 12 months did not effectively reduce MRSA infections in surgical wards with relatively low baseline MRSA rates.[10] Although this study did not detect any intervention effects of the hand hygiene promotion strategy on MRSA rates, cessation of this intervention was associated with an increase in MRSA rates, suggesting that discontinuing activities to optimize hand hygiene practices may be detrimental. Likewise, a three-year interrupted time series with multiple sequential interventions in a US teaching hospital demonstrated that hand hygiene compliance increased significantly, from 41% to 87%, during the initiative, with a sustained decline in the rates of HAIs and MRSA bacteremia. However, the rate of *S. aureus* infections attributable to the operating room rose against the general trend.[11]

Third, the additive effect of hand hygiene on MRSA reduction is unclear. In settings where compliance is already above about 50%, modeling studies suggest that further increases in compliance will have rapidly diminishing returns for reducing MRSA transmission (see also Chapter 5). The above-cited study from Ontario also supports the emerging evidence that once a high threshold level of hand hygiene compliance is achieved, there is little benefit in attempting to achieve higher rates of hand hygiene compliance among healthcare providers.[8] By contrast, in facilities with lower hand hygiene compliance or very high MRSA rates, a campaign promoting ABHRs may still be highly effective.

Fourth, it remains unclear whether contact precautions can be stopped in settings with relatively low MRSA prevalence and sufficient hand hygiene compliance. As mentioned above, glove misuse may decrease good hand hygiene practices and even increase MRSA transmission. Furthermore, several recent high-quality studies have questionned the value of patient isolation and contact precautions for effective MRSA control. Thus, some experts suggest that low MRSA rates can be sustained by implementing standard precautions only. This hypothesis needs to be tested in large clinical trials in which standard precautions and hand hygiene are tested alone, not as a part of a multimodal intervention as frequently done.

Finally, uncertainty persists about the role of hand hygiene in the control of community-associated MRSA transmission. Community-associated MRSA has distinct epidemiological features that raise multiple challenges with an impact also on healthcare settings; therefore, other measures such as improved surveillance,

contract tracing, general hygiene education, and active treatment and decolonization of infected cases and carriers may be as, if not more, important than hand
hygiene, but this remains to be elucidated.

RESEARCH AGENDA

Further research is necessary on the following unresolved issues:

- The quantitative association between increased hand hygiene compliance,
  ABHR use, and MRSA reduction effects remains unclear (e.g., nonlinear
  relationships; threshold effects).
- The role of improving hand hygiene only (independent of contact precau-
  tions) for sustained MRSA control needs to be elucidated.
- There is a lack of high-quality intervention studies to demonstrate the
  effectiveness of hand hygiene promotion on limiting community-associated
  MRSA acquisition and infection.

REFERENCES

1. Harbarth S, Control of endemic methicillin-resistant *Staphylococcus aureus* – recent advances
   and future challenges. *Clin Microbiol Infect* 2006;**12**:1154–1162.
2. Lee AS, Huttner B, Harbarth S, Control of methicillin-resistant *Staphylococcus aureus*. *Infect
   Dis Clin North Am* 2011;**25**:155–179.
3. Johnson PD, Martin R, Burrell LJ, et al., Efficacy of an alcohol/chlorhexidine hand
   hygiene program in a hospital with high rates of nosocomial MRSA infection. *Med J Aust*
   2005;**183**:509–514.
4. Grayson ML, Russo PL, Cruickshank M, et al., Outcomes from the first 2 years of the
   Australian National Hand Hygiene Initiative. *Med J Aust* 2011;**195**:615–619.
5. MacKenzie FM, Bruce J, Struelens MJ, et al., Antimicrobial drug use and infection control practices associated with the prevalence of methicillin-resistant *Staphylococcus aureus* in
   European hospitals. *Clin Microbiol Infect* 2007;**13**:269–276.
6. Stone SP, Fuller C, Savage J, et al., Evaluation of the national *CleanYourHands* campaign to
   reduce *Staphylococcus aureus* bacteraemia and *Clostridium difficile* infection in hospitals in England and Wales by improved hand hygiene: four year, prospective, ecological, interrupted
   time series study. *Br Med J* 2012;**344**:e3005.
7. Sroka S, Gastmeier P, Meyer E, Impact of alcohol hand-rub use on meticillin-resistant
   Staphylococcus aureus: an analysis of the literature. *J Hosp Infect* 2010;**74**:204–211.
8. DiDiodato G, Has improved hand hygiene compliance reduced the risk of hospital-acquired
   infections among hospitalized patients in Ontario? Analysis of publicly reported patient
   safety data from 2008 to 2011. *Infect Control Hosp Epidemiol* 2013;**34**:605–610.
9. Vernaz N, Sax H, Pittet D, et al., Temporal effects of antibiotic use and hand rub consumption
   on the incidence of MRSA and *Clostridium difficile*. *J Antimicrob Chemother* 2008;**62**:601–607.
10. Lee AS, Cooper BS, Malhotra-Kumar S, et al., Comparison of strategies to reduce
    meticillin-resistant *Staphylococcus aureus* rates in surgical patients: a controlled multicentre
    intervention trial. *BMJ Open* 2013;**3**:e003126.

11. Kirkland KB, Homa KA, Lasky RA, et al., Impact of a hospital-wide hand hygiene initiative on healthcare-associated infections: results of an interrupted time series. *BMJ Qual Saf* 2012;**21**:1019–1026.

Chapter 44B

Role of Hand Hygiene in *Clostridium difficile* Control

John M. Boyce[1] and Walter Zingg[2]

[1] Hospital Epidemiology and Infection Control, Yale-New Haven Hospital, and Yale University School of Medicine, New Haven, USA

[2] Infection Control Program and WHO Collaborating Centre on Patient Safety, University of Geneva Hospitals and Faculty of Medicine, Geneva, Switzerland

KEY MESSAGES

- Touching the skin of patients with *Clostridium difficile* colonization or diarrhea and touching environmental surfaces in the vicinity of patients with *C. difficile* diarrhea frequently results in contamination of the gloves and hands of healthcare personnel.

- Gloves should be worn routinely by healthcare personnel when caring for patients with *C. difficile* disease. Appropriate glove use deserves further research.

- If exposure to potential spore-forming pathogens such as *C. difficile* is strongly suspected or proven, in particular in outbreak situations, handwashing with soap and water is the preferred means.

Hand Hygiene: A Handbook for Medical Professionals, First Edition.
Edited by Didier Pittet, John M. Boyce and Benedetta Allegranzi.
© 2017 John Wiley & Sons, Inc. Published 2017 by John Wiley & Sons, Inc.

WHAT WE KNOW – THE EVIDENCE

Clostridum difficile has been recovered from the hands of healthcare workers (HCWs) in multiple studies, providing evidence that *C. difficile* transmission on the hands of HCWs is likely to be the most common mode of transmission.[1] Touching patients whose skin is colonized with *C. difficile* results in contamination of HCW gloves or hands. Although touching the groin or abdomen of a patient with *C. difficile* infection can result in heavy contamination of hands (Figure 44B.1), HCWs may also contaminate their gloves or hands by touching other parts of an affected patient's body.[2] Although *C. difficile* contaminates HCWs' hands more frequently when a patient is having diarrhea, contact with the patient's skin after diarrhea has resolved can still lead to hand contamination by the organism.[3]

Contaminated environmental surfaces also play a role in the spread of *C. difficile* in healthcare settings. The frequency of *C. difficile* hand contamination and transmission increases as the level of environmental contamination increases.[4] In one study, touching contaminated environmental surfaces in patient rooms was as likely to result in hand contamination as touching the skin of an affected patient (Figure 44B.2).[5]

Alcohol-based handrubs (ABHRs) and antiseptic agents used in antimicrobial soaps are effective against the vegetative (nonspore) form of *C. difficile*, but lack activity against *C. difficile* spores. As a result, ABHRs do not reduce the number of *C. difficile* spores on hands. Because ABHRs lack activity against spores, some

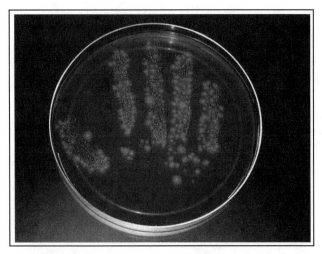

Figure 44B.1   Hand imprint culture of *Clostridium difficile* on sterile gloves after contact with a *C. difficile*–associated diarrhea-affected patient's groin. *Source*: Reprinted from Bobulsky G et al., with permission from C.J. Donskey.[2] *See plate section for color representation of this figure.*

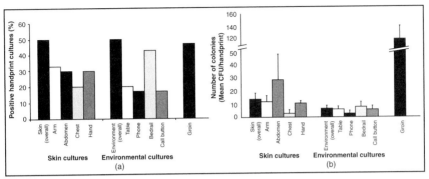

Figure 44B.2   Percentage of positive gloved hand imprint cultures (a) and the mean
(± standard error) number of colony-forming units (CFUs) acquired (b) after contact
with commonly examined skin sites of 30 patients with *Clostridium difficile* infection (CDI) and
commonly touched environmental surfaces in the CDI rooms. *Source*: Reprinted
from Bobulsky G et al. with permission from C.J. Donskey.[2]

experts have suggested that their increasing use in the past decade may have promoted the increase in *C. difficile* infections observed at the same time. However,
no formal link has been established between the hospital-wide use of ABHRs and
emerging *C. difficile* infection. There is some evidence that the increased use of soap
and water for hand hygiene reduces the incidence of *C. difficile* disease.[6] Indeed,
handwashing with soap (plain soap or antimicrobial soap) and water has been
shown to be the most effective way to reduce the number of *C. difficile* spores on
contaminated hands in laboratory testing conditions.[7] This is due to a combination of scrubbing and rinsing hands with water, and the use of paper towels, which
results in physical removal of the organism. Therefore, current guidelines recommend that handwashing with soap and water is the preferred means if exposure
to potential spore-forming pathogens such as *C. difficile* is strongly suspected or
proven.[1]

Routine use of gloves by healthcare personnel caring for patients with *C. difficile* infection is a key component of *C. difficile* control. In an early study of *C. difficile*
epidemiology, 47% of caregivers who did not wear gloves and did not wash their
hands after patient contact had *C. difficile* recovered from their hands.[8] In contrast,
none of four personnel who wore gloves had positive hand cultures. A prospective controlled trial of routine use of gloves by personnel caring for patients with *C.
difficile* infection demonstrated reduced transmission of *C. difficile* and a reduction
in *C. difficile* infection.[9] A randomized nonblinded trial found that daily disinfection of high-touch surfaces in the rooms of affected patients reduced acquisition
of *C. difficile* on the hands of personnel.[10] This finding may explain in part the fact
that multiple studies have found an association between improved disinfection of
environmental surfaces and reduction of *C. difficile* disease.

WHAT WE DO NOT KNOW – THE UNCERTAIN

Despite recent advances in our knowledge of the sources and mechanisms of *C. difficile* transmission, a number of unanswered questions remain. In patients with *C. difficile* infection, as well as in asymptomatic carriers, a significant proportion of *C. difficile* in the stool is in the vegetative form. The extent (if any) to which the vegetative form, which is susceptible to ABHRs and other antiseptic agents, contributes to the transmission of *C. difficile* is not known. Recent handwashing investigations have established that *C. difficile* spores are more difficult to remove from the hands than *Bacillus atrophaeus* or *Clostridium sporogenes* spores.[7] The reasons for this phenomenon are not clear.

RESEARCH AGENDA

Additional studies of the frequency and the level of *C. difficile* hand contamination after glove removal among HCWs caring for patients with *C. difficile* disease are needed. And additional data are needed on whether handwashing with soap and water provides any better protection against *C. difficile* transmission than hand hygiene using an ABHR when caregivers have used gloves to care for affected patients. Education of caregivers about the appropriate use of gloves (correct moment of donning and removal) deserves further attention (see also Chapter 23). Studies are needed to identify hand hygiene products that are more effective in removing *C. difficile* spores from HCWs' hands. Recent studies suggest that development of a sporicidal hand hygiene preparation may be feasible in the near future.[11]

REFERENCES

1. World Health Organization, *WHO Guidelines for Hand Hygiene in Health Care*. Geneva: WHO, 2009.
2. Bobulsky GS, Al-Nassir WN, Riggs MM, et al., *Clostridium difficile* skin contamination in patients with *C. difficile*-associated disease. *Clin Infect Dis* 2008;**46**:447–450.
3. Sethi AK, Al-Nassir WN, Nernandzic MM, et al., Persistence of skin contamination and environmental shedding of *Clostridium difficile* during and after treatment of *C. difficile* infection. *Infect Control Hosp Epidemiol* 2010;**31**:21–27.
4. Samore MH, Venkataraman L, Degirolami PC, et al., Clinical and molecular epidemiology of sporadic and clustered cases of nosocomial *Clostridium difficile* diarrhea. *Am J Med* 1996;**100**:32–40.
5. Guerrero DM, Nerandzic MM, Jury LA, et al., Acquisition of spores on gloved hands after contact with the skin of patients with Clostridium difficile infection and with environmental surfaces in their rooms. *Am J Infect Control* 2012;**40**:556–558.
6. Stone SP, Fuller C, Savage J, et al., Evaluation of the national *CleanYourHands* campaign to reduce *Staphylococcus aureus* bacteraemia and *Clostridium difficile* infection in hospitals in England and Wales by improved hand hygiene: four year, prospective, ecological, interrupted time series study. *Br Med J* 2012;**3**;344:e3005.

7. Edmonds SL, Zapka C, Kasper D, et al., Effectiveness of hand hygiene for removal of *Clostridium difficile* spores from hands. *Infect Control Hosp Epidemiol* 2013;**34**:302–305.
8. McFarland LV, Mulligan ME, Kwok RYY, et al., Nosocomial acquisition of *Clostridium difficile* infection. *N Engl J Med* 1989;**320**:204–210.
9. Johnson S, Gerding DN, Olson MM, et al., Prospective, controlled study of vinyl glove use to interrupt *Clostridium difficile* nosocomial transmission. *Am J Med* 1990;**88**:137–140.
10. Kundrapu S, Sunkesula V, Jury LA, et al., Daily disinfection of high-touch surfaces in isolation rooms to reduce contamination of healthcare workers' hands. *Infect Control Hosp Epidemiol* 2012;**33**:1039–1042.
11. Tomas ME, Nerandzic MM, Cadnum JL, et al., A novel, sporicidal formulation of ethanol for glove decontamination to prevent *Clostridium difficile* hand contamination during glove removal. *Inf Control Hosp Epidemiol* 2016;**37**:337–339.

Chapter 44C

Role of Hand Hygiene in Respiratory Diseases Including Influenza

Wing Hong Seto[1] and Benjamin J. Cowling[2]

[1] *World Health Organization Collaborating Centre for Infectious Disease, Epidemiology and Control, School of Public Health, Li Ka Shing Faculty of Medicine, The University of Hong Kong, Hong Kong, SAR, China*

[2] *Department of Pathology, Hong Kong Baptist Hospital, Kowloon Tong, Hong Kong, SAR, China*

KEY MESSAGES

- Hand hygiene is an integral part of standard and respiratory hygiene. They must be implemented together.

- As respiratory discharges can readily contaminate, it is critically important to integrate proper hand hygiene in the use of personal protective equipment (PPE).

- Respiratory droplets and aerosols could be important in the transmission of respiratory viruses, including influenza virus, and additional measures besides hand hygiene such as the donning of the proper respirator may also be important to control infection.

Hand hygiene is a vital component in preventing the spread of acute respiratory infections (ARI). This is understandable because these infections will result in the production of respiratory secretions leading to droplet transmission and contamination of the patient's skin. Furthermore, the accompanying symptoms, including cough, coryza, and sneezing, will enhance the excretion of infectious material into the environment. The proper practice of hand hygiene is therefore a fundamental measure to prevent the spread of ARI. The present chapter will discuss the place of hand hygiene in the hospital and in the community setting.

Hand Hygiene: A Handbook for Medical Professionals, First Edition.
Edited by Didier Pittet, John M. Boyce and Benedetta Allegranzi.
© 2017 John Wiley & Sons, Inc. Published 2017 by John Wiley & Sons, Inc.

WHAT WE KNOW – THE EVIDENCE

Virus Survival on Hands and in the Environment

A number of studies have shown the ability of respiratory viruses to survive on hands and surfaces. For example, Grayson et al. showed that influenza virus can survive on the hands of health care workers (HCWs) for more than an hour, while hand hygiene with soap and water or alcohol handrub can effectively decontaminate hands.[1] Larson et al. reported consistent findings on the efficacy of alternative approaches to hand antisepsis with an alcohol-based handrub (ABHR) or wipes.[2] Thomas et al. inoculated hands with influenza virus and reported some survival for up to 30 minutes.[3] Mukherjee et al. showed that individual coughs and sneezes deposited low concentrations of influenza virus on hands and household surfaces.[4] Other studies have shown that rhinovirus can survive on hands,[5] and can be transmitted via fomites.[6, 7] Other respiratory viruses are also presumed to spread through direct and indirect contact.

Hospital Settings

International guidelines, including those from the World Health Organization (WHO)[8] and the US Centers for Disease Control and Prevention (CDC),[9] have clearly mandated the proper practice of hand hygiene for the prevention of ARI, including influenza.

The WHO commissioned a systematic review and meta-analysis on the specific role of hand hygiene in the prevention of ARI; results are summarized in Figure 44C.1.[10] Due to a limited number of studies, this review mainly involves studies on severe acute respiratory syndrome (SARS), where hand hygiene was studied together with other preventive measures, generally droplet and/or contact precautions. However, these publications did include an analysis of hand hygiene as a separate component and found a statistically significant impact on prevention.

The *WHO Guideline for Hand Hygiene in Health Care* (2009) was the basis for the WHO infection control guideline for the 2009 H1N1 pandemic. Hand hygiene is a key component in this guideline, and it has been shown that WHO guideline application was indeed effective in preventing infections among HCWs during the pandemic.[11]

The Unique Place of Hand Hygiene in Respiratory Infections

Hand hygiene is integrated as a key component of control measures mandated in many infection control guidelines,[8,9] in particular with reference to ARI prevention.

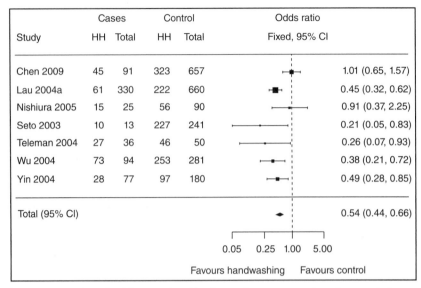

Figure 44C.1   The role of frequent hand hygiene to interrupt or reduce the spread of respiratory viruses; meta-analysis.[8] *Source*: Reproduced with permission from the World Health Organization.

- Respiratory hygiene/cough etiquette. It is now an integral part of standard precautions that patients with nasal discharges and cough should prevent the dispersion of such discharges with tissue or a medical mask. There is now a strong recommendation from the WHO that "respiratory hygiene (i.e. covering the mouth and nose during coughing or sneezing with a medical mask, tissue, or a sleeve or flexed elbow followed by hand hygiene) should be used in persons with ARIs to reduce the dispersal of respiratory secretions containing potentially infectious particles." According to CDC's respiratory hygiene/cough etiquette recommendations: "Perform hand hygiene (e.g., handwashing with non antimicrobial soap and water, ABHR, or antiseptic handwash) after having contact with respiratory secretions and contaminated objects/materials."

- In the proper wearing and removal of personal protective equipment (PPE), such as gloves and gowns, hand hygiene is an important element. In the removal of PPE, the most contaminated PPE items should be removed first. In general, a recommended sequence is: gloves (if gowns are disposable, gloves can be peeled off altogether with gown upon removal) (see also Chapter 23); hand hygiene; gown; eye protection; mask or respirator; and finally hand hygiene.

- The WHO has also recommended the "use of clinical triage for early identification of patients with ARIs to prevent the transmission of ARI pathogens to HCWs and other patients." In the flow diagram in the WHO guideline for such triage activities, hand hygiene is clearly an important component in the management of patients with ARIs.

- HCWs transporting ARI patients should also wear appropriate PPE, followed by hand hygiene.
- Hand hygiene is needed not just for caregivers, but also for visitors and family members accompanying and visiting patients in healthcare settings. Provide conveniently located ABHR dispensers; where sinks are available, ensure that supplies for handwashing (i.e., soap, disposable towels) or handrubbing with ABHR are consistently available.

Community Settings

Hand hygiene is also a valuable intervention in community settings.[19] A number of randomized controlled trials have been conducted in households, including one large study in households in Hong Kong where index cases with laboratory-confirmed influenza virus infection were identified at outpatient clinics, and their households were randomly allocated to hand hygiene without surgical face masks, hand hygiene plus surgical face masks, or a control arm.[20] That study reported a statistically significant effect of hand hygiene plus surgical face masks in prevention of transmission to family members, provided that the intervention was implemented within 36 hours of illness onset in the index case.[20] This illustrates the importance of early and rigorous intervention for a highly infectious disease such as influenza. A meta-analysis of studies conducted in community settings shows that there is marginally statistically significant efficacy of hand hygiene against laboratory-confirmed influenza with or without the addition of surgical face masks (Figure 44C.2). Hand hygiene was extremely efficacious in reducing confirmed influenza and respiratory illnesses in schools in Egypt.[21] An earlier systematic review found that hand hygiene is also an efficacious intervention against respiratory illnesses in general.[22]

WHAT WE DO NOT KNOW - THE UNCERTAIN

Controversy remains over the relative importance of contact, large respiratory droplets, and small particle aerosols in the transmission of influenza. One recent study estimated that aerosol transmission is responsible for around half of transmission in households in Hong Kong and Bangkok, which is indicative that hand hygiene alone may not be sufficient to control transmission in the household or perhaps in other community settings.[23] However, hand hygiene remains one of the most basic interventions against ARI that it is possible to implement in many different community settings where other measures (e.g., surgical face masks) may not be feasible.

Study	Hand hygiene Events	Total	Control Events	Total	Risk Ratio Fixed, 95% CI
Cowling 2008	5	84	12	205	1.02 (0.37, 2.80)
Cowling 2009	32	515	28	279	0.62 (0.38, 1.01)
Larson 2010	57	1884	26	904	1.05 (0.67, 1.66)
Aiello 2010	2	316	3	487	1.03 (0.17, 6.11)
Stebbins 2011	51	1695	53	1665	0.95 (0.65, 1.38)
Suess 2012	10	67	19	82	0.64 (0.32, 1.29)
Aiello 2012	6	349	16	370	0.40 (0.16, 1.00)
Total (95% CI)					0.82 (0.66, 1.02)

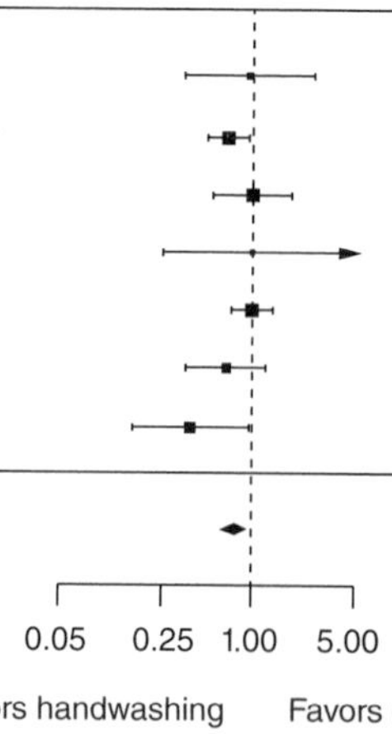

0.05   0.25   1.00   5.00

Favors handwashing   Favors control

Figure 44C.2   The efficacy of hand hygiene interventions with or without face masks to reduce the risk of laboratory-confirmed influenza in community settings; meta-analysis. *Source*: Reproduced with permission from the World Health Organization.

RESEARCH AGENDA

There are a number of areas for further research. One of the greatest gaps in our knowledge is the importance of alternative modes of transmission for respiratory viruses including influenza. It is established that in the practice of droplet and contact precautions, hand hygiene is indeed a vital component. However, studies are lacking to evaluate the contribution of hand hygiene when an alternative mode (such as transmission via hands following contact with environmental surfaces) is responsible for the transmission of the infection.

Another area for research is the patient's contribution for prevention of ARI. It is already clearly recommended under cough etiquette that the patient must perform hand hygiene after contamination by his/her own respiratory secretions, but the efficacy of this has not been studied. Perhaps regular hand hygiene by the patient will also reduce spread and can be applied also in the home context.

Finally, hand hygiene is already an integral part of standard precautions and respiratory hygiene. Hand hygiene compliance has been extensively studied, but not as an integral part of these preventive measures. The above are routine practices, and it is not known if hand hygiene is properly integrated. It will benefit from further research, especially in regard to how compliance can be further enhanced.

REFERENCES

1. Grayson ML, Melvani S, Druce J, et al., Efficacy of soap and water and alcohol-based hand-rub preparations against live H1N1 influenza virus on the hands of human volunteers. *Clin Infect Dis*. 2009;**48**:285–291.
2. Larson EL, Cohen B, Baxter KA, et al., Analysis of alcohol-based hand sanitizer delivery systems: efficacy of foam, gel, and wipes against influenza A (H1N1) virus on hands. *Am J Infect Control* 2012;**40**:806–809.
3. Thomas Y, Boquete-Suter P, Koch D, et al., Survival of influenza virus on human fingers. *Clin Microbiol Infect* 2014;**20**:58–64.
4. Mukherjee DV, Cohen B, Bovino ME, et al., Survival of influenza virus on hands and fomites in community and laboratory settings. *Am J Infect Control* 2012;**40**:590–594.
5. Winther B, McCue K, Ashe K, et al., Environmental contamination with rhinovirus and transfer to fingers of healthy individuals by daily life activity. *J Med Virol* 2007;**79**:1606–1610.
6. Gwaltney JM Jr, Hendley JO. Transmission of experimental rhinovirus infection by contaminated surfaces. *Am J Epidemiol* 1982;**116**:828–833.
7. Hendley JO, Wenzel RP, Gwaltney JM Jr. Transmission of rhinovirus colds by self-inoculation. *N Engl J Med* 1973;**288**:1361–1364.
8. World Health Organization, *WHO Infection prevention and control of epidemic- and pandemic-prone acute respiratory diseases in health care*. Available at www.who.int/csr/bioriskreduction/infection_control/publication/en/. Accessed March 7, 2017.
9. Centers for Disease Control and Prevention, *Prevention Strategies for Seasonal Influenza in Healthcare Settings*. Available at www.cdc.gov/flu/professionals/infectioncontrol/healthcaresettings.htm. Accessed March 7, 2017.
10. Seto WH, Conly JM, Pessoa-Silva CL, et al., Infection prevention and control measures for acute respiratory infections in healthcare settings: an update. *East Mediterr Health J* 2013;**19**(Suppl. 1):S39–S47.
11. Seto WH, Cowling BJ, Lam HS, et al., Clinical and nonclinical health care workers faced a similar risk of acquiring 2009 pandemic H1N1 infection. *Clin Infect Dis* 2011;**53**:280–283.
12. Chen WQ, Ling WH, Lu CY, et al., Which preventive measures might protect health care workers from SARS? *BMC Public Health* 2009;**9**:81.
13. Lau JT, Tsui H, Lau M, et al., SARS transmission, risk factors, and prevention in Hong Kong. *Emerg Infect Dis* 2004;**10**:587–592.
14. Nishiura H, Kuratsuji T, Quy T, et al., Rapid awareness and transmission of severe acute respiratory syndrome in Hanoi French Hospital, Vietnam. *Am J Trop Med Hyg* 2005;**73**:17–25.
15. Seto WH, Tsang D, Yung RW, et al., Effectiveness of precautions against droplets and contact in prevention of nosocomial transmission of severe acute respiratory syndrome (SARS). *Lancet* 2003;**361**:1519–1520.
16. Teleman MD, Boudville IC, Heng BH, et al., Factors associated with transmission of severe acute respiratory syndrome among health-care workers in Singapore. *Epidemiol Infect* 2004;**132**:797–803.
17. Wu J, Xu F, Zhou W, et al., Risk factors for SARS among persons without known contact with SARS patients, Beijing, China. *Emerg Infect Dis* 2004;**10**:210–216.

18. Yin WW, Gao LD, Lin WS, et al., Effectiveness of personal protective measures in prevention of nosocomial transmission of severe acute respiratory syndrome. *Zhonghua Liu Xing Bing Xue Za Zhi (Chinese Journal of Epidemiology)* 2004;**25**:18–22.
19. Aiello AE, Perez V, Coulborn RM, et al., Facemasks, hand hygiene, and influenza among young adults: a randomized intervention trial. *PLoS ONE* 2012;**7**:e29744.
20. Cowling BJ, Chan KH, Fang VJ, et al., Facemasks and hand hygiene to prevent influenza transmission in households: a cluster randomized trial. *Ann Intern Med* 2009;**151**:437–446.
21. Talaat M, Afifi S, Dueger E, et al., Effects of hand hygiene campaigns on incidence of laboratory-confirmed influenza and absenteeism in schoolchildren, Cairo, Egypt. *Emerg Infect Dis* 2011;**17**:619–625.
22. Aiello AE, Coulborn RM, Perez V, et al., Effect of hand hygiene on infectious disease risk in the community setting: a meta-analysis. *Am J Public Health* 2008;**98**:1372–1381.
23. Cowling BJ, Ip DK, Fang VJ, et al., Aerosol transmission is an important mode of influenza A virus spread. *Nat Commun* 2013;**4**:1935.

Chapter 44D

Handborne Spread of Noroviruses and its Interruption

Syed A. Sattar[1] and Yves Longtin[2]
[1] Department of Biochemistry, Microbiology and Immunology, Faculty of Medicine, University of Ottawa, Ottawa, Canada
[2] Infection Control and Prevention Unit, Jewish General Hospital, and McGill University, Montreal, Canada

KEY MESSAGES

- Human noroviruses (HuNoVs) continue to exert a heavy toll on human health worldwide, and their health impact appears to be rising due to a combination of ongoing societal changes.

- Proper and regular hand hygiene remains an important generic means of interrupting the spread of noroviral acute gastroenteritis, though further work is needed to address the concerns some have about the activity of alcohol-based handrubs (ABHRs) against HuNoVs.

- Concerted efforts are needed to improve the growth of HuNoVs in cell cultures. Such a breakthrough could greatly facilitate research and development to combat noroviral acute gastroenteritis.

Hand Hygiene: A Handbook for Medical Professionals, First Edition.
Edited by Didier Pittet, John M. Boyce and Benedetta Allegranzi.
© 2017 John Wiley & Sons, Inc. Published 2017 by John Wiley & Sons, Inc.

WHAT WE KNOW - THE EVIDENCE

The small size and modest chemistry of human noroviruses (HuNoVs) belie their profound impact on our health and economy. They are the most common cause of nonbacterial acute gastroenteritis (AGE) with more than 267 million clinical cases and over 200,000 fatalities annually around the world.[1] In the United States, HuNoVs were detected in more than 20% of young children, with AGE costing in excess of US$273 million/year for treatment alone.[2] The relative importance of HuNoVs is increasing with successful vaccination against rotaviral AGE.[2]

A blending of the attributes listed in Table 44D.1 makes HuNoVs truly unique as human pathogens. The HuNoVs disease incubation period – as short as 12 hours – is unmatched by any other infectious agent. The clinical symptoms of noroviral AGE are reminiscent of cholera, with virus being shed in both profuse diarrhea and projectile vomiting, resulting in widespread environmental contamination from an estimated 5 billion infectious units/g of feces.[3] The high levels of infectious particles excreted, together with a low minimal infective dose (~15 infectious particles) and environmental stability, may contribute to the contagiousness of HuNoVs leading to localized outbreaks as well as large epidemics. Community outbreaks and those in closed settings (e.g., homes for children and the aged, hospitals, and cruise ships) are common; severe ones in hospitals may lead to closure of the entire facility during cleanup. In the United States, HuNoVs cause ~50% of the recorded cases of AGE, with food handlers being incriminated the most.[1] No vaccination or specific chemotherapy is currently available against them.

While HuNoVs can spread in many ways, including possibly by droplets and droplet nuclei, hands are pivotal in their transmission (Figure 44D.1), and hand hygiene is essential for interrupting their environmental spread. However, since hands frequently interact with other potential vehicles, effective mitigation of HuNoV transmission must include a more comprehensive approach for success.

WHAT WE DO NOT KNOW - THE UNCERTAIN

The hand cleansing method of choice after caring for norovirus-affected patients remains unclear, and the relative efficacy of handwashing with soap and water versus handrubbing with an alcohol-based handrub (ABHR) is still debated. Neither plain nor medicated "antimicrobial" soaps show any discernible virucidal activity against HuNoVs.[4] Therefore, handwashing with soap and clean water is a generic way of mechanically ridding hands of HuNoVs provided the hands are properly lathered, rinsed, and dried.

In spite of the widening acceptance and use of ABHRs, some suggest that they may enhance the handborne spread of HuNoVs.[5] A combination of the following may form the genesis of this view: (a) much of the early testing of ABHRs against HuNoVs was based on using the more ethanol-resistant feline calicivirus (FCV) as

Table 44D.1   Basics of Human Noroviruses and the Diseases They Cause

Biology	• Non enveloped, icosahedral in shape with a virion diameter of ~30 nm • Genome single-stranded, nonsegmented, positive-sense RNA • Periodic genetic changes lead to new strains
Clinical picture	• Acute onset, nonbloody diarrhea, vomiting, nausea, abdominal cramps, low-grade fever with body aches; about 10% cases may require medical attention
Pathogenesis	• Exposure via fecal/vomitus-oral route; may also spread via droplets • Minimal infectious dose (MID) ~15 infectious particles[3] • Incubation period as short as 12 hrs • Clinical phase lasts 24–48 hrs; dehydration may be fatal in the very young and the aged • Subclinical infection in up to 5–16% of cases[6] • Primary attack rate ~40%; secondary attack rate >55% • Fecal shedding of virus up to three weeks post recovery; in the immunocompromised it may last for years and give rise to secondary cases • Recovery normally without any sequelae • No long-term immunity, and reinfections are common
Epidemiology	• Multiple strains may circulate simultaneously and cause infections • Worldwide distribution; no specific target age • No well-defined seasonality, though more common in winter • Sporadic cases to pandemics; outbreaks common in closed settings such as hospitals and cruise ships
Treatment	• No specific therapy; supportive therapy via rehydration
Prevention and control	• Vaccines using virus-like particles under trial • Control of food and water quality • Disinfection of high-touch environmental surfaces • Hand hygiene with either soap and water or an alcohol-based handrub (see text)

their surrogate;[6] (b) when HuNoVs were used, their viability was assessed using indirect and possibly inappropriate molecular means;[6] (c) wide variations exist in test protocols and interpretation of product effectiveness criteria; (d) field studies on hand hygiene sometimes fail to consider certain confounding factors.[7] Recent in vivo studies using the murine norovirus (MNV), which is more akin to HuNoVs,

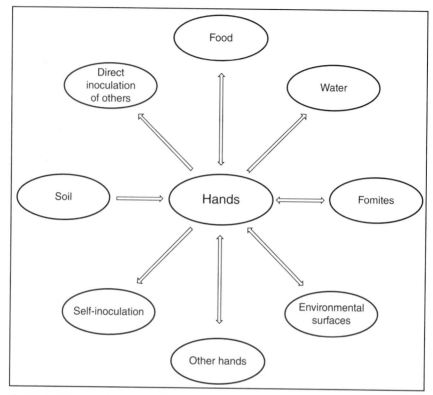

Figure 44D.1   The pivotal role of hands in the spread of human noroviruses.

reinforce the suitability of ABHRs in interrupting the spread of noroviral AGE.[8] However, for optimal effectiveness and safety, ABHRs must be selected and used considering the factors listed in Table 44D.2.

It is generally agreed that ABHRs can be used when caring for a patient affected by HuNoV in nonoutbreak settings[9] in combination with gloves. Some scientific societies recommend the preferential use of soap and water during HuNoV outbreaks.[10] This recommendation is based on limited evidence and must be carefully weighed against the lack of availability of sinks in many institutions.

RESEARCH AGENDA

HuNoVs have, until recently, remained refractory to in vitro culture, and there are no suitable small-animal models for them. This has seriously limited our understanding of these important pathogens. The recent successful in vitro culture could contribute immensely to our understanding of HuNoVs and lead to better environmental control as well as the development of vaccines and chemotherapy.[11]

Table 44D.2   Factors to Consider in Selecting and Using Alcohol-Based Handrubs against HuNoVs

Factors	Comments
Alcohol, type and concentration	Minimum ethanol concentration of 60% (vol/vol); other alcohols may be added but without any significant increase in activity.[8] Isopropanol at ≥70% has shown activity against MNV[13]
Need for other actives	Actives (e.g., triclosan, chlorhexidine gluconate, and *p*-chloro-metaxylenol) are ineffective against HuNoVs, thus not needed
Level of effectiveness desired	A minimum 2 $\log_{10}$ reduction in virus infectivity on hands is arbitrarily set by Health Canada for product registration[14]
Activity against other pathogens	Formulations containing ≥60% (vol/vol) ethanol show good activity against many bacterial, fungal, and viral nosocomial pathogens[8]
Duration of handrubbing	A thorough rubbing of hands together with the applied formulation for a minimum of 15–20 seconds is essential for optimal virus inactivation
Skin compatibility	Ethanol leaves no residue on the skin; excipients necessary to counter drying action of ethanol on skin
Residual activity	Thus far, no formulations are available with demonstrated residual activity on the skin
Environmental safety	Ethanol *per se* is readily biodegradable

The suboptimal compliance with hand hygiene, especially in healthcare, remains a perennial impediment to infection control and prevention in general. This factor alone will continue to limit the potential of hand hygiene in general even though many currently available handwash and handrub agents are sufficiently effective in dealing with major handborne pathogens including several types of non-enveloped viruses.[12,13] Any further improvements in the virucidal activity of ABHRs against small non-enveloped viruses would remain a challenge considering the compact size of such pathogens as well as the unavoidable requirements of safety and skin friendliness as well as speed of action.

Though the past three decades have seen much progress in our understanding of the basic biology of HuNoVs and their epidemiology, there remain major gaps in our knowledge on the relative importance of hands and other environmental vehicles in the spread of HuNoVs. We urgently require practical ways to culture lab-adapted as well as field strains of the viruses and also quantitate their infectivity in vitro for targeted advances in interrupting the environmental spread of noroviral infections. Such in vitro culture will also help in the development of specific chemotherapy and vaccines.

REFERENCES

1. Centers for Disease Control and Prevention. www.cdc.gov/ncidod/dvrd/revb/gastro/norovirus-factsheet.htm. Accessed March 7, 2017.
2. Payne DC, Vinjé J, Szilagyi PG, et al., Norovirus and medically attended gastroenteritis in U.S. children. *N Engl J Med.* 2013;**368**:1121–1130.
3. Teunis PF, Moe CL, Liu P, et al., Norwalk virus: how infectious is it? *J Med Virol* 2008;**80**:1468–1476.
4. Steinmann J, Paulmann D, Becker B, et al., Comparison of virucidal activity of alcohol-based hand sanitizers versus antimicrobial hand soaps in vitro and in vivo. *J Hosp Infect* 2012;**82**:277–280.
5. Blaney DD, Daly ER, Kirkland KB, et al., Use of alcohol-based hand sanitizers as a risk factor for norovirus outbreaks in long-term care facilities in northern New England: December 2006 to March 2007. *Am J Infect Control* 2011;**39**:296–301.
6. Hall AJ, Vinjé J, Lopman B, et al., Updated norovirus outbreak management and disease prevention guidelines. *Morbid Mortal Wkly Rep* 2011;**60**(RR03):1–15.
7. Longtin Y, Voss A, Allegranzi B, et al., Norovirus outbreaks and alcohol-based handrub solutions: association does not prove causation. *Am J Infect Control* 2012;**40**:191.
8. Sattar SA, Ali M, Tetro JA, *In vivo* comparison of two human norovirus surrogates for testing ethanol-based handrubs: the mouse chasing the cat! *PLoS ONE* 2011;**6**:e17340.
9. World Health Organization, *WHO Guidelines on Hand Hygiene in Health Care.* Geneva: WHO, 2009. Available at whqlibdoc.who.int/publications/2009/9789241597906_eng.pdf. Accessed March 7, 2017.
10. MacCannel T, Umscheid CA, Agarwal RK, et al., Guideline for the prevention and control of norovirus gastroenteritis outbreaks in healthcare settings. *Infect Control Hosp Epidemiol* 2011;**32**:939–969.
11. Jones MK, Watanabe M, Zhu S, et al., Enteric bacteria promote human and mouse norovirus infection of B cells. *Science* 2014;**346**:755–759.
12. Park GW, Barclay L, Macinga D, et al., Comparative efficacy of seven hand sanitizers against murine norovirus, feline calicivirus, and GII.4 norovirus. *J Food Prot* 2010;**73**:2232–2238.
13. Sattar SA, Abebe M, Bueti A, et al., Activity of an alcohol-based hand gel against human adeno-, rhino-, and rotaviruses using the fingerpad method. *Infect Control Hosp Epidemiol* 2000;**21**:516–519.
14. Health Canada, Guidance document human-use antiseptic drugs – Dec 2009. Available at www.hc-sc.gc.ca/dhp-mps/alt_formats/pdf/prodpharma/applic-demande/guide-ld/antiseptic_guide_ld-eng.pdf. Accessed on March 7, 2017.

Chapter 45

Conducting a Literature Review on Hand Hygiene

Daniela Pires, Fernando Bellissimo-Rodrigues, and Didier Pittet
Infection Control Program and WHO Collaborating Centre on Patient Safety, University of Geneva Hospitals and Faculty of Medicine, Geneva, Switzerland

KEY MESSAGES

- Hand hygiene is an expanding discipline of Infection Prevention and Control and Hospital Epidemiology.
- Literature search skills in MEDLINE®/PubMed® are crucial to any healthcare worker. **Hand hygiene** (entered since 2013), **hand disinfection** (since 1982), and **hand sanitizers** (since 2014) are the main MeSH vocabulary used by MEDLINE®/PubMed® to index the hand hygiene literature.
- Importantly, **handrub, handrubbing, handrubs,** or **alcohol-based handrubs** are not entry terms for any of the MeSH vocabulary referred; searching using these keywords only might miss important publications.

WHAT WE KNOW – THE EVIDENCE

Today, the global number of scientific publications and cited references in all disciplines grows at a rate of 8–9% per year.[1] Importantly, this vast knowledge base is mostly accessible to anyone connected to the Internet. However, this poses enormous challenges: how to find the answers to daily clinical problems amid all

Hand Hygiene: A Handbook for Medical Professionals, First Edition.
Edited by Didier Pittet, John M. Boyce and Benedetta Allegranzi.
© 2017 John Wiley & Sons, Inc. Published 2017 by John Wiley & Sons, Inc.

publications? How to keep up to date with the enormous flow of information? A nonfocused, nonstructured literature search can be frustrating. Fortunately, powerful tools exist to assist in these tasks. Of these, the most frequently used in biomedical literature are MEDLINE® and PubMed®. MEDLINE® is a database of citations and abstracts of life sciences journals from the US National Library of Medicine. PubMed® is a resource of the US National Center for Biotechnology Information that allows free access to MEDLINE®.[2]

The National Library of Medicine provides an excellent tutorial to improve your PubMed® search skills. In addition, some easy-to-read reviews on the subject are available.[3]

A few tips should be kept in mind when conducting your search. First, take a few seconds to formulate your clinical question and choose carefully the keywords for your search. If you have problems identifying the most relevant keywords, simply click on an important article in the field and, click on the down arrow next to the Abstract icon located on the upper left portion of the abstract display page, click on the MEDLINE button, and check for the MeSH (medical subject headings) vocabulary used for indexing the paper in question. Then you can conduct your search using similar keywords. MeSH is a uniform vocabulary used by MEDLINE® to index each unique publication. This vocabulary is arranged in a hierarchical manner (via the MeSH Tree structure) and is updated annually. Using MeSH is the most efficacious way to be specific in your search; it takes little practice to get used to its structure.

If you want to type freely on the search field, take a few seconds to understand what PubMed® is retrieving. For this, you should look carefully at the search details (on the right side column of PubMed® main page) after typing your keywords. For example, if you want to search for terms like **hand wash** and simply type – **hand wash** – you will find yourself amid titles and abstracts with the words **hand** and **wash** separately (which can take you to articles mentioning **on the other hand** and **wash out**, for example) and even worse, you will be redirected to the MeSH term **hand** (and find yourself amid **hand care** or **hand lotions** papers). In a PubMed® search, if you want to find titles and abstracts only with the terms you type together or as a phrase, you should use quotation marks (**"hand wash"**) or a dash (**hand-wash**). You can also type – **hand wash*** – ; in this case, in addition to conduct the search as a phrase, it will also allow different terminations to be searched for (e.g., **hand wash**_es_ and **hand wash**_ing_). However, by restricting your search on phrases (**"hand wash"** or **hand-wash** or **hand wash***) you will not be directed to any MeSH terms, and this can also compromise your search. Again, it is very important to look at the search details section and modify your search according to what you really are looking for.

Finally, you can make good use of the limits section, where you can constrain your research by type of clinical studies (as clinical trials, systematic reviews), date of publication, and so on.

Importantly, if your objective is to perform a more extensive academic literature review, a broader search is warranted; in this situation, using MEDLINE® only is certainly not sufficient. There are several other databases with different scopes that may complement the MEDLINE® search. Some examples of these are, but not restricted to, EMBASE® (a biomedical and pharmacological database, by Reed Elsevier Properties SA), CINAHL (Cumulative Index to Nursing and Allied Health Literature, by EBSCO Health SA), and SciELO (Scientific Electronic Library Online, by Brazilian National Council for Scientific and Technological Development and Pan-American Health Organization). Additionally, if you want to write a systematic review on the subject, it may be useful to consult the Cochrane Collaboration and the PRISMA statement for reporting systematic reviews and meta-analyses.[4]

Hand hygiene, **hand disinfection**, and **hand sanitizers** are the main MeSH vocabulary used by PubMed® to index the hand hygiene literature. In the MeSH Tree structure, **hand hygiene** is a broader term than **hand disinfection** and more specific than **Communicable Disease Control**. By searching by **hand hygiene** MeSH term you will find all the publications indexed under **hand hygiene** and **hand disinfection**. It is interesting to note that **hand hygiene** only became part of MeSH vocabulary in 2013. On the contrary, **hand disinfection** has been part of MeSH terminology since 1982. A **hand sanitizers** MeSH term was added in 2014, and placed in the MeSH Tree of **Chemicals and Drug categories**, so articles published before 2014 will only be retrieved if **hand sanitizer** was in the article title or abstract.

Another important concept in MeSH vocabulary is the entry terms. These are terms that PubMed® assumes as synonyms of the main MeSH vocabulary. For example, **hand washing** is an entry term for **hand disinfection**. So, if you type – **hand washing** – PubMed® will also automatically search for the MeSH term **hand disinfection**. **Hand disinfection** has the following entry terms: **disinfection**; **hand surgical scrubbing**; **scrubbing, surgical**; **hand sanitization**; **sanitization, hand**; **handwashing**; **hand washing**; **hand washings**; **washing, hand**; **washings, hand**. It is worth noting that some of the most widely used terms in the current hand hygiene literature, such as **handrub** (or **handrubbing** or **handrubs**) or **alcohol-based handrubs**, are not entry terms for any of the MeSH vocabulary referred. This is particularly important because if you search using the keywords that are not MeSH vocabulary or entry terms, PubMed® will retrieve some articles but you may miss important publications. Importantly, the fact that these are not entry terms currently does not mean that they will not be in the future. The preferred recourse to alcohol-based handrubs to clean hands in healthcare practices is only real since the early 2000s,[5,6] predicting a possible entry in the MeSH vocabulary in the near future, similarly to the very recent (2014) entry of the MeSH term **hand sanitizers**.

We conducted a literature search in PubMed®, using different keywords commonly used in the hand hygiene literature (Table 45.1). Furthermore, we looked at the relative frequency of these keywords in hand hygiene publications. Looking at all the terms combined, we found around 8,000 publications pertaining to the research of hand hygiene from 1921 to 2015 (August 23).

The MeSH vocabulary **hand hygiene** retrieved 4,932 publications, and the MeSH vocabulary **hand disinfection** found 4,572 publications. As explained above, this resulted from the higher position of **hand hygiene** in the MeSH Tree. In contrast, if instead of searching using MeSH vocabulary, we typed freely on the search field, we observed different results. **Hand disinfection** (typed as – **hand desinf*** – in PubMed® search box) retrieved almost twice the number of publications compared with **hand hygiene** (typed as – "**hand hygiene**" – in PubMed® search box), 4,826 versus 2,643, respectively. As stated before, this kind of search leaves out the indexing by PubMed® (MeSH vocabulary) and looks only for the search words in the titles and abstracts. The higher number of articles found under **hand disinfection** might reflect the more widespread use of this term by authors. However, the term **hand disinfection** is nowadays considered a misconception,[7] as **disinfection** is only correctly applied to inanimate surfaces. Furthermore, we can see that the third most frequently used term in the literature is hand washing (typed as – **hand wash*** – in PubMed® search box). Using a combination of hand hygiene, hand disinfection, and hand washing (both as MeSH terms, phrase search and several ending possibilities), we will retrieve 7,903 results (or 96% of the overall results). These are undoubtedly the most used terms to refer to the hand hygiene literature.

Additionally, we analyzed the evolution of hand hygiene publications over time and its relationship with the date of the publication of some landmark papers (Table 45.2 and Figure 45.1). A few years after the start of the SENIC (Study on the Efficacy of Nosocomial Infection Control) study, in 1974, we observe a small but consistent increase in the number of publications on hand hygiene. However, after that initial increase, the number of publications remains fairly constant from 1985 to 2000 (around 100 publications/year). It is at the turn of the millennium that we witness an exponential growth in the production of scientific articles in the field of hand hygiene. This is most probably related to two landmark studies on hand hygiene performed at the University of Geneva Hospitals (HUG)[5,6] (see also Chapter 1). These studies launched the basis for transatlantic collaboration and the publication of the US Centers for Disease Control and Prevention (CDC) guidelines for Hand Hygiene in Healthcare Settings in 2002.[7] Studies published at the beginning of the twenty-first century further assisted the globalization of the hand hygiene concept, for example through the launch of the World Health Organization (WHO) *Clean Care is Safer Care* campaign, and the publication of the WHO guidelines.[8,9] More recently, a video on hand hygiene produced by the *New England Journal of Medicine* and a study on the global implementation of WHO's multimodal strategy for hand hygiene improvement further helped to raise awareness of hand hygiene, fueling research activity worldwide.[10,11]

Table 45.1 Summary of Hand Hygiene Literature Commonly Used Terms, PubMed® Search Strategy, and Number of Publications

Hand Hygiene Literature Commonly Used Terms[1]	PubMed® Search Strategy[2]	Number of Articles	PubMed® Search Details
hand hygiene	hand hygiene[Mesh]	4932	Hand hygiene[Mesh]
	"hand hygiene"	2643	"hand hygiene"[All Fields]
hand disinfection	hand disinfection[Mesh]	4572	hand disinfection[Mesh]
	hand disinf*	4826	hand disinfectant[All Fields] OR hand disinfectants[All Fields] OR hand disinfection[All Fields] OR hand disinfections[All Fields]
hand sanitizers	hand sanitizers[Mesh]	27	hand sanitizers[Mesh]
	hand sanit*	247	hand sanitation[All Fields] OR hand sanitiser[All Fields] OR hand sanitisers[All Fields] OR hand sanitising[All Fields] OR hand sanitization[All Fields] OR hand sanitizer[All Fields] OR hand sanitizers[All Fields] OR hand sanitizing[All Fields]
hand washing	"hand washing" OR "handwashing" OR "hand wash"	3279	"hand washing"[All Fields] OR "handwashing"[All Fields] OR "hand wash"[All Fields]
hand rubbing	hand rub* OR handrubbing	470	(hand rub[All Fields] OR hand rubbing[All Fields] OR hand rubs[All Fields]) OR handrubbing[All Fields]
surgical scrubbing	surgical scrub*	257	surgical scrub[All Fields] OR surgical scrubbing[All Fields] OR surgical scrubs[All Fields]

hand cleansing	hand cleans*	89	hand cleanser[All Fields] OR hand cleansers[All Fields] OR hand cleansing[All Fields]
hand decontamination	hand deconta*	54	hand decontaminants[All Fields] OR hand decontaminating[All Fields] OR hand decontamination[All Fields]
hand cleaning	"hand cleaning"	30	"hand cleaning"[All Fields]
hand antisepsis	hand-antisep*	115	hand antisepsis[All Fields] OR hand antiseptic[All Fields] OR hand antiseptics[All Fields]
alcohol-based hand rub	alcohol-based hand rub*	281	alcohol based hand rub[All Fields] OR alcohol based hand rubbing[All Fields] OR alcohol based hand rubs[All Fields]
ALL keywords[3]	ALL keywords[3]	8233	4

Search performed on August 23, 2015.

[1]The terms used for search resulted from a consensus between the authors.

[2]The terms are stated as typed in PubMed®.

[3]The search strategy used was: (Hand Hygiene[MeSH] OR "hand hygiene" OR hand disinfection[MeSH] OR hand disinf* OR hand sanitizers[MeSH] OR hand sanit* OR "hand washing" OR "handwashing" OR "hand wash" OR hand rub* OR "handrubbing" OR hand cleans* OR hand deconta* OR "hand cleaning" OR alcohol-based hand rub* OR hand-antisep* OR surgical scrub*).

[4]The search details retrieved were: ("Hand Hygiene"[MeSH] OR "hand hygiene"[All Fields] OR "hand disinfection"[MeSH] OR (hand disinfectant[All Fields] OR hand disinfectants[All Fields] OR hand disinfection[All Fields] OR hand disinfections[All Fields]) OR "hand sanitizers"[MeSH] OR (hand sanitation[All Fields] OR hand sanitiser[All Fields] OR hand sanitisers[All Fields] OR hand sanitising[All Fields] OR hand sanitization[All Fields] OR hand sanitizer[All Fields] OR hand sanitizers[All Fields] OR (hand rub[All Fields] OR hand rubbing[All Fields] OR "hand washing"[All Fields] OR "handwashing"[All Fields] OR "hand wash"[All Fields] OR (hand rub[All Fields] OR hand rubbing[All Fields] OR "handrubbing"[All Fields] OR (hand cleanser[All Fields] OR hand cleansers[All Fields] OR hand cleansing[All Fields]) OR (hand decontaminants[All Fields] OR hand decontaminating[All Fields] OR hand decontamination[All Fields]) OR "hand cleaning"[All Fields] OR (alcohol based hand rub[All Fields] OR alcohol based hand rubbing[All Fields] OR alcohol based hand rubs[All Fields] OR (hand antisepsis[All Fields] OR hand antiseptic[All Fields] OR hand antiseptics[All Fields] OR (surgical scrub[All Fields] OR surgical scrubbing[All Fields] OR surgical scrubs[All Fields]).

Table 45.2   Selected Landmark Publications on Hand Hygiene

Year	Publication
1962	Mortimer EA et al., Transmission of staphylococci between newborns: importance of the hands to personnel. *Am J Dis Child*[12]
1974	Start of SENIC (Study on the Efficacy of Nosocomial Infection Control)
1985	Haley RW et al., The efficacy of infection surveillance and control programmes in preventing nosocomial infections in the US hospitals. *Am J Epidemiol*[13]
1985	CDC guidelines for the prevention and control of nosocomial infections. Guideline for handwashing and hospital environmental control[14]
1995	APIC guideline for handwashing and hand antisepsis in healthcare settings[15]
1999	Pittet D et al., Compliance with handwashing in a teaching hospital. *Ann Intern Med*[5]
2000	Pittet D et al., Effectiveness of a hospital-wide programme to improve compliance with hand hygiene. *Lancet*[6]
2002	Guideline for hand hygiene in healthcare settings: recommendations of the Healthcare Infection Control Practices Advisory Committee and the HICPAC/SHEA/APIC/IDSA Hand Hygiene Task Force[7]
2005	WHO *Clean Care is Safer Care* campaign
2007	Sax H et al., My Five Moments for Hand Hygiene: a user-centred design approach to understand, train, monitor and report hand hygiene. *J Hosp Infect*[16]
2009	WHO guidelines, Hand Hygiene in Healthcare and a Guide to the Implementation of the WHO Multimodal Hand Hygiene Improvement Strategy[8,9]
2011	Longtin Y et al., Hand hygiene. *N Engl J Med*[10]
2013	Allegranzi B et al., Global implementation of WHO's multimodal strategy for improvement of hand hygiene: a quasi-experimental study. *Lancet Infect Dis*[11]

APIC, Association for Professionals in Infection Control and Epidemiology; CDC, Centers for Disease Control and Prevention; HCW, healthcare workers; HICPAC, Healthcare Infection Control Practices Advisory Committee; IDSA, Infectious Diseases Society of America; SHEA, Society for Healthcare Epidemiology of America; WHO, World Health Organization.
The search was conducted on August 23, 2015.
Please refer to table II for the identification of the studies.

WHAT WE DO NOT KNOW AND RESEARCH AGENDA

Adding hand hygiene to the MeSH Tree Structure in 2013 was an important step for improving the PubMed® search capability on this topic. However, it would be desirable to further update entry terms. Furthermore, an effort to unify terminology between authors needs to be made.

   To conclude, it is relatively straightforward to assume that the exponential increase in hand hygiene publications is related to increasing interest in this field,

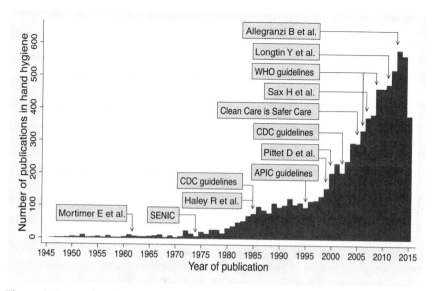

Figure 45.1   Number of publications on hand hygiene by year and main landmark publications. (Search conducted on August 23, 2015)

as well as with the academic and policy maker recognition of its importance. Raising awareness (both among healthcare workers, hospital administration, policy makers, and stakeholders) is a very important step in improving clinical practice. However, we cannot readily assume that this growing interest in research translates into proportionally better practice.

REFERENCES

1. Bornmann L, Mutz R, Growth rates of modern science: a bibliometric analysis based on the number of publications and cited references. *J Assoc Inf Sci Technol*. Available at onlinelibrary .wiley.com/doi/10.1002/asi.23329/full. Accessed March 7, 2017.
2. Smith R, Chalmers I, Britain's gift: a "Medline" of synthesised evidence: worldwide free access to evidence based resources could transform health care. *Br Med J* 2001;**323**:1437–1438.
3. Shojania KG, Olmsted RN, Searching the health care literature efficiently: from clinical decision-making to continuing education. *Am J Infect Control* 2002;**30**:187–195.
4. Liberati A, Altman DG, Tetzlaff J, et al., The PRISMA statement for reporting systematic reviews and meta-analyses of studies that evaluate healthcare interventions: explanation and elaboration. *Br Med J* 2009;**339**:b2700.
5. Pittet D, Mourouga P, Perneger TV, Compliance with handwashing in a teaching hospital. *Ann Intern Med* 1999;**130**:126–130.
6. Pittet D, Hugonnet S, Harbarth S, et al., Effectiveness of a hospital-wide programme to improve compliance with hand hygiene. *Lancet* 2000;**356**:1307–1312.

 7. Boyce JM, Pittet D, Guideline for Hand Hygiene in Health-Care Settings: recommendations of the Healthcare Infection Control Practices Advisory Committee and the HICPAC/SHEA/APIC/IDSA Hand Hygiene Task Force. *Am J Infect Control* 2002;**30**:S1–S46.

 8. World Health Organization, *WHO Guidelines on Hand Hygiene in Health Care: first global patient safety challenge: Clean Care is Safer Care*. Geneva: WHO, 2009.

 9. World Health Organization, *WHO A guide to the implementation of the WHO Multimodal Hand Hygiene Improvement Strategy*. Geneva: WHO, 2009.

10. Longtin Y, Sax H, Allegranzi B, et al., Videos in clinical medicine. Hand hygiene. *N Engl J Med* 2011;**364**:e24.

11. Allegranzi B, Gayet-Ageron A, Damani N, et al., Global implementation of WHO's multimodal strategy for improvement of hand hygiene: a quasi-experimental study. *Lancet Infect Dis* 2013;**13**:843–851.

12. Mortimer EA, Lipsitz PJ, Wolinsky E, et al., Transmission of staphylococci between newborns: importance of the hands to personnel. *Am J Dis Child* 1962;**104**:289–295.

13. Haley RW, Culver DH, White JW, et al., The efficacy of infection surveillance and control programs in preventing nosocomial infections in US hospitals. *Am J Epidemiol* 1985;**121**:182–205.

14. Garner JS, Favero MS, CDC guideline for handwashing and hospital environmental control, 1985. *Infect Control* 1986;**7**:231–243.

15. Larson EL, APIC guideline for handwashing and hand antisepsis in health care settings. *Am J Infect Control* 1995;**23**:251–269.

16. Sax H, Allegranzi B, Uçkay I, et al., "My five moments for hand hygiene": a user-centred design approach to understand, train, monitor and report hand hygiene. *J Hosp Infect* 2007;**67**:9–21.

Appendix

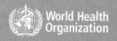

Hand Hygiene Self-Assessment Framework 2010
Introduction and user instructions

The Hand Hygiene Self-Assessment Framework is a systematic tool with which to obtain a situation analysis of hand hygiene promotion and practices within an individual health-care facility.

What is its purpose?

While providing an opportunity to reflect on existing resources and achievements, the Hand Hygiene Self-Assessment Framework also helps to focus on future plans and challenges. In particular, it acts as a diagnostic tool, identifying key issues requiring attention and improvement. The results can be used to facilitate development of an action plan for the facility's hand hygiene programme. Repeated use of the Hand Hygiene Self-Assessment Framework will also allow documentation of progress with time.

Overall, this tool should be a catalyst for implementing and sustaining a comprehensive hand hygiene programme within a health-care facility.

Who should use the Hand Hygiene Self-Assessment Framework?

This tool should be used by professionals in charge of implementing a strategy to improve hand hygiene within a health-care facility. If no strategy is being implemented yet, then it can also be used by professionals in charge of infection control or senior managers at the facility directorate. The framework can be used globally, by health-care facilities at any level of progress as far as hand hygiene promotion is concerned.

How is it structured?

The Hand Hygiene Self-Assessment Framework is divided into five components and 27 indicators. The five components reflect the five elements of the WHO Multimodal Hand Hygiene Improvement Strategy (http://www.who.int/gpsc/5may/tools/en/index.html) and the indicators have been selected to represent the key elements of each component. These indicators are based on evidence and expert consensus and have been framed as questions with defined answers (either "Yes/No" or multiple options) to facilitate self-assessment. Based on the score achieved for the five components, the facility is assigned to one of four levels of hand hygiene promotion and practice: Inadequate, Basic, Intermediate and Advanced.

Inadequate: hand hygiene practices and hand hygiene promotion are deficient. Significant improvement is required.

Basic: some measures are in place, but not to a satisfactory standard. Further improvement is required.

Intermediate: an appropriate hand hygiene promotion strategy is in place and hand hygiene practices have improved. It is now crucial to develop long-term plans to ensure that improvement is sustained and progresses.

Advanced: hand hygiene promotion and optimal hand hygiene practices have been sustained and/or improved, helping to embed a culture of safety in the health-care setting.

Leadership criteria have also been identified to recognise facilities that are considered a reference centre and contribute to the promotion of hand hygiene through research, innovation and information sharing. The assessment according to leadership criteria should only be undertaken by facilities having reached the Advanced level.

How does it work?

While completing each component of the Hand Hygiene Self-Assessment Framework, you should circle or highlight the answer appropriate to your facility for each question. Each answer is associated with a score. After completing a component, add up the scores for the answers you have selected to give a subtotal for that component. During the interpretation process these subtotals are then added up to calculate the overall score to identify the hand hygiene level to which your health-care facility is assigned.

The assessment should not take more than 30 minutes, provided that the information is easily available.

Within the Framework you will find a column called "WHO implementation tools" listing the tools made available from the WHO First Global Patient Safety Challenge to facilitate the implementation of the WHO Multimodal Hand Hygiene Improvement Strategy (http://www.who.int/gpsc/5may/tools/en/index.html). These tools are listed in relation to the relevant indicators included in the Framework and may be useful when developing an action plan to address areas identified as needing improvement.

Is the Hand Hygiene Self-Assessment Framework suitable for inter-facility comparison?

Health-care facilities or national bodies may consider adopting this tool for external comparison or benchmarking. However, this was not a primary aim during the development of this tool. In particular, we would draw attention to the risks inherent in using a self-reported evaluation tool for external benchmarking and also advise the use of caution if comparing facilities of different sizes and complexity, in different socioeconomic settings. It would be essential to consider these limitations if inter-facility comparison is to be undertaken.

Hand Hygiene: A Handbook for Medical Professionals, First Edition.
Edited by Didier Pittet, John M. Boyce and Benedetta Allegranzi.
© 2017 John Wiley & Sons, Inc. Published 2017 by John Wiley & Sons, Inc.

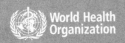

Hand Hygiene Self-Assessment Framework 2010

1. System Change

Question	Answer	Score	WHO improvement tools
1.1 How easily available is alcohol-based handrub in your health-care facility? Choose one answer	Not available	0	→ Ward Infrastructure Survey → Protocol for Evaluation of Tolerability and Acceptability of Alcohol-based Handrub in Use or Planned to be Introduced:Method 1 → Guide to Implementation II.1
	Available, but efficacy[1] and tolerability[2] have not been proven	0	
	Available only in some wards or in discontinuous supply (with efficacy[1] and tolerability[2] proven)	5	
	Available facility-wide with continuous supply (with efficacy[1] and tolerability[2] proven)	10	
	Available facility-wide with continuous supply, and at the point of care[3] in the majority of wards (with efficacy[1] and tolerability[2] proven)	30	
	Available facility-wide with continuous supply at each point of care[3] (with efficacy[1] and tolerability[2] proven)	50	
1.2 What is the sink:bed ratio? Choose one answer	Less than 1:10	0	→ Ward Infrastructure Survey → Guide to Implementation II.1
	At least 1:10 in most wards	5	
	At least 1:10 facility-wide and 1:1 in isolation rooms and in intensive care units	10	
1.3 Is there a continuous supply of clean, running water[4]?	No	0	→ Ward Infrastructure Survey → Guide to Implementation II.1
	Yes	10	
1.4 Is soap[5] available at each sink?	No	0	→ Ward Infrastructure Survey → Guide to Implementation II.1
	Yes	10	
1.5 Are single-use towels available at each sink?	No	0	→ Ward Infrastructure Survey → Guide to Implementation II.1
	Yes	10	
1.6 Is there dedicated/available budget for the continuous procurement of hand hygiene products (e.g. alcohol-based handrubs)?	No	0	→ Guide to Implementation II.1
	Yes	10	

Extra Question: Action plan

Answer this question ONLY if you scored less than 100 for questions 1.1 to 1.6: Is there realistic plan in place to improve the infrastructure[6] in your health-care facility?	No	0	→ Alcohol-based Handrub Planning and Costing Tool → Guide to Local Production: WHO-recommended Handrub Formulations → Guide to Implementation II.1
	Yes	5	
	System Change subtotal	**/100**	

1. Efficacy: The alcohol-based handrub product used should meet recognised standards of antimicrobial efficacy for hand antisepsis (ASTM or EN standards). Alcohol-based handrubs with optimal antimicrobial efficacy usually contain 75 to 85% ethanol, isopropanol, or n-propanol, or a combination of these products. The WHO-recommended formulations contain either 75% v/v isopropanol, or 80% v/v ethanol.

2. Skin tolerability: The alcohol-based handrub product is well tolerated by health-care workers skin (i.e. it does not harm or irritate the skin) when used in clinical care, as demonstrated by reliable data. The WHO Protocol for Evaluation of Tolerability and Acceptability of Alcohol-based Handrub in Use or Planned to be Introduced can be used as a reference.

3. Point of care: The place where three elements come together: the patient, the health-care worker, and care or treatment involving contact with the patient or his/her surroundings (within the patient zone). Point-of-care products should be accessible without having to leave the patient zone (ideally within arms reach of the health-care worker or within 2 meters).

4. Clean, running water: A water supply that is either piped in (or where this is not available, from onsite storage with appropriate disinfection) that meets appropriate safety standards for microbial and chemical contamination. Further details can be found in Essential environmental health standards in health care (Geneva, World Health Organization, 2008, http://whqlibdoc.who.int/publications/2008/9789241547239_eng.pdf).

5. Soap: Detergent-based products that contain no added antimicrobial agents, or may contain these solely as preservatives. They are available in various forms including bar soap, tissue, leaf, and liquid preparations.

6. Infrastructure: The "infrastructure" here referred to includes facilities, equipment, and products that are required to achieve optimal hand hygiene practices within the facility. Specifically, it refers to the indicators included in questions 1.1-1.5 and detailed in the WHO Guidelines on Hand Hygiene in Health Care 2009, Part I, Chapter 23.5 (e.g. availability of alcohol based handrub at all points of care, a continuous supply of clean, running water and a sink:bed ratio of at least 1:10, with soap and single-use towels at each sink).

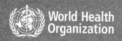

Hand Hygiene Self-Assessment Framework 2010

2. Training and Education

Question	Answer	Score	WHO improvement tools
2.1 Regarding training of health-care workers in your facility:			
2.1a How frequently do health-care workers receive training regarding hand hygiene¹ in your facility? **Choose one answer**	Never	0	→ Slides for Education Session for Trainers, Observers and Health-care Workers
	At least once	5	
	Regular training for medical and nursing staff, or all professional categories (at least annually)	10	→ Hand Hygiene Training Films → Slides Accompanying the Training Films
	Mandatory training for all professional categories at commencement of employment, then ongoing regular training (at least annually)	20	→ Slides for the Hand Hygiene Co-ordinator → Hand Hygiene Technical Reference Manual
2.1b Is a process in place to confirm that all health-care workers complete this training?	No	0	→ Hand Hygiene Why, How and When Brochure
	Yes	20	→ Guide to Implementation II.2
2.2 Are the following WHO documents (available at www.who.int/gpsc/5may/tools), or similar local adaptations, easily available to all health-care workers?			→ Guide to Implementation II.2
2.2a The 'WHO Guidelines on Hand Hygiene in Health-care: A Summary'	No	0	→ WHO Guidelines on Hand Hygiene in Health Care: A Summary
	Yes	5	
2.2b The WHO 'Hand Hygiene Technical Reference Manual'	No	0	→ Hand Hygiene Technical Reference Manual
	Yes	5	
2.2c The WHO 'Hand Hygiene: Why, How and When' Brochure	No	0	→ Hand Hygiene Why, How and When Brochure
	Yes	5	
2.2d The WHO 'Glove Use Information' Leaflet	No	0	→ Glove Use Information Leaflet
	Yes	5	
2.3 Is a professional with adequate skills⁸ to serve as trainer for hand hygiene educational programmes active within the health-care facility?	No	0	→ WHO Guidelines on Hand Hygiene in Health Care → Hand Hygiene Technical Reference Manual
	Yes	15	→ Hand Hygiene Training Films
2.4 Is a system in place for training and validation of hand hygiene compliance observers?	No	0	→ Slides Accompanying the Training Films → Guide to Implementation II.2
	Yes	15	
2.5 Is there is a dedicated budget that allows for hand hygiene training?	No	0	→ Template Letter to Advocate Hand Hygiene to Managers → Template Letter to communicate Hand Hygiene Initiatives to Managers
	Yes	10	→ Template Action Plan → Guide to Implementation II.2 and III.1 (page 33)
	Training and Education subtotal	/100	

7. Training in hand hygiene: This training can be done using different methods but the information conveyed should be based on the WHO multimodal hand hygiene improvement strategy or similar material. Training should include the following:
• The definition, impact and burden of health care-associated infection (HCAI)
• Major patterns of transmission of health care-associated pathogens
• Prevention of HCAI and the critical role of hand hygiene
• Indications for hand hygiene (based on the WHO 'My 5 Moments for Hand Hygiene' approach)
• Correct technique for hand hygiene (refer to 'How to Handrub' and 'How to Hand Wash')

8. A professional with adequate skills: Medical staff or nursing staff trained in Infection Control or Infectious Diseases, whose tasks formally include dedicated time for staff training. In some settings, this could also be medical or nursing staff involved in clinical work, with dedicated time to acquire thorough knowledge of the evidence for and correct practice of hand hygiene (the minimum required knowledge can be found in the WHO Guidelines on Hand Hygiene in Health Care and the Hand Hygiene Technical Reference Manual).

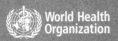

World Health Organization | **Patient Safety** A World Alliance for Safer Health Care | **SAVE LIVES** Clean **Your** Hands

Hand Hygiene Self-Assessment Framework 2010

3. Evaluation and Feedback

Question	Answer	Score	WHO improvement tools
3.1 Are regular (at least annual) ward-based audits undertaken to assess the availability of handrub, soap, single use towels and other hand hygiene resources?	No	0	→ Ward Infrastructure Survey → Guide to Implementation II.3
	Yes	10	
3.2 Is health care worker knowledge of the following topics assessed at least annually (e.g. after education sessions)?			
3.2a. The indications for hand hygiene	No	0	→ Hand Hygiene Knowledge Questionnaire for Health-Care Workers
	Yes	5	
3.2b. The correct technique for hand hygiene	No	0	→ Guide to Implementation II.3
	Yes	5	
3.3 Indirect Monitoring of Hand Hygiene Compliance			
3.3a Is consumption of alcohol-based handrub monitored regularly (at least every 3 months)?	No	0	→ Soap/Handrub Consumption Survey
	Yes	5	→ Guide to Implementation II.3
3.3b Is consumption of soap monitored regularly (at least every 3 months)?	No	0	
	Yes	5	
3.3c Is alcohol based handrub consumption at least 20L per 1000 patient-days?	No (or not measured)	0	
	Yes	5	
3.4 Direct Monitoring of Hand Hygiene Compliance Only complete section 3.4 if hand hygiene compliance observers in your facility have been trained and validated and utilise the WHO 'My 5 Moments for Hand Hygiene' (or similar) methodology			
3.4a How frequently is direct observation of hand hygiene compliance performed using the WHO Hand Hygiene Observation tool (or similar technique)? **Choose one answer**	Never	0	→ WHO Hand Hygiene Observation form → Hand Hygiene Technical Reference Manual → Guide to Implementation II.3
	Irregularly	5	
	Annually	10	
	Every 3 months or more often	15	
3.4b What is the overall hand hygiene compliance rate according to the WHO Hand Hygiene Observation tool (or similar technique) in your facility? **Choose one answer**	≤ 30%	0	→ Guide to Implementation II.3 → Observation form → Data Entry Analysis tools → Instructions for Data Entry and Analysis → Epi Info™ software[9] → Data Summary Report Framework
	31 – 40%	5	
	41 – 50%	10	
	51 – 60%	15	
	61 – 70%	20	
	71 – 80%	25	
	≥ 81%	30	
3.5 Feedback			
3.5a **Immediate feedback** Is immediate feedback given to health-care workers at the end of each hand hygiene observation session?	No	0	→ Guide to Implementation II.3 → Observation and Basic Compliance Calculation forms
	Yes	5	
3.5b **Systematic feedback** Is regular (at least 6 monthly) feedback of data related to hand hygiene indicators with demonstration of trends over time given to:			→ Data Summary Report Framework → Guide to Implementation II.3
3.5b.i Health-care workers?	No	0	
	Yes	7.5	
3.5b.ii Facility leadership?	No	0	
	Yes	7.5	
	Evaluation and Feedback subtotal	**/100**	

9. Epi Info™: This software can be downloaded free of charge from the CDC website (http://www.cdc.gov/epiinfo/)

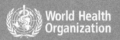

Hand Hygiene Self-Assessment Framework 2010

4. Reminders in the Workplace

Question	Answer	Score	WHO improvement tools
4.1 Are the following posters (or locally produced equivalent with similar content) displayed?			→ Guide to Implementation II.4
4.1a Poster explaining the indications for hand hygiene Choose one answer	Not displayed	0	→ Your 5 Moments for Hand Hygiene (Poster)
	Displayed in some wards/treatment areas	15	
	Displayed in most wards/treatment areas	20	
	Displayed in all wards/treatment areas	25	
4.1b Poster explaining the correct use of handrub Choose one answer	Not displayed	0	→ How to Handrub (Poster)
	Displayed in some wards/treatment areas	5	
	Displayed in most wards/treatment areas	10	
	Displayed in all wards/treatment areas	15	
4.1c Poster explaining correct hand-washing technique Choose one answer	Not displayed	0	→ How to Handwash (Poster)
	Displayed in some wards/treatment areas	5	
	Displayed in most wards/treatment areas	7.5	
	Displayed at every sink in all wards/treatment areas	10	
4.2 How frequently does a systematic audit of all posters for evidence of damage occur, with replacement as required? Choose one answer	Never	0	→ Guide to Implementation II.4
	At least annually	10	
	Every 2-3 months	15	
4.3 Is hand hygiene promotion undertaken by displaying and regularly updating posters other than those mentioned above?	No	0	→ Guide to Implementation II.4
	Yes	10	
4.4 Are hand hygiene information leaflets available on wards?	No	0	→ Hand Hygiene: When and How Leaflet
	Yes	10	→ Guide to Implementation II.4
4.5 Are other workplace reminders located throughout the facility? (e.g. hand hygiene campaign screensavers, badges, stickers, etc)	No	0	→ SAVE LIVES: Clean Your Hands Screensaver → Guide to Implementation II.4
	Yes	15	
	Reminders in the Workplace subtotal	**/100**	

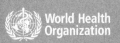

Patient Safety
A World Alliance for Safer Health Care

SAVE LIVES
Clean **Your** Hands

Hand Hygiene Self-Assessment Framework 2010

5. Institutional Safety Climate for Hand Hygiene

Question	Answer	Score	WHO improvement tools
5.1 With regard to a hand hygiene team[10] that is dedicated to the promotion and implementation of optimal hand hygiene practice in your facility:			→ Guide to Implementation II.5
5.1a Is such a team established?	No	0	
	Yes	5	
5.1b Does this team meet on a regular basis (at least monthly)?	No	0	
	Yes	5	
5.1c Does this team have dedicated time to conduct active hand hygiene promotion? (e.g. teaching monitoring hand hygiene performance, organizing new activities)	No	0	
	Yes	5	
5.2 Have the following members of the facility leadership made a clear commitment to support hand hygiene improvement? (e.g. a written or verbal commitment to hand hygiene promotion received by the majority of health-care workers)			→ Template Letter to Advocate Hand Hygiene to Managers → Template Letter to communicate Hand Hygiene Initiatives to Managers → Guide to Implementation II.5
5.2a Chief executive officer	No	0	
	Yes	10	
5.2b Medical director	No	0	
	Yes	5	
5.2c Director of nursing	No	0	
	Yes	5	
5.3 Has a clear plan for the promotion of hand hygiene throughout the entire facility for the 5 May (Save Lives Clean Your Hands Annual Initiative) been established ?	No	0	→ Sustaining Improvement – Additional Activities for Consideration by Health-Care Facilities → Guide to Implementation II.5
	Yes	10	
5.4 Are systems for identification of Hand Hygiene Leaders from all disciplines in place?			
5.4a A system for designation of Hand Hygiene champions[11]	No	0	
	Yes	5	
5.4b A system for recognition and utilisation of Hand Hygiene role models[12]	No	0	
	Yes	5	
5.5 Regarding patient involvement in hand hygiene promotion:			→ Guidance on Engaging Patients and Patient Organizations in Hand Hygiene Initiatives → Guide to Implementation II.5
5.5a Are patients informed about the importance of hand hygiene? (e.g. with a leaflet)	No	0	
	Yes	5	
5.5b Has a formalised programme of patient engagement been undertaken?	No	0	
	Yes	10	
5.6 Are initiatives to support local continuous improvement being applied in your facility, for example:			→ Sustaining Improvement – Additional Activities for Consideration by Health-Care Facilities → Guide to Implementation II.5
5.6a Hand hygiene E-learning tools	No	0	
	Yes	5	
5.6b A hand hygiene institutional target to be achieved is established each year	No	0	
	Yes	5	
5.6c A system for intra-institutional sharing of reliable and tested local innovations	No	0	
	Yes	5	
5.6d Communications that regularly mention hand hygiene e.g. facility newsletter, clinical meetings	No	0	
	Yes	5	
5.6e System for personal accountability[13]	No	0	
	Yes	5	
5.6f A Buddy system[14] for new employees	No	0	
	Yes	5	
Institutional Safety Climate subtotal		**/100**	

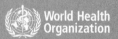

Hand Hygiene Self-Assessment Framework 2010

10. Hand hygiene team: The make-up of this team will vary. It is likely to most frequently consist of an infection control unit, but may range (depending on resources available) from a single person with the role of managing the hand hygiene programme, to a group of staff members from various departments within the facility with meetings dedicated to the hand hygiene programme.

11. Hand hygiene champion: A person who is an advocate for the causes of patient safety and hand hygiene standards and takes on responsibility for publicizing a project in his/her ward and/or facility-wide.

12. Hand hygiene role model: A person who serves as an example, whose behaviour is emulated by others. In particular, a hand hygiene role model should have a hand hygiene compliance rate of at least 80%, be able to remind others to comply, and be able to teach practically about the WHO 5 Moments for Hand Hygiene concept.

13. System for personal accountability: explicit actions are in place to stimulate health-care workers to be accountable for their behaviour with regard to hand hygiene practices. Examples are notification by observers or infection control professionals, reproaches by peers, and reports to higher level facility authorities, with possible consequences on the individual evaluation.

14. Buddy system: A programme in which each new health-care worker is coupled with an established, trained health-care worker who takes responsibility for introducing them to the hand hygiene culture of the health-care setting (including practical training on indications and technique for performing hand hygiene, and explanation of hand hygiene promotion initiatives within the facility).

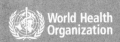

World Health Organization | **Patient Safety** A World Alliance for Safer Health Care | **SAVE LIVES** Clean **Your** Hands

Hand Hygiene Self-Assessment Framework 2010

Interpretation: **A Four Step Process**

1.
Add up your points.

Score	
Component	Subtotal
1. System Change	
2. Education and Training	
3. Evaluation and Feedback	
4. Reminders in the Workplace	
5. Institutional Safety Climate	
Total	

2.
Determine the assigned 'Hand Hygiene Level' for your facility.

Total Score (range)	Hand Hygiene Level
0 - 125	Inadequate
126 - 250	Basic
251 - 375	Intermediate (or Consolidation)
376 - 500	Advanced (or Embedding)

3.
If your facility has reached the Advanced level, then complete the Leadership section overleaf.

(otherwise go to Step 4).

4.
Review the areas identified by this evaluation as requiring improvement in your facility and develop an action plan to address them (starting with the relevant WHO improvement tools listed). Keep a copy of this assessment to compare with repeated uses in the future.

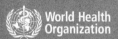

World Health Organization	Patient Safety	SAVE LIVES

Hand Hygiene Self-Assessment Framework 2010

Leadership Criteria	Answer (circle one)	
System Change		
Has a cost-benefit analysis of infrastructure changes required for the performance of optimal hand hygiene at the point of care been performed?	Yes	No
Does alcohol-based handrubbing account for at least 80% of hand hygiene actions performed in your facility?	Yes	No
Training and Education		
Has the hand hygiene team undertaken training of representatives from other facilities in the area of hand hygiene promotion?	Yes	No
Have hand hygiene principles been incorporated into local medical and nursing educational curricula?	Yes	No
Evaluation and Feedback		
Are specific healthcare associated infections (HCAIs) monitored? (eg. *Staphylococcus aureus* bacteremia, Gram negative bacteremia, device-related infections)	Yes	No
Is a system in place for monitoring of HCAI in high risk-settings? (e.g. intensive care and neonatal units)	Yes	No
Is a facility-wide prevalence survey of HCAI performed (at least) annually?	Yes	No
Are HCAI rates presented to facility leadership and to health-care workers in conjunction with hand hygiene compliance rates?	Yes	No
Is structured evaluation undertaken to understand the obstacles to optimal hand hygiene compliance and the causes of HCAI at the local level, and results reported to the facility leadership?	Yes	No
Reminders in the Workplace		
Is a system in place for creation of new posters designed by local health-care workers?	Yes	No
Are posters created in your facility used in other facilities?	Yes	No
Have innovative types of hand hygiene reminders been developed and tested at the facility?	Yes	No
Institutional Safety Climate		
Has a local hand hygiene research agenda addressing issues identified by the WHO Guidelines as requiring further investigation been developed?	Yes	No
Has your facility participated actively in publications or conference presentations (oral or poster) in the area of hand hygiene?	Yes	No
Are patients invited to remind health-care workers to perform hand hygiene?	Yes	No
Are patients and visitors educated to correctly perform hand hygiene?	Yes	No
Does your facility contribute to and support the national hand hygiene campaign (if existing)?	Yes	No
Is impact evaluation of the hand hygiene campaign incorporated into forward planning of the infection control programme?	Yes	No
Does your facility set an annual target for improvement of hand hygiene compliance facility-wide?	Yes	No
If the facility has such a target, was it achieved last year?	Yes	No
Total	**/20**	

Your facility has reached the Hand Hygiene Leadership level if you answered "yes" to at least one leadership criteria per category and its total leadership score is 12 or more. Congratulations and thank you!

Index

Hand Hygiene: A Handbook for Medical Professionals, First Edition.
Edited by Didier Pittet, John M. Boyce and Benedetta Allegranzi.
© 2017 John Wiley & Sons, Inc. Published 2017 by John Wiley & Sons, Inc.